Pharmacology
for Anaesthesia and Intensive
Care

Pharmacology for Anaesthesia and Intensive Care

Tom Peck
Consultant Anaesthetist, Royal Hampshire County Hospital, Winchester; Honorary Consultant, University Hospital Southampton

Benjamin Harris
Consultant Anaesthetist and Intensivist, Basingstoke and North Hampshire Hospital, Hampshire Hospitals NHS Foundation Trust

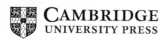

CAMBRIDGE
UNIVERSITY PRESS

University Printing House, Cambridge CB2 8BS, United Kingdom

One Liberty Plaza, 20th Floor, New York, NY 10006, USA

477 Williamstown Road, Port Melbourne, VIC 3207, Australia

314–321, 3rd Floor, Plot 3, Splendor Forum, Jasola District Centre,
New Delhi – 110025, India

79 Anson Road, #06–04/06, Singapore 079906

Cambridge University Press is part of the University of Cambridge.

It furthers the University's mission by disseminating knowledge in the pursuit of
education, learning, and research at the highest international levels of excellence.

www.cambridge.org
Information on this title: www.cambridge.org/9781108710961
DOI: 10.1017/9781108591317

Tom Peck and Benjamin Harris © 2021

First published 2000
Second edition 2003
Third edition 2008
Fourth edition 2014
8th printing 2019
Fifth edition 2021

A catalogue record for this publication is available from the British Library.

Library of Congress Cataloging-in-Publication Data
Names: Peck, T. E., author. | Harris, Benjamin (Consultant Anaesthetist), author.
Title: Pharmacology for anaesthesia and intensive care / Tom Peck, Consultant Anaesthetist, Royal Hampshire County
Hospital, Winchester; Honorary Consultant, University Hospital Southampton, Benjamin Harris, Consultant
Anaesthetist, Hampshire Hospitals NHS Trust.
Description: Fifth edition. | Cambridge, United Kingdom ; New York, NY : Cambridge University Press, 2021. | Includes index.
Identifiers: LCCN 2020039003 (print) LCCN 2020039004 (ebook) | ISBN 9781108710961 (paperback) |
ISBN 9781108591317 (ebook)
Subjects: LCSH: Pharmacology. | Anesthetics.
Classification: LCC RM300 .P396 2021 (print) | LCC RM300 (ebook) | DDC 615.1–dc23
LC record available at https://lccn.loc.gov/2020039003
LC ebook record available at https://lccn.loc.gov/2020039004

ISBN 978-1-108-71096-1 Paperback

....

Contents

Preface

This fifth edition continues to push down what seems to be a successful avenue. The overall size and feel remains the same with changes limited to depth and scope of information rather than simply expanding the number of drugs discussed, especially in Sections III and IV. Applied kinetics and total intravenous anaesthesia content has been expanded and new information on the environmental impact of anaesthetic agents has been added where relevant.

This edition also welcomes a new co-author, Dr Ben Harris, who brings a welcome depth of knowledge to the intensive care content which has been expanded and re-written in places.

It should be noted that this is the only edition without the direct involvement of Dr Sue Hill. Although not listed as an author in the first edition she was the wise head who guided, shaped and encouraged two ambitious trainees in what seemed an impossible venture. Her input into this book over the past 20 years is hard to overestimate. She is currently enjoying a well-earned retirement.

Thank you Sue.

Foreword

"Pharmacology for Anaesthesia and Intensive Care" has already been an essential reference work for anaesthetists and intensivists for several years, and so I was delighted when Dr. Tom Peck asked me to write a foreword for the 5th edition.

Drs. Tom Peck and Ben Harris are gifted and highly respected clinicians, and between them have a wealth of experience in training and education with a particular emphasis on pharmacology. This foundation has served them well in maintaining a nice balance between the level of detail, and the clarity of the text. Where necessary – such as in the first section on the basic principles of pharmacology and medicinal chemistry – they dive into the details, but are able to guide the reader to a clear understanding of complex concepts.

In sections II to IV the authors discuss the drugs used in anaesthetic and intensive care practice, as well as most of the other drugs to which their patients might already be exposed. Each chapter focusses on one drug or drug family, starting off with a very useful summary of the relevant physiology, followed by a comprehensive description of the clinical pharmacology of that drug or drug family. These sections contain frequent brief references to the underlying pharmacological principles which serve to reinforce the understanding and relevance of these principles. All information provided is placed in a clinical context, and all sections have been thoroughly updated.

I am convinced that this book will continue to be a useful reference, not only for trainees preparing for the UK or European (fellowship/EDAIC/EDIC) examinations in anaesthesia and intensive care, but also for consultants wishing to refresh and update their knowledge. Moreover, I believe that the readability and clarity of the writing will appeal to other groups of healthcare professionals wishing to enhance their understanding and knowledge of pharmacology (nurses, medical students, and trainees and consultants in other medical specialties).

I took a galley proof version of this book on holiday with me, but only expected to read the first few chapters before the end of the holiday. This soon changed, and I found myself reading it from cover-to-cover within a few days. I have no doubt that all who read it will find it similarly compelling and informative.

Anthony Absalom
Professor of Anesthesiology, University of Groningen
Consultant Anaesthetist, University Medical Center Groningen
Editor, British Journal of Anaesthesia
Immediate past-present, UK Society for Intravenous Anaesthesia

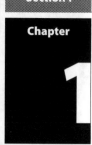

Drug Passage across the Cell Membrane

Many drugs need to pass through one or more cell membranes to reach their site of action. A common feature of all cell membranes is a phospholipid bilayer, about 10 nm thick, arranged with the hydrophilic heads on the outside and the lipophilic chains facing inwards. This gives a sandwich effect, with two hydrophilic layers surrounding the central hydrophobic one. Spanning this bilayer or attached to the outer or inner leaflets are glycoproteins, which may act as ion channels, receptors, intermediate messengers (G-proteins) or enzymes. The cell membrane has been described as a 'fluid mosaic' as the positions of individual phosphoglycerides and glycoproteins are by no means fixed (Figure 1.1). An exception to this is a specialised membrane area such as the neuromuscular junction, where the array of postsynaptic receptors is found opposite a motor nerve ending.

The general cell membrane structure is modified in certain tissues to allow more specialised functions. Capillary endothelial cells have fenestrae, which are regions of the endothelial cell where the outer and inner membranes are fused together, with no intervening cytosol. These make the endothelium of the capillary relatively permeable; fluid in particular can pass rapidly through the cell by this route. In the case of the renal glomerular endothelium, gaps or clefts exist between cells to allow the passage of larger molecules as part of filtration. Tight junctions exist between endothelial cells of brain blood vessels, forming the blood–brain barrier, intestinal mucosa and renal tubules. These limit the passage of polar molecules and also prevent the lateral movement of glycoproteins within the cell membrane, which may help to keep specialised glycoproteins at their site of action (e.g. transport glycoproteins on the luminal surface of intestinal mucosa) (Figure 1.2).

Methods of Crossing the Cell Membrane

Passive Diffusion

This is the commonest method for crossing the cell membrane. Drug molecules move down a concentration gradient, from an area of high concentration to one of low concentration, and the process requires no energy to proceed. Many drugs are weak acids or weak bases and can exist in either the unionised or ionised form, depending on the pH. The unionised form of a drug is lipid-soluble and diffuses easily by dissolution in the lipid bilayer. Thus the rate at which transfer occurs depends on the pK_a of the drug in question. Factors influencing the rate of diffusion are discussed below.

In addition, there are specialised **ion channels** in the membrane that allow intermittent passive movement of selected ions down a concentration gradient. When opened, ion channels allow rapid ion flux for a short time (a few milliseconds) down relatively large

Extracellular

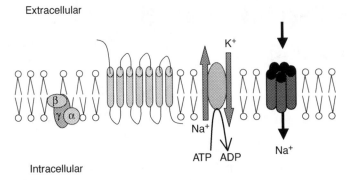

Intracellular

Figure 1.1 Representation of the cell membrane structure. The integral proteins embedded in this phospholipid bilayer are G-protein, G-protein-coupled receptors, transport proteins and ligand-gated ion channels. Additionally, enzymes or voltage-gated ion channels may also be present.

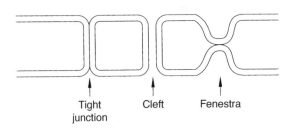

Figure 1.2 Modifications of the general cell membrane structure.

concentration and electrical gradients, which makes them suitable to propagate either ligand- or voltage-gated action potentials in nerve and muscle membranes.

The acetylcholine (ACh) receptor has five subunits (pentameric) arranged to form a central ion channel that spans the membrane (Figure 1.3). Of the five subunits, two (the α subunits) are identical. The receptor requires the binding of two ACh molecules to open the ion channel, allowing ions to pass at about 10^7 s^{-1}. If a threshold flux is achieved, depolarisation occurs, which is responsible for impulse transmission. The ACh receptor demonstrates selectivity for small cations, but it is by no means specific for Na^+. The $GABA_A$ receptor is also a pentameric, ligand-gated channel, but selective for anions, especially the chloride anion. The NMDA (N-methyl D-aspartate) receptor belongs to a different family of ion channels and is a dimer; it favours calcium as the cation mediating membrane depolarisation.

Ion channels may have their permeability altered by endogenous compounds or by drugs. Local anaesthetics bind to the internal surface of the fast Na^+ ion channel and prevent the conformational change required for activation, while non-depolarising muscle relaxants prevent receptor activation by competitively inhibiting the binding of ACh to its receptor site.

Facilitated Diffusion

Facilitated diffusion refers to the process where molecules combine with membrane-bound carrier proteins to cross the membrane. The rate of diffusion of the molecule–protein complex is still down a concentration gradient but is faster than would be expected by

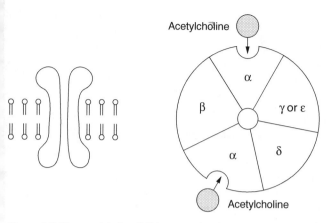

Figure 1.3 The acetylcholine (ACh) receptor has five subunits and spans the cell membrane. ACh binds to the α subunits, causing a conformational change and allowing the passage of small cations through its central ion channel. The ε subunit replaces the fetal-type γ subunit after birth once the neuromuscular junction reaches maturity.

diffusion alone. An example of this process is the absorption of glucose, a highly polar molecule, which would be relatively slow if it occurred by diffusion alone. There are several transport proteins responsible for facilitated glucose diffusion; they belong to the solute carrier (SLC) family 2. The SLC proteins belonging to family 6 are responsible for transport of neurotransmitters across the synaptic membrane. These are specific for different neurotransmitters: SLC6A3 for dopamine, SLC6A4 for serotonin and SLC6A5 for noradrenaline. They are the targets for certain antidepressants; serotonin-selective re-uptake inhibitors (SSRIs) inhibit SLC6A4.

Active Transport

Active transport is an energy-requiring process. The molecule is transported against its concentration gradient by a molecular pump, which requires energy to function. Energy can be supplied either directly to the ion pump, primary active transport, or indirectly by coupling pump-action to an ionic gradient that is actively maintained, secondary active transport. Active transport is encountered commonly in gut mucosa, the liver, renal tubules and the blood–brain barrier.

Na^+/K^+ ATPase is an example of primary active transport – the energy in the high-energy phosphate bond is lost as the molecule is hydrolysed, with concurrent ion transport against the respective concentration gradients. It is an example of an antiport, as sodium moves in one direction and potassium in the opposite direction. The Na^+/amino acid symport (substances moved in the same direction) in the mucosal cells of the small bowel or on the luminal side of the proximal renal tubule is an example of secondary active transport. Here, amino acids will only cross the mucosal cell membrane when Na^+ is bound to the carrier protein and moves down its concentration gradient (which is generated using Na^+/K^+ ATPase). So, directly and indirectly, Na^+/K^+ ATPase is central to active transport (Figure 1.4).

Primary active transport proteins include the ABC (ATP-binding cassette) family, which are responsible for transport of essential nutrients into and toxins out of cells. An important protein belonging to this family is the multi-drug resistant protein transporter, also known

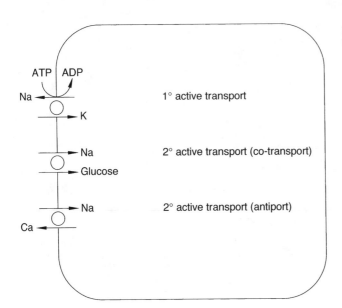

Figure 1.4 Mechanisms of active transport across the cell membrane.

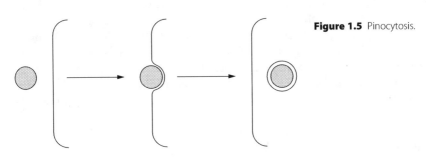

Figure 1.5 Pinocytosis.

as p-glycoprotein (PGP), which is found in gut mucosa and the blood–brain barrier. Many cytotoxic, antimicrobial and other drugs are substrates for PGP and are unable to penetrate the blood–brain barrier.

The anticoagulant dabigatran is a substrate for PGP and co-administration of PGP inhibitors, such as amiodarone and verapamil, will increase dabigatran bioavailability and therefore the risk of adverse haemorrhagic complications. PGP inducers, such as rifampicin, will reduce dabigatran bioavailability and lead to inadequate anticoagulation.

Inhibitors and inducers of PGP are commonly also inhibitors and inducers of CYP3A4 and will interact strongly with drugs that are substrates for both PGP and CYP3A4.

Pinocytosis

Pinocytosis is the process by which an area of the cell membrane invaginates around the (usually large) target molecule and moves it into the cell. The molecule may then be released into the cell or may remain in the vacuole so created, until the reverse process occurs on the opposite side of the cell.

The process is usually used for molecules that are too large to traverse the membrane easily via another mechanism (Figure 1.5).

Factors Influencing the Rate of Diffusion

Molecular Size

The rate of passive diffusion is inversely proportional to the square root of molecular size (Graham's law). In general, small molecules will diffuse much more readily than large ones. The molecular weights of anaesthetic agents are relatively small and anaesthetic agents diffuse rapidly through lipid membranes to exert their effects.

Concentration Gradient

Fick's law states that the rate of transfer across a membrane is proportional to the concentration gradient across the membrane. Thus increasing the plasma concentration of the unbound fraction of the drug will increase its rate of transfer across the membrane and will accelerate the onset of its pharmacological effect. This is the basis of Bowman's principle, applied to the onset of action of non-depolarising muscle relaxants. The less potent the drug, the more required to exert an effect – but this increases the concentration gradient between plasma and active site, so the onset of action is faster.

Ionisation

The lipophilic nature of the cell membrane only permits the passage of the uncharged fraction of any drug. The degree to which a drug is ionised in a solution depends on the molecular structure of the drug and the pH of the solution in which it is dissolved and is given by the Henderson–Hasselbalch equation.

The pK_a is the pH at which 50% of the drug molecules are ionised – thus the concentrations of ionised and unionised portions are equal. The value for pK_a depends on the molecular structure of the drug and is independent of whether it is acidic or basic.

The Henderson–Hasselbalch equation is most simply expressed as:

$$pH = pK_a + \log\left\{ \frac{[\text{proton acceptor}]}{[\text{proton donor}]} \right\}.$$

Hence, for an acid (XH), the relationship between the ionised and unionised forms is given by:

$$pH = pK_a + \log\left\{ \frac{[X^-]}{[XH]} \right\},$$

with X^- being the ionised form of an acid.

For a base (X), the corresponding form of the equation is:

$$pH = pK_a + \log\left\{ \frac{[X]}{[XH^+]} \right\},$$

with XH^+ being the ionised form of a base.

Using the terms 'proton donor' and 'proton acceptor' instead of 'acid' or 'base' in the equation avoids confusion and the degree of ionisation of a molecule may be readily established if its pK_a and the ambient pH are known. At a pH below their pK_a weak acids will be more unionised; at a pH above their pK_a they will be more ionised. The reverse is true for weak bases, which are more ionised at a pH below their pK_a and more unionised at a pH above their pK_a.

Bupivacaine is a weak base with a tertiary amine group in the piperidine ring. The nitrogen atom of this amine group is a proton acceptor and can become ionised, depending on pH. With a pK_a of 8.1, it is 83% ionised at physiological pH.

Aspirin is an acid with a pK_a of 3.0. It is almost wholly ionised at physiological pH, although in the highly acidic environment of the stomach it is essentially unionised, which therefore increases its rate of absorption. However, because of the limited surface area within the stomach more is absorbed in the small bowel.

Lipid Solubility

The lipid solubility of a drug reflects its ability to pass through the cell membrane; this property is independent of the pK_a of the drug as lipid solubility is quoted for the unionised form only. However, high lipid solubility alone does not necessarily result in a rapid onset of action. Alfentanil is nearly seven times less lipid-soluble than fentanyl, yet it has a more rapid onset of action. This is a result of several factors. First, alfentanil is less potent and has a smaller distribution volume and therefore initially a greater concentration gradient exists between effect site and plasma. Second, both fentanyl and alfentanil are weak bases and alfentanil has a lower pK_a than fentanyl (alfentanil = 6.5; fentanyl = 8.4), so that at physiological pH a much greater fraction of alfentanil is unionised and available to cross membranes.

Lipid solubility affects the rate of absorption from the site of administration. Fentanyl is suitable for transdermal application as its high lipid solubility results in effective transfer across the skin. Intrathecal diamorphine readily dissolves into, and fixes to, the local lipid tissues, whereas the less lipid-soluble morphine remains in the cerebrospinal fluid longer, and is therefore liable to spread cranially, with an increased risk of respiratory depression.

Protein Binding

Only the unbound fraction of any drug in plasma is free to cross the cell membrane; drugs vary greatly in the degree of plasma protein binding. In practice, the extent of this binding is of importance only if the drug is highly protein-bound (more than 90%). In these cases, small changes in the bound fraction produce large changes in the amount of unbound drug. In general, this increases the rate at which the drug is metabolised, so a new equilibrium is re-established with little change in free drug concentration. For a very small number of highly protein-bound drugs where metabolic pathways are close to saturation (such as phenytoin) this cannot happen and plasma concentration of the unbound drug will increase and possibly reach toxic levels.

Both albumin and globulins bind drugs; each has many binding sites, the number and characteristics of which are determined by the pH of plasma. In general, albumin binds neutral or acidic drugs (e.g. barbiturates), and globulins (in particular, α_1 acid glycoprotein) bind basic drugs (e.g. morphine).

Albumin has two important binding sites: the warfarin and diazepam sites. Binding is usually readily reversible, and competition for binding at any one site between different drugs can alter the active unbound fraction of each. Binding is also possible at other sites on the molecule, which may cause a conformational change and indirectly influence binding at the diazepam and warfarin sites.

Although α_1 acid glycoprotein binds basic drugs, other globulins are important in binding individual ions and molecules, particularly the metals. Thus, iron is bound to β_1 globulin and copper to α_2 globulin.

Protein binding is altered in a range of pathological conditions. Inflammation changes the relative proportions of the different proteins and albumin concentration falls in any acute infective or inflammatory process. This effect is independent of any reduction in synthetic capacity resulting from liver impairment and is not due to protein loss. In conditions of severe hypoalbuminaemia (e.g. in end-stage liver cirrhosis or burns), the proportion of unbound drug increases markedly such that the same dose will have a greatly exaggerated pharmacological effect. The magnitude of these effects may be hard to estimate and drug dose should be titrated against clinical effect.

2 Absorption, Distribution, Metabolism and Excretion

Absorption

Drugs may be given by a variety of routes; the route chosen depends on the desired site of action and the type of drug preparations available. Routes used commonly by the anaesthetist include inhalation, intravenous, oral, intramuscular, rectal, epidural and intrathecal. Other routes, such as transdermal, subcutaneous and sublingual, can also be used. The rate and extent of absorption after a particular route of administration depends on both drug and patient factors.

Not all drugs need to reach the systemic circulation to exert their effects, for example, oral vancomycin used to treat pseudomembranous colitis; antacids also act locally in the stomach. In such cases, systemic absorption may result in unwanted side effects.

Intravenous administration provides a direct, and therefore more reliable, route of systemic drug delivery. No absorption is required, so plasma levels are independent of such factors as gastrointestinal (GI) absorption and adequate skin or muscle perfusion. However, there are disadvantages in using this route. Pharmacological preparations for intravenous therapy are generally more expensive than the corresponding oral medications, and the initially high plasma level achieved with some drugs may cause undesirable side effects. In addition, if central venous access is used, this carries its own risks. Nevertheless, most drugs used in intensive care are given by intravenous infusion.

Oral

After oral administration, absorption must take place through the gut mucosa. For drugs without specific transport mechanisms, only the unionised fraction passes readily through the lipid membranes of the gut. Because the pH of the GI tract varies along its length, the physicochemical properties of the drug will determine from which part of the GI tract the drug is absorbed.

Acidic drugs (e.g. aspirin) are unionised in the highly acidic medium of the stomach and therefore are absorbed more rapidly than basic drugs. Although weak bases (e.g. propranolol) are ionised in the stomach, they are relatively unionised in the duodenum, so are absorbed from this site. The salts of permanently charged drugs (e.g. vecuronium, glycopyrrolate) remain ionised at all times and are therefore not absorbed from the GI tract.

In practice, even acidic drugs are predominantly absorbed from the small bowel, as the surface area for absorption is so much greater due to the presence of mucosal villi.

However, acidic drugs, such as aspirin, have some advantages over basic drugs in that absorption is initially rapid, giving a shorter time of onset from ingestion, and will continue even in the presence of GI tract stasis.

Bioavailability

Bioavailability is generally defined as the fraction of a drug dose reaching the systemic circulation, compared with the same dose given intravenously. In general, the oral route has the lowest bioavailability of any route of administration. Bioavailability can be determined from the ratio of the areas under the concentration–time curves for an identical bolus dose given both orally and intravenously (Figure 2.1).

Factors Influencing Bioavailability

- *Pharmaceutical preparation* – the way in which a drug is formulated affects its rate of absorption. If a drug is presented with a small particle size or as a liquid, dispersion is rapid. If the particle size is large, or binding agents prevent drug dissolution in the stomach (e.g. enteric-coated preparations), absorption may be delayed.
- *Physicochemical interactions* – other drugs or food may interact and inactivate or bind the drug in question (e.g. the absorption of tetracyclines is reduced by the concurrent administration of Ca^{2+} such as in milk).
- *Patient factors* – various patient factors affect absorption of a drug. The presence of congenital or acquired malabsorption syndromes, such as coeliac disease or tropical sprue, will affect absorption, and gastric stasis, whether as a result of trauma or drugs, slows the transit time through the gut.
- *Pharmacokinetic interactions and first-pass metabolism* – drugs absorbed from the gut (with the exception of the buccal and rectal mucosa) pass via the portal vein to the liver where they may be subject to first-pass metabolism. Metabolism at either the gut wall (e.g. glyceryl trinitrate (GTN)) or liver will reduce the amount reaching the circulation.

Therefore, an adequate plasma level may not be achieved orally using a dose similar to that needed intravenously. So, for an orally administered drug, the bioavailable fraction (F_B) is given by:

$$F_B = F_A \times F_G \times F_H$$

Here F_A is the fraction absorbed, F_G the fraction remaining after metabolism in the gut mucosa and F_H the fraction remaining after hepatic metabolism. Therefore, drugs with

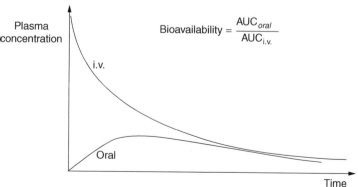

$$\text{Bioavailability} = \frac{AUC_{oral}}{AUC_{i.v.}}$$

Figure 2.1 Bioavailability may be estimated by comparing the areas under the curves.

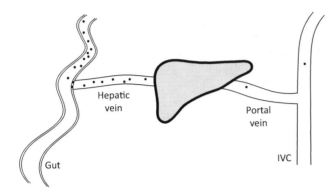

Figure 2.2 First-pass metabolism may occur in the gut wall or in the liver to reduce the amount of drug reaching the circulation.

Hepatic vein

Portal vein

Gut

IVC

a high oral bioavailability are stable in the GI tract, are well absorbed and undergo minimal first-pass metabolism (Figure 2.2). First-pass metabolism may be increased and oral bioavailability reduced through the induction of hepatic enzymes (e.g. phenobarbital induces hepatic enzymes, reducing the bioavailability of warfarin). Conversely, hepatic enzymes may be inhibited and bioavailability increased (e.g. cimetidine may increase the bioavailability of propranolol).

Extraction Ratio

The extraction ratio (ER) is that fraction of drug removed from blood by the liver. ER depends on hepatic blood flow, uptake into the hepatocyte and enzyme metabolic capacity within the hepatocyte. The activity of an enzyme is described by its Michaelis constant, which is the concentration of substrate at which it is working at 50% of its maximum rate. Those enzymes with high metabolic capacity have Michaelis constants very much higher than any substrate concentrations likely to be found clinically; those with low capacity will have Michaelis constants close to clinically relevant concentrations. Drugs fall into three distinct groups:

Drugs for which the hepatocyte has rapid uptake and a high metabolic capacity, for example, propofol and lidocaine. Free drug is rapidly removed from plasma, bound drug is released to maintain equilibrium and a concentration gradient is maintained between plasma and hepatocyte because drug is metabolised very quickly. Because protein binding has rapid equilibration, the total amount of drug metabolised will be independent of protein binding but highly dependent on liver blood flow.

Drugs that have low metabolic capacity and high level of protein binding (>90%). This group includes phenytoin and diazepam. Their ER is limited by the metabolic capacity of the hepatocyte and not by blood flow. If protein binding is altered (e.g. by competition) then the free concentration of drug increases significantly. This initially increases uptake into the hepatocyte and rate of metabolism and plasma levels of free drug do not change significantly. However, if the intracellular concentration exceeds maximum metabolic capacity (saturates the enzyme) drug levels within the cell remain high, so reducing uptake (reduced concentration gradient) and ER. Those drugs with a narrow therapeutic index may then show significant toxic effects; hence the need for regular checks on plasma concentration, particularly when other medication is altered. Therefore for this group of drugs extraction is influenced by changes in protein binding more than by changes in hepatic blood flow.

Drugs that have low metabolic capacity and low level of protein binding. The total amount of drug metabolised for this group of drugs is unaffected by either hepatic blood flow or by changes in protein binding.

Sublingual

The sublingual, nasal and buccal routes have two advantages – they are rapid in onset and, by avoiding the portal tract, have a higher bioavailability. This is advantageous for drugs where a rapid effect is essential, for example, GTN spray for angina or sublingual nifedipine for the relatively rapid control of high blood pressure.

Rectal

The rectal route can be used to avoid first-pass metabolism, and may be considered if the oral route is not available. Drugs may be given rectally for their local (e.g. steroids for inflammatory bowel disease), as well as their systemic effects (e.g. diclofenac suppositories for analgesia). There is little evidence that the rectal route is more efficacious than the oral route; it provides a relatively small surface area, and absorption may be slow or incomplete.

Intramuscular

The intramuscular route avoids the problems associated with oral administration and the bioavailable fraction approaches 1. The speed of onset is generally more rapid compared with the oral route, and for some drugs approaches that for the intravenous route.

The rate of absorption depends on local perfusion at the site of intramuscular injection. Injection at a poorly perfused site may result in delayed absorption and for this reason the well-perfused muscles deltoid, quadriceps or gluteus are preferred. If muscle perfusion is poor as a result of systemic hypotension or local vasoconstriction then an intramuscular injection will not be absorbed until muscle perfusion is restored. Delayed absorption will have two consequences. First, the drug will not be effective within the expected time, which may lead to further doses being given. Second, if perfusion is then restored, plasma levels may suddenly rise into the toxic range. For these reasons, the intravenous route is preferred if there is any doubt as to the adequacy of perfusion.

Not all drugs can be given intramuscularly, for example, phenytoin. Intramuscular injections may be painful (e.g. cyclizine) and may cause a local abscess or haematoma, so should be avoided in patients with abnormal clotting. There is also the risk of inadvertent intravenous injection of drug intended for the intramuscular route.

Subcutaneous

Certain drugs are well absorbed from the subcutaneous tissues and this is the favoured route for low-dose heparin therapy. A further indication for this route is where patient compliance is a problem and depot preparations may be useful. Anti-psychotic medication and some contraceptive formulations have been used in this way. Co-preparation of insulin with zinc or protamine can produce a slow absorption profile lasting several hours after subcutaneous administration.

As with the intramuscular route, the kinetics of absorption are dependent on local and regional blood flow, and may be markedly reduced in shock. Again, this has the dual effect of rendering the (non-absorbed) drug initially ineffective, and then subjecting the patient to a bolus once the perfusion is restored.

Transdermal

Drugs may be applied to the skin either for local topical effect, such as steroids, but also may be used to avoid first-pass metabolism and improve bioavailability. Thus, fentanyl and nitrates may be given transdermally for their systemic effects. Factors favouring transdermal absorption are high lipid solubility and a good regional blood supply to the site of application (therefore, the thorax and abdomen are preferred to limbs). Special transdermal formulations (patches) are used to ensure slow, constant release of drug for absorption and provide a smoother pharmacokinetic profile. Only small amounts of drug are released at a time, so potent drugs are better suited to this route of administration if systemic effects are required.

Local anaesthetics may be applied topically to anaesthetise the skin before venepuncture, skin grafts or minor surgical procedures. The two most common preparations are topical eutectic mixture of local anaesthetic (EMLA) and topical amethocaine. The first is a eutectic mixture (each agent lowers the boiling point of the other forming a gel-phase) of lidocaine and prilocaine. Amethocaine is an ester-linked local anaesthetic, which may cause mild, local histamine release producing local vasodilatation, in contrast to the vasoconstriction seen with EMLA. Venodilatation may be useful when anaesthetising the skin prior to venepuncture.

Inhalation

Inhaled drugs may be intended for local or systemic action. The particle size and method of administration are significant factors in determining whether a drug reaches the alveolus and, therefore, the systemic circulation, or whether it only reaches the upper airways. Droplets of less than 1 micron diameter (which may be generated by an ultrasonic nebuliser) can reach the alveolus and hence the systemic circulation. However, a larger droplet or particle size reaches only airway mucosa from the larynx to the bronchioles (and often is swallowed from the pharynx) so that virtually none reaches the alveolus.

Local Site of Action

The bronchial airways are the intended site of action for inhaled or nebulised bronchodilators. However, drugs given for a local or topical effect may be absorbed resulting in unwanted systemic effects. Chronic use of inhaled steroids may lead to Cushingoid side effects, whereas high doses of inhaled β_2-agonists (e.g. salbutamol) may lead to tachycardia and hypokalaemia. Nebulised adrenaline, used for upper airway oedema causing stridor, may be absorbed and can lead to significant tachycardia, arrhythmias and hypertension, although catecholamines are readily metabolised by lung tissue. Similarly, sufficient quantities of topical lidocaine applied prior to fibreoptic intubation may be absorbed and cause systemic toxicity.

Inhaled nitric oxide reaches the alveolus and dilates the pulmonary vasculature. It is absorbed into the pulmonary circulation but does not produce unwanted systemic effects as it has a short half-life, as a result of binding to haemoglobin.

Systemic Site of Action

The large surface area of the lungs (70 m^2 in an adult) available for absorption can lead to a rapid increase in systemic concentration and hence rapid onset of action at distant effect sites. Volatile anaesthetic agents are given by the inhalation route with their ultimate site of action the central nervous system.

The kinetics of the inhaled anaesthetics are covered in greater detail in Chapter 9.

Epidural

The epidural route is used to provide regional analgesia and anaesthesia. Epidural local anaesthetics, opioids, ketamine and clonidine have all been used to treat acute pain, whereas steroids are used for diagnostic and therapeutic purposes in patients with chronic pain. Drug may be given as a single-shot bolus or through a catheter placed in the epidural space as a series of boluses or by infusion.

The speed of onset of block is determined by the proportion of unionised drug available to penetrate the cell membrane. Local anaesthetics are bases with pK_as greater than 7.4 so are predominantly ionised at physiological pH (see Chapter 1). Local anaesthetics with a low pK_a, such as lidocaine, will be less ionised and onset of the block will be faster than for bupivacaine, which has a higher pK_a. Thus lidocaine rather than bupivacaine is often used to 'top up' an existing epidural before surgery. Adding sodium bicarbonate to a local anaesthetic solution increases pH and the unionised fraction, further reducing the onset time. Duration of block depends on tissue binding; bupivacaine has a longer duration of action than lidocaine. The addition of a vasoconstrictor, such as adrenaline or felypressin, will also increase the duration of the block by reducing loss of local anaesthetic from the epidural space.

Significant amounts of drug may be absorbed from the epidural space into the systemic circulation especially during infusions. Local anaesthetics and opioids are both commonly administered via the epidural route and carry significant morbidity when toxic systemic levels are reached.

Intrathecal

Compared with the epidural route, the amount of drug required when given intrathecally is very small; little reaches the systemic circulation and this rarely causes unwanted systemic effects. The extent of spread of a subarachnoid block with local anaesthetic depends on volume and type of solution used. Appropriate positioning of the patient when using hyperbaric solutions, such as with 'heavy' bupivacaine, can limit the spread of block.

Distribution

Drug distribution depends on factors that influence the passage of drug across the cell membrane (see Chapter 1) and on regional blood flow. Physicochemical factors include: molecular size, lipid solubility, degree of ionisation and protein binding. Drugs fall into one of three general groups:

- *Those confined to the plasma* – certain drugs (e.g. dextran 70) are too large to cross the vascular endothelium. Other drugs (e.g. warfarin) may be so intensely protein-bound that the unbound fraction is tiny, so that the amount available to leave the circulation is immeasurably small.

- *Those with limited distribution* – the non-depolarising muscle relaxants are polar, poorly lipid-soluble and bulky. Therefore, their distribution is limited to tissues supplied by capillaries with fenestrae (i.e. muscle) that allow their movement out of the plasma. They cannot cross cell membranes but work extracellularly.
- *Those with extensive distribution* – these drugs are often highly lipid-soluble. Providing their molecular size is relatively small, the extent of plasma protein binding does not restrict their distribution due to the weak nature of such interactions. Other drugs are sequestered by tissues (amiodarone by fat; iodine by the thyroid; tetracyclines by bone), which effectively removes them from the circulation.

Those drugs that are not confined to the plasma are initially distributed to tissues with the highest blood flow (brain, lung, kidney, thyroid, adrenal) then to tissues with a moderate blood flow (muscle), and finally to tissues with a very low blood flow (fat). These three groups of tissues provide a useful model when explaining how plasma levels decline after drug administration.

Blood–Brain Barrier

The blood–brain barrier (BBB) is an anatomical and functional barrier between the circulation and the central nervous system (see Chapter 1).

Active transport and facilitated diffusion are the predominant methods of molecular transfer, which in health is tightly controlled. Glucose and hormones, such as insulin, cross by active carrier transport, while only lipid-soluble, low molecular weight drugs can cross by simple diffusion. Thus inhaled and intravenous anaesthetics can cross readily whereas the larger, polar muscle relaxants cannot and have no central effect. Similarly, glycopyrrolate has a quaternary, charged nitrogen and does not cross the BBB readily. This is in contrast to atropine, a tertiary amine, which may cause centrally mediated effects such as confusion or paradoxical bradycardia. The presence of ABC transport proteins protect the brain from toxins as well as certain antibiotics and cytotoxics (see Chapter 1).

As well as providing an anatomical barrier, the BBB contains enzymes such as monoamine oxidase. Therefore, monoamines are converted to non-active metabolites by passing through the BBB. Physical disruption of the BBB may lead to central neurotransmitters being released into the systemic circulation and may help explain the marked circulatory disturbance seen with head injury and subarachnoid haemorrhage.

In the healthy subject penicillin penetrates the BBB poorly. However, in meningitis, the nature of the BBB alters as it becomes inflamed, and permeability to penicillin (and other drugs) increases, so allowing therapeutic access.

Drug Distribution to the Fetus

The placental membrane that separates fetal and maternal blood is initially derived from adjacent placental syncytiotrophoblast and fetal capillary membranes, which subsequently fuse to form a single membrane. Being phospholipid in nature, the placental membrane is more readily crossed by lipid-soluble than polar molecules. It is much less selective than the BBB and even molecules with only moderate lipid solubility appear to cross with relative ease and significant quantities may appear in cord (fetal) blood. Placental blood flow and the free drug concentration gradient between maternal and fetal blood determine the rate at which drug equilibration takes place. The pH of fetal blood is lower than that of the mother and fetal plasma protein binding may therefore differ. High protein binding in the fetus increases drug transfer across the placenta since fetal free drug levels are low. In contrast, high protein binding in the mother reduces the rate of drug transfer since maternal free drug levels are low. The fetus also may metabolise some drugs; the rate of metabolism increases as the fetus matures.

The effects of maternal pharmacology on the fetus may be divided into those effects that occur in pregnancy, especially the early first trimester when organogenesis occurs, and at birth.

Drugs during Pregnancy

The safety of any drug in pregnancy must be evaluated, but interspecies variation is great and animal models may not exclude the possibility of significant human teratogenicity. In addition, teratogenic effects may not be apparent for some years; stilboestrol taken during pregnancy predisposes female offspring to ovarian cancer at puberty. Wherever possible drug therapy should be avoided throughout pregnancy; if treatment is essential drugs with a long history of safety should be selected.

There are conditions, however, in which the risk of not taking medication outweighs the theoretical or actual risk of teratogenicity. Thus, in epilepsy the risk of hypoxic damage to the fetus secondary to fitting warrants the continuation of anti-epileptic medication during pregnancy. Similarly, the presence of an artificial heart valve mandates the continuation of anticoagulation despite the attendant risks.

Drugs at the Time of Birth

The newborn may have anaesthetic or analgesic drugs in their circulation depending on the type of analgesia for labour and whether delivery was operative. Drugs with a low molecular weight that are lipid-soluble will be present in higher concentrations than large polar molecules.

Bupivacaine is the local anaesthetic most commonly used for epidural analgesia. It crosses the placenta less readily than does lidocaine as its higher pK_a makes it more ionised than lidocaine at physiological pH. However, the fetus is relatively acidotic with respect to the mother, and if the fetal pH is reduced further due to placental insufficiency, the phenomenon of ion trapping may become significant. The fraction of ionised bupivacaine within the fetus increases as the fetal pH falls, its charge preventing it from leaving the fetal circulation, so that levels rise toward toxicity at birth.

Pethidine is used commonly for analgesia during labour. The high lipid solubility of pethidine enables significant amounts to cross the placenta and reach the fetus. It is metabolised to norpethidine, which is less lipid-soluble and can accumulate in the fetus, levels peaking about 4 hours after the initial maternal intramuscular dose. Owing to reduced fetal clearance the half-lives of both pethidine and norpethidine are prolonged up to three times.

Thiopental crosses the placenta rapidly, and experimentally it has been detected in the umbilical vein within 30 seconds of administration to the mother. Serial samples have shown that the peak umbilical artery (and hence fetal) levels occur within 3 minutes of maternal injection. There is no evidence that fetal outcome is affected with an 'injection to delivery' time of up to 20 minutes after injection of a sleep dose of thiopental to the mother.

The non-depolarising muscle relaxants are large polar molecules and essentially do not cross the placenta. Therefore, the fetal neuromuscular junction is not affected. Only very small amounts of suxamethonium cross the placenta, though again this usually has little effect. However, if the mother has an inherited enzyme deficiency and cannot metabolise suxamethonium, then maternal levels may remain high and a significant degree of transfer may occur. This may be especially significant if the fetus has also inherited the enzyme defect, in which case there may be a degree of depolarising blockade at the fetal neuromuscular junction.

Metabolism

While metabolism usually reduces the activity of a drug, activity may be designed to increase; a prodrug is defined as a drug that has no inherent activity before metabolism but that is converted by the body to an active moiety. Examples of prodrugs are enalapril (metabolised to enalaprilat), diamorphine (metabolised to 6-monoacylmorphine), and parecoxib (metabolised to valdecoxib). Metabolites may also have equivalent activity to the parent compound, in which case duration of action is not related to plasma levels of the parent drug.

In general, metabolism produces a more polar (water soluble) molecule that can be excreted in the bile or urine – the chief routes of drug excretion. There are two phases of metabolism, I and II.

Phase I (Functionalisation or Non-synthetic)

- Oxidation
- Reduction
- Hydrolysis.

Many phase I reactions, particularly oxidative pathways, occur in the liver due to a non-specific mixed-function oxidase system in the endoplasmic reticulum. These enzymes form the cytochrome P450 system, named after the wavelength (in nm) of their maximal absorption of light when the reduced state is combined with carbon monoxide. However, this cytochrome system is not unique to the liver; these enzymes are also found in gut mucosa, lung, brain and kidney. Methoxyflurane is metabolised by CYP2E1 in the kidney, generating a high local concentration of fluoride ions, which was the cause of renal failure seen with this agent (see sevoflurane metabolism, p. 120).

The enzymes of the cytochrome P450 system are classified into families and sub-families by their degree of shared amino acid sequences – families and subfamilies share 40% and 55% respectively of the amino acid sequence. In addition, the subfamilies are further divided into isoforms. Families are labelled CYP1, CYP2, and so on, the sub-families CYP1A, CYP1B, and so on, and the isoforms CYP1A1, CYP1A2, and so on. Table 2.1 summarises isoenzymes of particular importance in the metabolism of drugs relevant to the anaesthetist. Many drugs are metabolised by more than one isoenzyme (e.g. midazolam by CYP3A4 and CYP3A5). Genetic variants are also found, in particular CYP2D6 and CYP2C9; variants of CYP2D6 are associated with defective metabolism of codeine.

In addition to abnormal alleles, some people have multiple copies of the CYP2D6 gene – all of which are expressed. As a result, these ultrafast metabolisers convert codeine to morphine very rapidly and experience unpleasant side effects of morphine rather than an effective analgesic effect.

Table 2.1 Metabolism of drugs by cytochrome P450 system. CYP2C9, CYP2C19 and CYP2D6 all demonstrate significant genetic polymorphism; other cytochromes also have variants, but these three are clinically important.

CYP2B6	CYP2C9	CYP2C19	CYP2D6	CYP2E1	CYP3A4	CYP3A5
propofol	propofol	losartan	codeine	sevoflurane	diazepam	diazepam
	parecoxib	diazepam	flecainide	halothane	temazepam	
	losartan	phenytoin	metoprolol	isoflurane	midazolam	
	S-warfarin	omeprazole		paracetamol	fentanyl	
		clopidogrel			alfentanil	
					lidocaine	
					vecuronium	

The P450 system is not responsible for all phase I metabolism. The monoamines (adrenaline, noradrenaline, dopamine) are metabolised by the mitochondrial enzyme monoamine oxidase. Individual genetic variation, or the presence of exogenous inhibitors of this breakdown pathway, can result in high levels of monoamines in the circulation, with severe cardiovascular effects. Ethanol is metabolised by the cytoplasmic enzyme alcohol dehydrogenase to acetaldehyde, which is then further oxidised to acetic acid. This enzyme is one that is readily saturated, leading to a rapid increase in plasma ethanol if consumption continues. Esterases are also found in the cytoplasm of a variety of tissues, including liver and muscle, and are responsible for the metabolism of esters, such as etomidate, aspirin, atracurium and remifentanil. The lung also contains an angiotensin-converting enzyme that is responsible for AT1 to AT2 conversion; this enzyme is also able to break down bradykinin.

In addition, some metabolic processes take place in the plasma: cisatracurium breaks down spontaneously in a pH- and temperature-dependent manner – Hofmann degradation – and suxamethonium is hydrolysed by plasma cholinesterase.

Phase II (Conjugation or Synthetic)

- Glucuronidation (e.g. morphine, propofol)
- Sulfation (e.g. quinol metabolite of propofol)
- Acetylation (e.g. isoniazid, sulfonamides)
- Methylation (e.g. catechols, such as noradrenaline).

Although many drugs are initially metabolised by phase I processes followed by a phase II reaction, some drugs are modified by phase II reactions only. Phase II reactions increase the water solubility of the drug or metabolite to allow excretion into the bile or urine. They occur mainly in the hepatic endoplasmic reticulum but other sites, such as the lung, may also be involved. This is especially true in the case of acetylation, which also occurs in the lung and spleen.

In liver failure, phase I reactions are generally affected before phase II, so drugs with a predominantly phase II metabolism, such as lorazepam, are less affected.

Genetic Polymorphism

There are inherited differences in enzyme structure that alter the way drugs are metabolised in the body. The genetic polymorphisms of particular relevance to anaesthesia are those of plasma cholinesterase, those involved in acetylation and the CYP2D6 variants mentioned above.

Suxamethonium is metabolised by hydrolysis in the plasma, a reaction that is catalysed by the relatively non-specific enzyme plasma cholinesterase. Certain individuals have an unusual variant of the enzyme and metabolise suxamethonium much more slowly. Several autosomal recessive genes have been identified, and these may be distinguished by the degree of enzyme inhibition demonstrated in vitro by substances such as fluoride and the local anaesthetic dibucaine. Muscle paralysis due to suxamethonium may be prolonged for individuals with an abnormal form of the enzyme. This is discussed in greater detail in Chapter 11.

Acetylation is a phase II metabolic pathway in the liver. Drugs metabolised by N-acetyltransferase type 2 (NAT2) include hydralazine and isoniazid. There are genetically different isoenzymes of NAT2 that acetylate at a slow or fast rate. The pharmacokinetic and hence pharmacodynamic profile seen with these drugs depends on the acetylator status of the individual.

Enzyme Inhibition and Induction

Some drugs (see Table 2.2) induce the activity of the hepatic microsomal enzymes. The rate of metabolism of the enzyme-inducing drug as well as other drugs is increased and may lead to reduced plasma levels. Other drugs, especially those with an imidazole structure (e.g. cimetidine), inhibit the activity of hepatic microsomal enzymes and may result in increased plasma levels.

Table 2.2 Effects of various drugs on hepatic microsomal enzymes

	Inducing	Inhibiting
Antibiotics	rifampicin	metronidazole, isoniazid, chloramphenicol
Alcohol	chronic abuse	acute use
Inhaled anaesthetics	enflurane, halothane	
Barbiturates	phenobarbital, thiopental	
Anticonvulsants	phenytoin, carbamazepine	
Hormones	glucocorticoids	
MAOIs		phenelzine, tranylcypromine
H_2 antagonists		cimetidine
Others	cigarette smoking	amiodarone, grapefruit juice

Excretion

Elimination refers to the processes of removal of the drug from the plasma and includes distribution and metabolism, while excretion refers to the removal of drug from the body. The chief sites of excretion are in the urine and the bile (and hence the GI tract), although traces of drug are also detectable in tears and breast milk. The chief route of excretion for the volatile anaesthetic agents is via the lungs; however, metabolites are detectable in urine, and indeed the metabolites of agents such as methoxyflurane may have a significant effect on renal function.

The relative contributions from different routes of excretion depend upon the structure and molecular weight of a drug. In general, high molecular weight compounds (>30,000 Da) are not filtered or secreted by the kidney and are therefore preferentially excreted in the bile. A significant fraction of a drug carrying a permanent charge, such as pancuronium, may be excreted unchanged in urine.

Renal Excretion

Filtration at the Glomerulus

Small, non-protein-bound, poorly lipid-soluble but readily water-soluble drugs are excreted into the glomerular ultrafiltrate. Only free drug present in that fraction of plasma that is filtered is removed at the glomerulus. The remaining plasma will have the same concentration of free drug as that fraction filtered and so there is no change in the extent of plasma protein binding. Thus highly protein-bound drugs are not extensively removed by filtration – but may be excreted by active secretory mechanisms in the tubule.

Secretion at the Proximal Tubules

There are active energy-requiring processes in the proximal convoluted tubules by which a wide variety of molecules may be secreted into the urine against their concentration gradients. Different carrier systems exist for acidic and basic drugs that are each capacity-limited for their respective drug type (i.e. maximal clearance of one acidic drug will result in a reduced clearance of another acidic drug but not of a basic drug). Drug secretion may also be inhibited, for example, probenecid blocks the secretion of penicillin.

Diffusion at the Distal Tubules

At the distal tubule, passive diffusion may occur down the concentration gradient. Acidic drugs are preferentially excreted in an alkaline urine as this increases the fraction present in the ionised form, which cannot be reabsorbed. Conversely, basic drugs are preferentially excreted in acidic urine where they are trapped as cations.

Biliary Excretion

High molecular weight compounds, such as the steroid-based muscle relaxants, are excreted in bile. Secretion from the hepatocyte into the biliary canaliculus takes place against a concentration gradient, and is therefore active and energy-requiring, and subject to inhibition and competition for transport. Certain drugs are excreted unchanged in bile (e.g. rifampicin), while others are excreted after conjugation (e.g. morphine metabolites are excreted as glucuronides).

Enterohepatic Circulation

Drugs excreted in the bile such as glucuronide conjugates may be hydrolysed in the small bowel by glucuronidase secreted by bacteria. Lipid-soluble, active drugs may result and be reabsorbed, passing into the portal circulation to the liver where the extracted fraction is reconjugated and re-excreted in the bile, and the rest passes into the systemic circulation. This process may continue many times. Failure of the oral contraceptive pill while taking broad-spectrum antibiotics has been blamed on a reduced intestinal bacterial flora causing a reduced enterohepatic circulation of oestrogen and progesterone.

Effect of Disease

Renal Disease

In the presence of renal disease, those drugs that are normally excreted via the renal tract may accumulate. This effect will vary according to the degree to which the drug is dependent upon renal excretion – in the case of a drug whose clearance is entirely renal a single dose may have a very prolonged effect. This was true of gallamine, a non-depolarising muscle relaxant, which, if given in the context of renal failure, required dialysis or haemofiltration to reduce the plasma level and hence reverse the pharmacological effect.

If it is essential to give a drug that is highly dependent on renal excretion in the presence of renal impairment, a reduction in dose must be made. If the apparent volume of distribution remains the same, the loading dose also remains the same, but repeated doses may need to be reduced and dosing interval increased. However, due to fluid retention the volume of distribution is often increased in renal failure, so loading doses may be higher than in health.

Knowledge of a patient's creatinine clearance is very helpful in estimating the dose reduction required for a given degree of renal impairment. As an approximation, the dose, D, required in renal failure is given by:

$$D = \text{Usual dose} \times (\text{impaired clearance/normal clearance})$$

Tables contained in the *British National Formulary* give an indication of the appropriate reductions in mild, moderate and severe renal impairment.

Liver Disease

Hepatic impairment alters many aspects of the pharmacokinetic profile of a drug. Protein synthesis is decreased (hence decreased plasma protein levels and reduced protein binding). Both phase I and II reactions are affected, and thus the metabolism of drugs is reduced. The presence of ascites increases the volume of distribution and the presence of portocaval shunts increases bioavailability by reducing hepatic clearance of drugs.

There is no analogous measure of hepatic function compared with creatinine clearance for renal function. Liver function tests in common clinical use may be divided into those that measure the synthetic function of the liver – the international normalised ratio (INR) or prothrombin time and albumin – and those that measure inflammatory damage of the hepatocyte. It is possible to have a markedly inflamed liver with high transaminase levels, with retention of reasonable synthetic function. In illness, the profile of protein synthesis shifts toward acute phase proteins; albumin is not an acute phase protein so levels are reduced in any acute illness.

Patients with severe liver failure may suffer hepatic encephalopathy as a result of a failure to clear ammonia and other molecules. These patients are very susceptible to the effects of benzodiazepines and opioids, which should therefore be avoided if possible. For patients requiring strong analgesia in the perioperative period a coexisting coagulopathy will often rule out a regional technique, leaving few other analgesic options other than careful intravenous titration of opioid analgesics, accepting the risk of precipitating encephalopathy.

The Extremes of Age

Neonate and Infant

In the newborn and young, the pharmacokinetic profiles of drugs are different for a number of reasons. These are due to qualitative, as well as quantitative, differences in the neonatal anatomy and physiology.

Fluid Compartments

The volume and nature of the pharmacokinetic compartments is different, with the newborn being relatively overhydrated and losing volume through diuresis in the hours and days after birth. As well as the absolute proportion of water being higher, the relative amount in the extracellular compartment is increased. The relative sizes of the organs and regional blood flows are also different from the adult; the neonatal liver is relatively larger than that of an adult although its metabolising capacity is lower and may not be as efficient.

Distribution

Plasma protein levels and binding are less than in the adult. In addition, the pH of neonatal blood tends to be lower, which alters the relative proportions of ionised and unionised drug. Thus, both the composition and acid-base value of the blood affect plasma protein binding.

Metabolism and Excretion

While the neonate is born with several of the enzyme systems functioning at adult levels, the majority of enzymes do not reach maturity for a number of months. Plasma levels of cholinesterase are reduced, and in the liver the activity of the cytochrome P450 family of enzymes is markedly reduced. Newborns have a reduced rate of excretion via the renal tract. The creatinine clearance is less than 10% of the adult rate per unit body weight, with nephron numbers and function not reaching maturity for some months after birth.

Though the implications of many of these differences may be predicted, the precise doses of drugs used in the newborn has largely been determined clinically. Preferred drugs should be those that have been used safely for a number of years, and in which the necessary dose adjustments have been derived empirically. In addition, there is wide variation between individuals of the same post-conceptual age.

Elderly

A number of factors contribute to pharmacokinetic differences observed in the elderly. The elderly have a relative reduction in muscle mass, with a consequent increase in the proportion of fat, altering volume of distribution. This loss of muscle mass is of great importance in determining the sensitivity of the elderly to remifentanil, which is significantly metabolised by muscle esterases. There is a reduction in the activity of hepatic enzymes with increasing age, leading to a relative decrease in hepatic drug clearance. Creatinine clearance diminishes steadily with age, reflecting reduced renal function.

As well as physiological changes with increasing age, the elderly are more likely to have multiple coexisting diseases. The implications of this are two-fold. First, the disease processes may directly alter drug pharmacokinetics and second, polypharmacy may produce drug interactions that alter both pharmacokinetics and pharmacodynamic response.

Chapter
3

Drug Action

Mechanisms of Drug Action

Drugs may act in a number of ways to exert their effect. These range from relatively simple non-specific actions that depend on the physicochemical properties of a drug to highly specific and stereoselective actions on proteins in the body, namely enzymes, voltage-gated ion channels and receptors.

Actions Dependent on Chemical Properties

The antacids exert their effect by neutralising gastric acid. The chelating agents are used to reduce the concentration of certain metallic ions within the body. Dicobalt edetate chelates cyanide ions and may be used in cyanide poisoning or following a potentially toxic dose of sodium nitroprusside. The reversal agent sugammadex (a γ-cyclodextrin) selectively chelates rocuronium and reversal is possible from deeper levels of neuromuscular block than can be effected with the anticholinesterases.

Enzymes

Enzymes are biological catalysts, and most drugs that interact with enzymes are inhibitors. The results are two-fold: the concentration of the substrate normally metabolised by the enzyme is increased and that of the product(s) of the reaction is decreased. Enzyme inhibition may be competitive (edrophonium for anticholinesterase), non-competitive or irreversible (aspirin for cyclo-oxygenase and omeprazole for the Na^+/H^+ ATPase). Angiotensin-converting enzyme (ACE) inhibitors such as ramipril prevent the conversion of angiotensin I to II and bradykinin to various inactive fragments. Although reduced levels of angiotensin II are responsible for the therapeutic effects when used in hypertension and heart failure, raised levels of bradykinin may cause an intractable cough.

Voltage-gated Ion Channels

Voltage-gated ion channels are involved in conduction of electrical impulses associated with excitable tissues in muscle and nerve. Several groups of drugs have specific blocking actions at these ion channels. Local anaesthetics act by inhibiting sodium channels in nerve membrane, several anticonvulsants block similar channels in the brain, calcium channel blocking agents act on vascular smooth muscle ion channels and anti-arrhythmic agents block myocardial ion channels. These actions are described in the relevant chapters in Sections II and III.

Receptors

A receptor is a protein, often integral to a membrane, containing a region to which a natural ligand binds specifically to bring about a response. A drug acting at a receptor binds to a recognition site where it may elicit an effect (an agonist), prevent the action of a natural ligand (an inhibitor), or reduce a constitutive effect of a receptor (an inverse agonist). Natural ligands may also bind to more than one receptor and have a different mechanism of action at each (e.g. ionotropic and metabotropic actions of γ-aminobutyric acid (GABA) at $GABA_A$ and $GABA_B$ receptors).

Receptors are generally protein or glycoprotein in nature and may be associated with or span the cell membrane, be present in the membranes of intracellular organelles or be found in the cytosol or nucleus. Those in the membrane are generally for ligands that do not readily penetrate the cell, whereas those within the cell are for lipid-soluble ligands that can diffuse through the cell wall to their site of action, or for intermediary messengers generated within the cell itself.

Receptors may be grouped into three classes depending on their mechanism of action: (1) altered ion permeability; (2) production of intermediate messengers; and (3) regulation of gene transcription (Figure 3.1).

Altered Ion Permeability: Ion Channels

Receptors of this type are part of a membrane-spanning complex of protein subunits that have the potential to form a channel through the membrane. When opened, such a channel allows the passage of ions down their concentration and electrical gradients. Here, ligand binding causes a conformational change in the structure of this membrane protein complex, allowing the channel to open and so increasing the permeability of the membrane to certain ions (ionotropic). There are three important ligand-gated ion channel families: the pentameric, the ionotropic glutamate and the ionotropic purinergic receptors.

The Pentameric Family

The pentameric family of receptors has five membrane-spanning subunits. The best-known example of this type of ion channel receptor is the nicotinic acetylcholine receptor at the neuromuscular junction. It consists of one β, one ε, one δ and two α subunits. Two acetylcholine molecules bind to the α subunits, resulting in a rapid increase in Na^+ flux through the ion channel formed, leading to membrane depolarisation.

Another familiar member of this family is the $GABA_A$ receptor, in which GABA is the natural ligand. Conformational changes induced when the agonist binds cause a chloride-selective ion channel to form, leading to membrane hyperpolarisation. The benzodiazepines (BDZs) can influence GABA activity at this receptor but augment chloride ion conductance by an allosteric mechanism (see below for explanation).

The $5\text{-}HT_3$ receptor is also a member of this pentameric family; it is the only serotonin receptor to act through ion-channel opening.

Ionotropic Glutamate

Glutamate is an excitatory neurotransmitter in the central nervous system (CNS) that works through several receptor types, of which N-Methyl-D-aspartate (NMDA), α-amino-3-hydroxy-5-methyl-4-isoxazolepropionic acid (AMPA) and kainate are ligand-gated ion

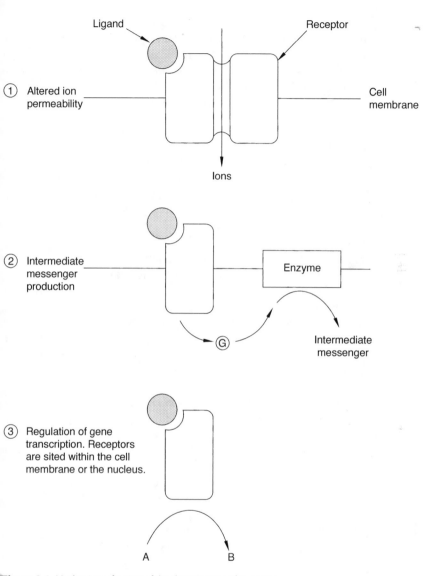

Figure 3.1 Mechanism of action of the three groups of receptors.

channels. The NMDA receptors are comprised of two subunits, one pore-forming (NR1) and one regulatory that binds the co-activator, glycine (NR2). In vivo, it is thought that the receptors dimerise, forming a complex with four subunits. Each NR1 subunit has three membrane-spanning helices, two of which are separated by a re-entrant pore-forming loop. NMDA channels are equally permeable to Na^+ and K^+ but have a particularly high permeability to the divalent cation, Ca^{2+}. Ketamine, xenon and nitrous oxide are non-competitive antagonists at these receptors.

Ionotropic Purinergic Receptors

This family of receptors includes PX1 and PX2. Each has two membrane-spanning helices and no pore-forming loops. They form cationic channels that are equally permeable to Na^+ and K^+ but are also permeable to Ca^{2+}. These purinergic receptors are activated by ATP and are involved in mechanosensation and pain. These are not to be confused with the two G-protein coupled receptor forms of purinergic receptors, which are distinguished by selectivity for adenosine or ATP.

Production of Intermediate Messengers

There are several membrane-bound systems that transduce a ligand-generated signal presented on one side of the cell membrane into an intracellular signal transmitted by intermediate messengers. The most common is the G-protein coupled receptor system but there are others including the tyrosine kinase and guanylyl cyclase systems.

G-protein Coupled Receptors and G-proteins

G-protein coupled receptors (GPCRs) are membrane-bound proteins with a serpentine structure consisting of seven helical regions that traverse the membrane. G-proteins are a group of heterotrimeric (three different subunits, α, β and γ) proteins associated with the inner leaflet of the cell membrane that act as universal transducers involved in bringing about an intracellular change from an extracellular stimulus. The GPCR binds a ligand on its extracellular side and the resultant conformational change increases the likelihood of coupling with a particular type of G-protein resulting in activation of intermediate messengers at the expense of guanylyl triphosphate (GTP) breakdown. This type of receptor interaction is sometimes known as **metabotropic** in contrast with ionotropic for ion-channel forming receptors. As well as transmitting a stimulus across the cell membrane the G-protein system produces signal amplification, whereby a modest stimulus may have a much greater intracellular response. This amplification occurs at two levels: a single activated GPCR can stimulate multiple G-proteins and each G-protein can activate several intermediate messengers.

G-proteins bind GDP and GTP, hence the name 'G-protein'. In the inactive form GDP is bound to the α subunit but on interaction with an activated GPCR, GTP replaces GDP, giving a complex of α-GTP-βγ. The α-GTP subunit then dissociates from the βγ dimer and activates or inhibits an effector protein, either an enzyme, such as **adenylyl cyclase** or **phospholipase C** (Figure 3.2) or an ion channel. For example, β-adrenergic agonists activate adenylyl cyclase and opioid receptor agonists, such as morphine, depress transmission of pain signals via inhibition of N-type Ca^{2+} channels through G-protein mechanisms. In some systems, the βγ dimer can also activate intermediary mechanisms.

The α-subunit itself acts as a GTPase enzyme, splitting the GTP attached to it to regenerate an inactive α-GDP subunit. This then reforms the entire inactive G-protein complex by recombination with another βγ dimer.

The α subunit of the G-proteins shows marked variability, with at least 17 molecular variants arranged into three main classes. G_s type G-proteins have α subunits that activate adenylyl cyclase, G_i have α subunits that inhibit adenylyl cyclase and G_q have α subunits that activate phospholipase C. Each GPCR will act via a specific type of G-protein complex and this determines the outcome from

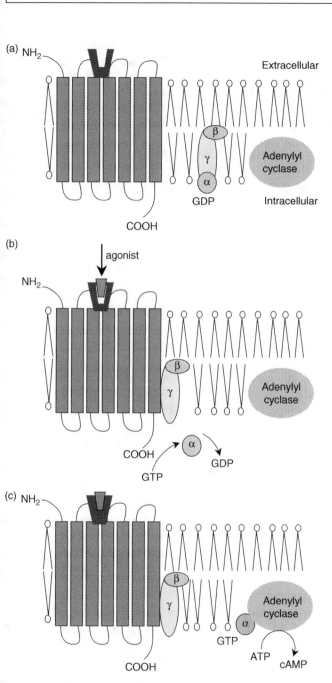

Figure 3.2 Effect of ligand-binding to G-protein coupled receptor (GPCR). Ligand binding to the 7-TMD GPCR favours association with the G-Protein, which allows GTP to replace GDP. The α unit then dissociates from the G-protein complex to mediate enzyme and ion-channel activation/inhibition.

ligand-receptor coupling. It is known that the ratio of G-protein to GPCR is in favour of the G-proteins in the order of about 100 to 1, permitting signal amplification. Regulation of GPCR activity involves phosphorylation at the intracellular carboxyl-terminal that encourages binding of a protein, β-arrestin, which is the signal for removal of the receptor protein from the cell membrane. The binding of an agonist may increase phosphorylation and so regulate its own effect, accounting for tachyphylaxis seen with β-adrenergic agonists.

Adenylyl cyclase catalyses the formation of cAMP, which acts as a final common pathway for a number of extracellular stimuli. All β-adrenergic effects are mediated through G_s and opiate effects through G_i. The cAMP so formed acts by stimulating protein kinase A, which has two regulatory (R) and two catalytic (C) units. cAMP binds to the R unit, revealing the active C unit, which is responsible for the biochemical effect, and it may cause either protein synthesis, gene activation or changes in ionic permeability.

cAMP formed under the regulation of G-proteins is broken down by the action of the phosphodiesterases (PDEs). The PDEs are a family of five isoenzymes, of which PDE III is the most important in heart muscle. PDE inhibitors, such as theophylline and enoximone, prevent the breakdown of cAMP so that intracellular levels rise. Therefore, in the heart, positive inotropy is possible by either increasing cAMP levels (with a β-adrenergic agonist or a non-adrenergic inotrope such as glucagon), or by reducing the breakdown of cAMP (with a PDE III inhibitor such as milrinone).

Phospholipase C is also under the control of G-proteins, but the α subunit is of the G_q type. Activation of G_q-proteins by formation of an active ligand–receptor complex promotes the action of phospholipase C. This breaks down a membrane lipid, phosphatidylinositol 4,5-bisphosphate (PIP_2), to form inositol triphosphate (IP_3) and diacylglycerol (DAG).

The two molecules formed have specific actions; IP_3 causes calcium release in the endoplasmic reticulum, and DAG causes activation of protein kinase C, with a variety of biochemical effects specific to the nature of the cell in question. Increased calcium levels act as a trigger to many intracellular events, including enzyme action and hyperpolarisation. Again, the common messenger will cause specific effects according to the nature of the receiving cellular subcomponent.

$α_1$-Adrenoceptors, the muscarinic cholinergic types 1, 3 and 5 as well as angiotensin II type 1 receptors exert their effects by activation of G_q-proteins.

Membrane guanylyl cyclase. Some hormones such as atrial natriuretic peptide mediate their actions via membrane-bound receptors with intrinsic guanylyl cyclase activity. As a result cGMP levels increase and it acts as a secondary messenger by phosphorylation of intracellular enzymes.

Nitric oxide exerts its effects by increasing the levels of intracellular cGMP by stimulating a cytosolic guanylyl cyclase rather than a membrane-bound enzyme.

Membrane tyrosine kinase. Insulin and growth factor act through the tyrosine kinase system, which is contained within the cell membrane, resulting in a wide range of physiological effects. Insulin, epidermal growth factor and platelet-derived growth factor all activate such tyrosine kinase-linked receptors.

The insulin receptor consists of two α- and two β-subunits, the latter span the cell membrane. When a ligand binds to the α-subunits, intracellular tyrosine residues on its β-subunits are phosphorylated, so activating their tyrosine kinase activity. The activated enzyme catalyses phosphorylation of other protein targets, which generate the many effects of insulin. These effects include the intracellular metabolic effects, the insertion of glucose transport protein into the cell membrane as well as those actions involving gene transcription.

Regulation of Gene Transcription

Steroids and thyroid hormones act through intracellular receptors to alter the expression of DNA and RNA. They indirectly alter the production of cellular proteins so their effects are necessarily slow. These cytoplasmic receptors act as ligand-regulated transcription factors; they are normally held in an inactive form by association with inhibitory proteins. The binding of an appropriate hormone induces a conformational change that activates the receptor and permits translocation to the nucleolus, which leads to association with specific DNA promoter sequences and production of mRNA.

Adrenosteroid Hormones

There are two types of corticosteroid receptor: the mineralocorticoid receptor, MR, and the glucocorticoid receptor, GR. The GR receptor is wide spread in cells, including the liver where corticosteroids alter the hepatic production of proteins during stress to favour the so-called acute-phase reaction proteins. The MR is restricted to epithelial tissue such as renal collecting tubules and colon, although these cells also contain GR receptors. Selective MR receptor activation occurs due to the presence of 11-β hydroxysteroid dehydrogenase, which converts cortisol to cortisone: cortisone is inactive at the GR receptor.

Other Nuclear Receptors

The antidiabetic drug pioglitazone is an agonist at a nuclear receptor, peroxisome proliferator-activated receptor, which controls protein transcription associated with increased sensitivity to insulin in adipose tissue.

Dynamics of Drug–Receptor Binding

The binding of a ligand (L) to its receptor (R) is represented by the equation:

$$L + R \leftrightarrow LR.$$

This reaction is reversible. The law of mass action states that the rate of a reaction is proportional to the concentrations of the reacting components. Thus, the velocity of the forward reaction is given by:

$$V_1 = k_1 \cdot [L] \cdot [R],$$

where k_1 is the rate constant for the forward reaction (square brackets indicate concentration).

The velocity of the reverse reaction is given by:

$$V_2 = k_2 \cdot [LR],$$

where k_2 is the rate constant for the reverse reaction.

At equilibrium, the reaction occurs at the same rate in both directions ($V_1 = V_2$), and the equilibrium dissociation constant, K_D, is given by the equation:

$$K_D = [L] \cdot [R]/[LR] = k_2/k_1.$$

Its reciprocal, K_A, is the equilibrium association constant and is a reflection of the strength of binding between the ligand and receptor. Note that these constants do not have the same units; the units for K_D are $mmol.L^{-1}$ whereas those for K_A are $L.mmol^{-1}$ (when reading pharmacology texts take careful note of which of these two constants is being described). It was Ariens who first suggested that response is proportional to receptor occupancy and this was the basis of pharmacodynamic modelling. However, the situation is not as straightforward as this may imply and we need to explain the existence of partial agonists and inverse agonists as well as the phenomenon of spare receptors.

Receptor proteins can exist in a number of conformations that are in equilibrium, in particular the active and inactive forms; in the absence of an agonist the equilibrium favours the inactive form. Antagonists bind equally to both forms of the receptor and do not alter the equilibrium. Agonists bind to the receptor and push this equilibrium toward the active conformation. The active conformation then triggers the series of molecular events that result in the observed effect.

Types of Drug–Receptor Interaction

The two properties of a drug that determine the nature of its pharmacological effect are affinity and intrinsic activity.

- Affinity refers to how well or avidly a drug binds to its receptor – in the analogy of the lock and key, this is how well the key fits the lock. The avidity of binding is determined by the K_D or K_A of the drug.
- Intrinsic activity (IA) or efficacy refers to the magnitude of effect the drug has once bound; IA takes a value between 0 and 1, although inverse agonists can have an IA between -1 and 0.

It is important to distinguish these properties. A drug may have a high affinity, but no activity, and thus binding will produce no pharmacological response. If such a drug prevents the binding of a more active ligand, this ligand will be unable to exert its effect – so the drug is demonstrating receptor antagonism. However, if a drug binds well but only induces a fractional response, never a full response, then the maximum possible response can never be achieved. This is the situation with partial agonists. Therefore:

- An agonist has significant receptor affinity and full intrinsic activity (IA = 1).
- An antagonist has significant receptor affinity but no intrinsic activity (IA = 0).

- A partial agonist has significant receptor affinity but only fractional intrinsic activity (0 < IA < 1).
- An inverse agonist can be full or partial with $-1 \leq IA < 0$.

Receptor Agonism

Full Agonists

Full agonists are drugs able to generate a maximal response from a receptor. Not only do they have a high affinity for the receptor, but also they have a high IA. In clinical terms, the potency of the drug is determined by its K_D; the lower the K_D the higher the potency. For many drugs, the ED_{50} (the dose producing 50% of the maximum response) corresponds to the K_D.

Partial Agonists

If an agonist drug has an intrinsic activity less than 1, such that it occupies receptors, but produces a submaximal effect compared with the full agonist, it is termed a partial agonist. The distinguishing feature of partial agonists is that they fail to achieve a maximal effect even in very high dose (i.e. with full receptor occupancy) (Figure 3.3c). An example of a partial agonist is buprenorphine acting at the μ-opioid receptor. Partial agonists may act as either agonists or antagonists depending on circumstances. If used alone, they are agonists. When combined with a full agonist they produce additive effects at low doses of the full agonist, but this switches to competitive antagonism as the dose of full agonist increases; the full agonist needs to displace the partial agonist in order to restore maximum effect. In the case of partial agonists the equilibrium between active and inactive receptor forms can never be entirely in favour of the active conformation, so the link between activation of receptor and effect is only a fraction of that seen with full agonists.

Inverse Agonists

It is possible for a drug to bind and exert an effect opposite to that of the endogenous agonist. Such a drug is termed an inverse agonist and may have high or moderate affinity. The mechanism of inverse agonism is related to a constitutive action of receptors; some receptors can show a low level of activity even in the absence of a ligand, since the probability of taking up an active conformation is small but measurable. Inverse agonists bind to these receptors and greatly reduce the incidence of the active conformation responsible for this constitutive activity; as a result, inverse agonists appear to exert an opposite effect to the agonist. The difference between an inverse agonist and a competitive antagonist is important – an inverse agonist will favour a shift of equilibrium toward inactive receptors whereas a competitive antagonist binds equally to active and inactive receptors and simply prevents the agonist from binding. Inverse agonism was first described at benzodiazepine binding sites, but such convulsant agents have no clinical relevance, however, ketanserin is an inverse agonist at $5HT_{2c}$ receptors.

Receptor Antagonism

Antagonists exhibit affinity but no intrinsic activity. Their binding may be either reversible or irreversible.

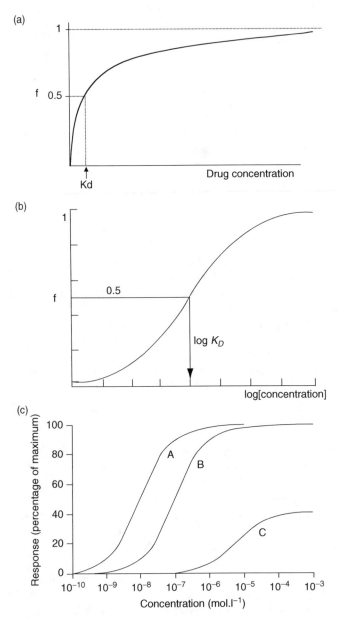

Figure 3.3 Dose–response curves. (a) Normal agonist dose–response curve, which is hyperbolic. (b) This curve is plotted using a log scale for dose and produces the classical sigmoid shape. (c) A and B are full agonists; B is less potent than A; C is a partial agonist that is unable to elicit a maximal response.

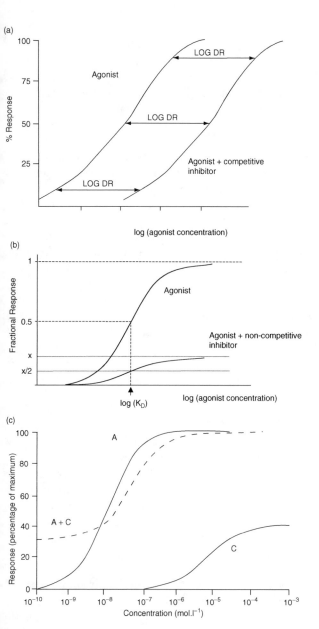

Figure 3.4 Reversible antagonists. (a) Competitive inhibition. Note the parallel shift to the right in the presence of competitive inhibitor, with preservation of maximum response. DR represents dose-ratio (see text). (b) Non-competitive inhibition. This time maximum possible response is given as a fraction. In the presence of the non-competitive inhibitor the curve is not shifted to the right, but the maximum obtainable response is reduced. K_D is the dissociation constant and is unaltered by the inhibitor. (c) Partial agonist acting as competitive inhibitor. In this scenario A is a full agonist; C is a partial agonist. The dotted line, A + C, shows the dose-response curve for A in the presence of a sub-maximal dose of C. At low concentration of A the combination results in a greater effect than with A alone but as the dose of A is increased there comes a point at which the effect of A + C is less than with A alone. This is because at the crossover point the only way A can increase the response is by competing for receptors occupied by C. C therefore appears to act as a competitive inhibitor.

Reversible

Reversible antagonists may either be competitive or non-competitive.

Competitive Antagonists

For competitive antagonists the effect of the antagonist may be overcome by increasing the concentration of the agonist – the two molecules are competing for the same site and the relative amounts of each (combined with receptor affinity) determine the ratios of receptor occupation. In the presence of a competitive inhibitor the log[dose] versus response curve is shifted to the right along the x-axis; the extent of this shift is known as the dose ratio (Figure 3.4a). It defines the factor by which agonist concentration must be increased in order to produce equivalent responses in the presence and absence of a competitive inhibitor. The pA_2 value, the negative logarithm of the concentration of antagonist required to produce a dose ratio of 2, is used to compare the efficiency of competitive antagonism for different antagonists at a given receptor.

Examples of competitive inhibition include the non-depolarising muscle relaxants competing with acetylcholine for cholinergic binding sites at the nicotinic receptor of the neuromuscular junction, and β-blockers competing with noradrenaline at β-adrenergic receptor sites in the heart.

As a general principle, first postulated by Bowman, weaker antagonists at the neuromuscular junction have a more rapid onset of action. This is because they are given in a higher dose for the same maximal effect so that more molecules are available to occupy receptors, and the receptor occupancy required for full effect is achieved more rapidly. Rocuronium, a non-depolarising muscle relaxant, has only one-fifth of the potency of vecuronium, and therefore is given at five times the dose for the same effect. The flooding of the receptors means that the threshold receptor occupancy is achieved more rapidly, with a clear clinical benefit.

Non-competitive Antagonists

Non-competitive antagonists do not bind to the same site as the agonist, and classically they do not alter the binding of the agonist. Their antagonism results from preventing receptor activation through conformational distortion. Their action cannot be overcome by increasing the concentration of an agonist. An example is the non-competitive antagonism of glutamate by ketamine at NMDA receptors in the CNS. Recent classification of antagonists now groups non-competitive inhibitors and negative allosteric modulators (see below) together. This is because most non-competitive inhibitors, when investigated carefully, do alter agonist binding.

Allosteric Modulation of Receptor Binding

Not all drugs with reversible activity will produce effects that fit neatly into either the competitive or non-competitive category. Some drugs can bind to sites distant from the agonist receptor site, yet still alter the binding characteristics of the agonist. Such drugs are called allosteric modulators and may either reduce (negative allosteric modulators) or enhance (positive allosteric modulators) the activity of a given dose of agonist without having any discernible effects of their own. An example of a positive allosteric modulator is the effect of benzodiazepines on the activity of GABA at the $GABA_A$ receptor complex.

Irreversible

Irreversible antagonists may either bind irreversibly to the same site as the agonist or at a distant site. Whatever the nature of the binding site, increasing agonist concentration will not overcome the blockade. There are several examples of clinically useful drugs with irreversible actions on receptors. Phenoxybenzamine irreversibly binds to and antagonises the effects of catecholamines at α-adrenoceptors. The antiplatelet agent, clopidogrel, is a prodrug, the active metabolite of which binds irreversibly to G_i-protein coupled ADP $PY2Y_{12}$ receptors.

Spare Receptors

The neuromuscular junction contains acetylcholine (ACh) receptors, which when occupied by ACh cause depolarisation of the motor end plate. However, only a fraction of these receptors need to be occupied to produce a maximal pharmacological effect. Occupancy of only a small proportion of the receptors ensures that a small quantity of ACh produces a maximal response. As a result there are 'spare receptors', which provide some protection against failure of transmission in the presence of toxins. This can be demonstrated as follows: if a small dose of an irreversible inhibitor is given then a proportion of the receptors are bound by the inhibitor and rendered unavailable so the log[dose] versus response curve for ACh is shifted to the right because a higher fraction of the remaining receptors must be occupied to produce the original response. If a further irreversible antagonist is used more receptors are made unavailable and results in a further right-shift of the log[dose] versus response curve. When more than three-quarters of the receptors are occupied by irreversible antagonist then whatever the dose of ACh, a maximum response cannot occur and the shape of the curve changes so that both the maximum response and the slope is reduced.

Tachyphylaxis, Desensitisation and Tolerance

Repeated doses of a drug may lead to a change in the pharmacological response, which may be increased or decreased for the same dose.

Tachyphylaxis

Tachyphylaxis is defined as a rapid decrease in response to repeated doses over a short time period. The most common mechanism is the decrease of stores of a transmitter before resynthesis can take place. An example is the diminishing response to repeated doses of ephedrine, an indirectly acting sympathomimetic amine, caused by the depletion of noradrenaline.

Desensitisation

Desensitisation refers to a chronic loss of response over a longer period and may be caused by a structural change in receptor morphology or by an absolute loss of receptor numbers. The term is often used synonymously with tachyphylaxis. An example is the loss of β-adrenergic receptors from the myocardial cell surface in the continued presence of adrenaline and dobutamine.

Tolerance

Tolerance refers to the phenomenon whereby larger doses are required to produce the same pharmacological effect, such as occurs in chronic opioid use or abuse. This reflects an altered sensitivity of the receptors of the CNS to opioids – the mechanism may be a reduction of receptor density or a reduction of receptor affinity. Tolerance occurs if nitrates are given by continuous infusion for prolonged periods as the sulfhydryl groups on vascular smooth muscle become depleted. A drug holiday of a few hours overnight when the need for vasodilatation is likely to be at its lowest allows replenishment of the sulfhydryl groups and restoration of the pharmacological effect.

Drug Interaction

Interactions occur when one drug modifies the action of another. This interaction may either increase or decrease the second drug's action. Sometimes these interactions result in unwanted effects, but some interactions are beneficial and can be exploited therapeutically.

Drug interaction can be described as physicochemical, relating to the properties of the drug or its pharmaceutical preparation, pharmacokinetic due to alterations in the way the body handles the drug or pharmacodynamic where the activity of one drug is affected. The chance of a significant interaction increases markedly with the number of drugs used and the effects of any interaction are often exaggerated in the presence of disease or coexisting morbidity.

Historically, up to one in six drug charts contained a significant drug interaction, but modern electronic prescribing systems are programmed with warnings. An uncomplicated general anaesthetic may use ten or more different agents that may interact with one another or, more commonly, with the patient's concurrent medication.

Pharmaceutical

These interactions occur because of a chemical or physical incompatibility between the preparations being used. Sodium bicarbonate and calcium will precipitate out of solution as calcium carbonate when co-administered in the same giving set. However, one agent may inactivate another without such an overt indication to the observer; insulin may be denatured if prepared in solutions of dextrose and may, therefore, lose its pharmacological effect. Drugs may also react with the giving set or syringe and therefore need special equipment for delivery, such as a glass syringe for paraldehyde administration. Glyceryl trinitrate is absorbed by polyvinyl chloride; therefore, special polyethylene administration sets are preferred.

Pharmacokinetic

Absorption

In the case of drugs given orally, this occurs either as a result of one drug binding another in the lumen of the gastrointestinal (GI) tract or by altering the function of the GI tract as a whole. Charcoal can adsorb drugs in the stomach, preventing absorption through the GI tract (charcoal is activated by steam to cause fissuring, thereby greatly increasing the surface area for adsorption). Metoclopramide when given as an adjunct for the treatment of migraines reduces GI stasis, which is a feature of the disease, and speeds the absorption of co-administered analgesics. This is an example of a favourable interaction.

P-glycoprotein transport protein (PGP) is an efflux transporter and responsible for transporting a wide range of drugs out of intestinal cells. It is located in the luminal membrane of the entire intestinal membrane and reduces oral bioavailability of many drugs by pumping them back into the lumen of the gut. Drugs which induce PGP, such as rifampicin and phenytoin, may reduce drug bioavailability. Conversely, inhibitors of PGP, such as amiodarone and verapamil, may increase the bioavailability of susceptible drugs.

Distribution

Drugs that decrease cardiac output (such as β-blockers) reduce the flow of blood carrying absorbed drug to its site of action. The predominant factor influencing the time to onset of fasciculation following the administration of suxamethonium is cardiac output, which may be reduced by the prior administration of β-blockers. In addition, drugs that alter cardiac output may have a differential effect on regional blood flow and may cause a relatively greater reduction in hepatic blood flow, so slowing drug elimination.

Chelating agents are used therapeutically in both the treatment of overdose and of iron overload in conditions such as haemochromatosis. The act of chelation combines the drug with the toxic element and prevents tissue damage. Sodium calcium edetate chelates the heavy metal lead and is used as a slow intravenous infusion in the treatment of lead poisoning. Dicobalt edetate chelates cyanide ions and is used in the treatment of cyanide poisoning, which may occur following the prolonged infusion of sodium nitroprusside.

Competition for binding sites to plasma proteins has been suggested to account for many important drug interactions. This is not generally true; it is of importance only for highly protein-bound drugs when enzyme systems are close to saturation at therapeutic levels. One possible exception is the displacement of phenytoin, which is 90% protein-bound, from binding sites by a co-administered drug when therapeutic levels are already at the upper end of normal. In this case a 10% reduction in binding, to 81%, almost doubles the free phenytoin level. Although hepatocytes will increase their metabolism as a result, the enzyme system is readily saturated and this leads to zero-order kinetics and the plasma level remains high instead of re-equilibrating. Most so-called 'protein-binding' interactions are actually due to an alteration in metabolic capacity of one drug by the other. The commonest example seen in practice is the administration of amiodarone to a patient taking warfarin. Amiodarone inhibits the metabolism of S-warfarin by CYP2C9, which can significantly increase plasma levels of the active form of warfarin and produce iatrogenic coagulopathy. A similar interaction occurs with the NSAID phenylbutazone.

Metabolism

Enzyme induction will increase the breakdown of drugs metabolised by the cytochrome P450 family. Anticonvulsants and dexamethasone reduce the duration of action of vecuronium by inducing CYP3A4. Rifampicin can induce a number of the isoenzymes including 2B6, 2C9, 2D6 and 3A4. Conversely, drugs may inhibit enzyme activity, leading to a decrease in metabolism and an increase in plasma levels (see Table 2.1); cimetidine is much more potent than ranitidine at inhibiting 1A2, 2D6 and 3A4.

Prodrugs such as losartan and clopidogrel require activation by CYP450 enzymes and therefore the consequences of induction and inhibition are the reverse of those for drugs that are inactivated by metabolism. The proposed interaction between omeprazole and clopidogrel involves inhibition of CYP2C19 by omeprazole preventing conversion of clopidogrel to its active metabolite and so reducing its antiplatelet activity. Food and drink can also influence the activity of the cytochrome system; grapefruit juice inhibits CYP3A4, broccoli induces 1A2 and ethanol induces 2E1.

Excretion

Sodium bicarbonate will make the urine more alkaline, which enhances the excretion of weak acids such as aspirin or barbiturates. Thus, aspirin overdose has been treated with infusions of fluid to produce a diuresis, together with sodium bicarbonate, to alkalinise the urine and to promote its renal excretion.

Pharmacodynamic

Pharmacodynamic interactions may be direct (same receptor system) or indirect (different mechanisms, same end-effect).

Direct Interactions

Flumazenil is used therapeutically to reverse the effects of benzodiazepines and naloxone to reverse the effects of opioids. This competitive antagonism is useful in treating drug over-dose from these agents.

One common direct interaction that may be overlooked is that between phenylephrine and α_1-adrenergic blockers used for the treatment of benign prostatic hyperplasia (BHP). Drugs used for BHP that act through this mechanism include alfuzosin, doxazosin, indor-amin, prazosin, tamsulosin and terazosin. It is important to identify these drugs to know when α-adrenergic agonists will be ineffective in the treatment of anaesthesia-related hypotension.

The interaction between monoamine oxidase inhibitors (MAOI) and pethidine is a classic example of an indirect interaction. The increase in noradrenaline caused by MAOIs is potentiated when re-uptake is inhibited by pethidine. MAOIs will also increase serotonin and therefore interact with selective serotonin reuptake inhibitors (SSRIs) and high-dose fentanyl with the possibility of precipitating serotonin syndrome.

Indirect Interactions

There are many potentially important indirect interactions of relevance to anaesthetists and intensivists. It is important to recognise the mechanisms of all prescribed drug actions so both beneficial and unwanted interactions can be identified. The use of neostigmine in the presence of non-depolarising muscle relaxants (NDMRs) is an example of an indirect interaction that is used therapeutically. Neostigmine inhibits acetylcholinesterase and so increases acetylcholine concentration in the synaptic cleft that can then compete for nicotinic receptors and displace the NDMR.

Both milrinone and adrenaline are positive inotropic agents with different mechanisms of action that can interact indirectly to improve contractility. Adrenaline works via a GPCR whereas milrinone acts intracellularly by inhibiting phosphodiesterase but both actions result in an increase in intracellular cAMP levels. Ramipril and β-blockers act additively to lower blood pressure by an indirect interaction; one via the renin–angiotensin system and the other via adrenoceptors.

Diuretics through their action on the levels of potassium may indirectly cause digoxin toxicity.

Summation

Summation refers to the action of the two drugs being additive, with each drug having an independent action in the absence of the other. Therefore, the co-administration of midazolam and propofol at the induction of anaesthesia reduces the amount of propofol necessary for the same anaesthetic effect.

Potentiation

Potentiation results from an interaction between two drugs in which one drug has no independent action of its own, yet their combined effect is greater than that of the active drug alone. For example, probenecid reduces the renal excretion of penicillin, such that the effect of a dose of penicillin is enhanced without itself having antibiotic activity.

Synergism

Synergy occurs when the combined action of two drugs is greater than would be expected from purely an additive effect. Often this is because the drugs exert similar effects, but through different mechanisms. Propofol and remifentanil act synergistically when used to maintain anaesthesia.

Isobologram

The nature of interactions between different agents may be studied by use of an isobologram (Greek *isos*, equal; *bolus*, effect). An isobologram describes the combined effect of two different drugs. Consider two drugs A and B, each of which individually produce the required effect at concentrations a and b mmol.L^{-1}, respectively. A curve may be constructed from the fractional concentrations of each, plotted on the x- and y-axes, that produce the target effect. A straight line from 1 on the x-axis (drug A) to 1 on the y-axis (drug B) describes a purely additive effect where half the concentrations of each drug combine to produce the original target effect. When the resultant curve is not linear, some interaction between the drugs is occurring. Consider what happens when we have a concentration a/2 of drug A. If we can combine it with a concentration b/2 of drug B and the result is the same as with either drug alone, then the point A (½, ½) can be marked, and there is a straight line indicating addivity. If however we need to combine a concentration a/2 of drug A with only a concentration of b/4 of drug B to elicit the same response, the point (½, ¼) can be marked, which describes a curve that is concave, suggesting synergism between drugs A and B. Similarly, if we needed a concentration greater than b/2 of drug B the curve would be convex, indicating some antagonistic interaction between the two drugs, point C (½, ¾) (see Figure 4.1).

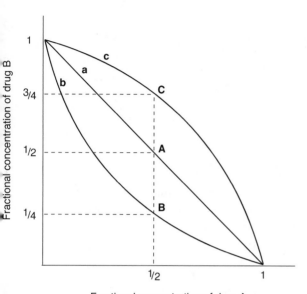

Figure 4.1 Isobolograms with lines of equal activity: (a) additive; (b) synergistic; (c) antagonistic (see text for explanation).

There are some combinations of drugs where combined activity is less than predicted from individual doses. This might seem an irrational form of drug combination, but could be useful if full doses of either drug cause an unacceptable adverse reaction. An example is the use of an ACE inhibitor in combination with an ATII (angiotensin II) receptor antagonist. For some patients the combination of these drugs works in the management of hypertension.

Chapter 5

Isomerism

Isomerism is the phenomenon by which molecules with the same atomic formulae have different structural arrangements – the component atoms of the molecule are the same, but they are arranged in a different configuration. There are two broad classes of isomerism:

- **Structural isomerism**
- **Stereoisomerism.**

Structural Isomerism

Molecules that are structural isomers have identical chemical formulae, but the order of atomic bonds differs. Depending on the degree of structural similarity between the isomers, comparative pharmacological effects may range from identical to markedly different. Isoflurane and enflurane are both volatile anaesthetic agents; prednisolone and aldosterone have significantly different activities, with the former having glucocorticoid and mineralo-corticoid actions but the latter being predominantly a mineralocorticoid. Isoprenaline and methoxamine have different cardiovascular effects, with methoxamine acting predominantly via α-adrenoceptors and isoprenaline acting via β-adrenoceptors. Dihydrocodeine and dobutamine are structural isomers with very different pharmacological effects; it is little more than coincidence that their chemical formulae are identical (Figure 5.1).

Tautomerism

Tautomerism refers to the dynamic interchange between two forms of a molecular structure, often precipitated by a change in the physical environment. For example, midazolam, which is ionised in solution at pH 4, changes structure by forming a seven-membered unionised ring at physiological pH 7.4, rendering it lipid-soluble, which favours passage through the blood–brain barrier (BBB) and increases speed of access to its active sites in the central nervous system (CNS) (see Figure 18.1). Another common form of isomerism is the keto-enol transformation seen in both morphine and thiopental.

Stereoisomerism

Stereoisomers have both the same chemical constituents and bond structure as each other but a different three-dimensional configuration. There are two forms of stereoisomerism:

- **Geometric**
- **Optical.**

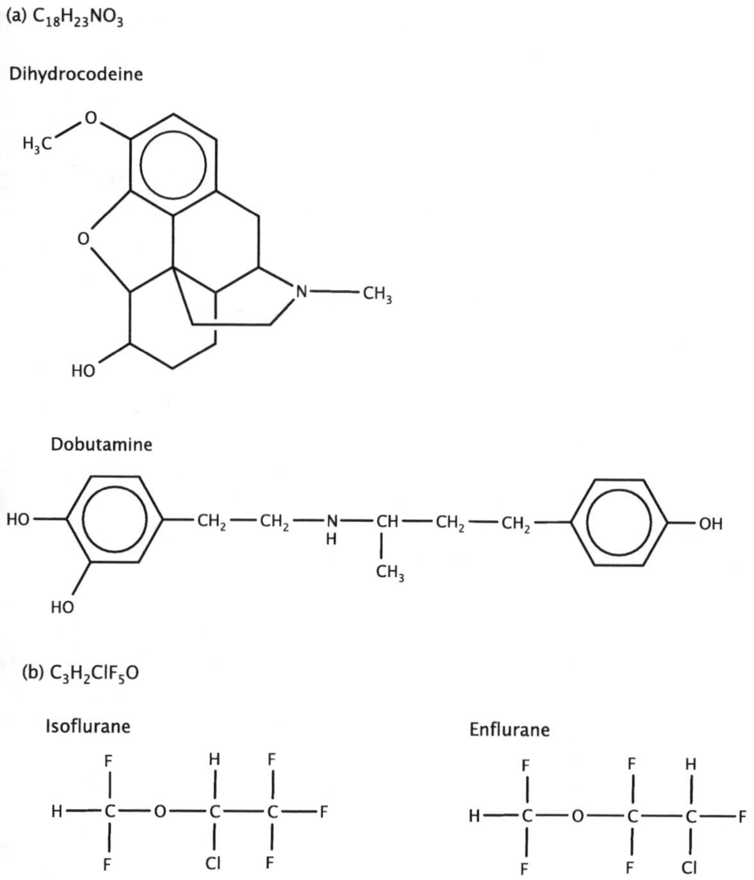

(a) $C_{18}H_{23}NO_3$

Dihydrocodeine

Dobutamine

(b) $C_3H_2ClF_5O$

Isoflurane

Enflurane

**Figure
5.1** Structural
isomers: (a) $C_{18}H_{23}$
NO_3;
(b) $C_3H_2ClF_5O$.

Geometric Isomerism

This exists when a molecule has dissimilar groups attached to two atoms (often carbon) linked either by a double bond or in a ring structure. The free rotation of groups is restricted and so the groups may either be on the same side of the plane of the double bond or ring, or on opposite sides. If the groups are on the same side the conformation is called cis- and if on opposite sides trans-. The bis-benzylisoquinolinium muscle relaxants, such as mivacurium, have two identical heterocyclic groups linked through an ester-containing carbon chain. Each of the heterocyclic groups contains a planar ring with groups that may be arranged in either the cis- or trans- conformation. So each of these compounds needs two prefixes describing their geometrical conformation, one for each heterocyclic group, hence cis-cis- in cisatracurium. Mivacurium contains three such geometric isomers, trans-trans- (58%), cis-trans- (36%) and cis-cis- (6%).

Optical Stereoisomers

Optical stereoisomers may have one or more chiral centres. A chiral centre is a carbon atom or a quaternary nitrogen surrounded by four different chemical groups. The bonds are so arranged that in three dimensions they point to the vertices of a tetrahedron; thus, there are two mirror image conformations that could occur but which cannot be superimposed.

A Single Chiral Centre

The absolute spatial arrangement of the four groups around a single chiral centre (Figure 5.2), either carbon or quaternary nitrogen, is now used to distinguish isomers as it unambiguously defines these spatial relationships. In the past the two isomers were distinguished by the direction in which they rotated plane polarised light (dextro- and laevo-, d- and l-, + and −), but now their absolute configurations are designated R or S. This is determined by the absolute arrangement of the atoms of the four substituent groups directly attached to the chiral atom. First, the atom of lowest atomic number is identified and the observer imagines this group lying behind the plane of the page. The other three atoms now lie in this plane and their atomic numbers are identified; if their atomic numbers descend in a clockwise fashion then this is the R (rectus) form, if anticlockwise it is the S (sinister) form. The R and S structures are mirror images of each other and they are referred to as **enantiomers**. There is no link between the R and S classification and the laevo and dextro classification, and an S structure may be laevo- or dextro-rotatory to plane polarised light.

In general, the three-dimensional conformation of a drug determines its pharmacodynamic actions at a molecular level. If the drug acts via a receptor, then conformation is of importance and there may be a marked difference in activity between enantiomers. However, if drug activity depends upon a physicochemical property then enantiomers would be expected to show similar activity.

There are many examples of optical isomers with a single chiral centre:

- S-warfarin and R-warfarin
- S-ketamine and R-ketamine
- S-etomidate and R-etomidate
- S-isoflurane and R-isoflurane
- S-halothane and R-halothane

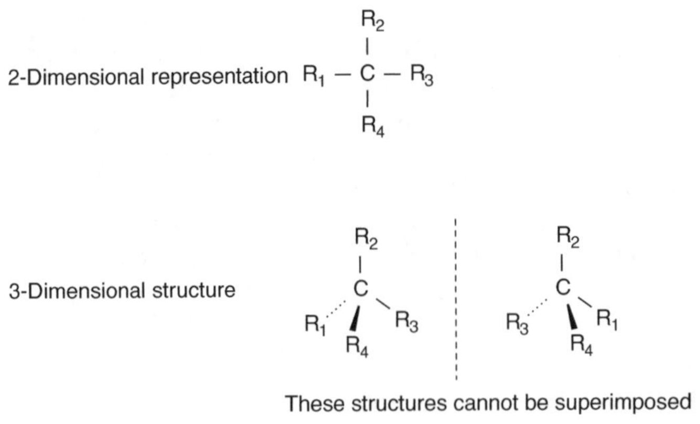

Figure 5.2 Chiral centres.

2-Dimensional representation $R_1 - \underset{\underset{R_4}{|}}{\overset{\overset{R_2}{|}}{C}} - R_3$

3-Dimensional structure

These structures cannot be superimposed

- S-bupivacaine and R-bupivacaine
- S-ropivacaine and R-ropivacaine.

The relative potencies of the two isomers may be similar, such as those of isoflurane, or very different, such as those of etomidate.

Diastereoisomers

When more than one chiral centre is present there are multiple possible stereoisomers. These are not all mirror images of each other, so they cannot be called enantiomers, instead the term diastereoisomers is used.

If a molecule contains more than one chiral atom, then with n such chiral centres n^2 stereoisomers are possible. Although the maximum number of possible isomers is n^2, if the molecule exhibits internal symmetry some of the possible configurations are duplicates. For example, atracurium has four chiral centres (two carbon atoms, two quaternary nitrogen atoms) with 16 theoretically possible isomers, but it is a symmetric molecule, so only 10 distinct three-dimensional structures actually exist.

Drug Preparations

Not all anaesthetic drugs have isomeric forms as they have neither a chiral centre nor any structural feature giving rise to geometric isomers. Examples include:

- sevoflurane
- propofol
- dopamine.

Racemic Mixtures

Many anaesthetic drugs are presented as a mixture of isomers. If the drug has a single chiral centre the different enantiomers are present in equal proportions and known as a racemic mixture. Examples include:

- isoflurane
- warfarin
- bupivacaine
- ketamine
- adrenaline.

In nature, molecules with chiral centres normally exist as single isomers (e.g. D-glucose) as enzymes selectively produce just one conformation. If natural agents are used for medicinal purposes, the purification process often results in racemisation so both isomers will be present in the pharmaceutical preparation (e.g. atropine).

While the mixture may contain equal amounts of the two isomers, the contribution to activity, both pharmacodynamic and pharmacokinetic, may be very different and, indeed, one may be responsible for undesirable toxicity or side effects.

Enantiopure Preparations

The pharmaceutical industry has identified the most active or least toxic isomer and produced a number of drugs as a single isomer preparation. There may be a clinical advantage in selecting the more desirable moiety and producing it as a single isomer, known as an enantiopure preparation. Examples include:

- R-etomidate
- S-bupivacaine (levobupivacaine)
- S-ropivacaine
- S-ketamine
- S-ketoprofen (dexketoprofen)
- S-medetomidine (dexmedetomidine)
- R-noradrenaline.

Mixtures of Multiple Isomers

Many of the drugs we use have complex carbon structures with multiple isomeric forms – both geometric and optical. The medical preparations of these drugs may contain all or only some of the possible isomers. The relative proportions of the isomers present is determined by their synthetic processes. Examples include:

- vecuronium
- pancuronium
- atracurium
- ephedrine
- morphine
- fentanyl
- remifentanil.

Pharmacokinetic Modelling

Pharmacokinetics is the study of the way in which the body handles administered drugs. The use of mathematical models allows us to predict how plasma concentration changes with time when the dose and interval between doses are changed, or when infusions of a drug are used. Because there is an association between plasma concentration of a drug and its pharmacodynamic effect, models allow us to predict the extent and duration of clinical effects. Mathematical models may therefore be used to programme computers to deliver a variable rate infusion to achieve a predetermined plasma level and hence a desired therapeutic effect.

It should be remembered that these pharmacokinetic models make a number of assumptions. Compartmental models make general assumptions based on virtual volumes without attempting to model 'real-life' volumes such as plasma or extracellular fluid volumes. Therefore, although convenient and useful to associate the virtual compartments with various tissue groups such as 'well perfused' or 'poorly perfused', this remains only an approximation of the physiological state.

Mathematical Concepts

Compartmental models are mathematical equations used to predict plasma concentrations of drugs based on experimental observations. The parameters described for models used in clinical application are based on small numbers of patients and infusion times shorter than the longest used clinically. Calculation of infusion rates for a given model involve the exponential function, the logarithmic function and calculus (integration and differentiation).

The Exponential Function

A function defines a unique value for the dependent variable, y, given a value for the independent variable, x. We write this as:

$$y = f(x)$$

For pharmacokinetics, we are interested in drug concentration (C) as a function of time (t). We can write:

$$C = f(t)$$

Observation tells us that after a single dose, plasma concentration falls with time and the rate at which that concentration falls is proportional to the concentration itself. This describes an exponential relationship, the simplest of which involves a single exponential. The general form of an exponential function is:

$$y = An^{ax}$$

In this relationship n is the *base* and x the *exponent*; A and a are constants. Although it is possible to use any base for our exponential function, the natural number e is chosen for its mathematical properties. The exponential function, $y = e^x$, is the only function that integrates and differentiates to itself, making manipulation of relationships involving exponentials much easier than if another base were chosen. The transcendental number *e* is irrational, it cannot be expressed as a fraction, and takes the value 2.716 ... where there is an infinite number of digits following the decimal point.

The rate at which a function changes is represented graphically by the tangent to the graph of y against x. Exponentials are positive if the *rate* at which y changes *increases* as x increases or negative if the *rate* at which y changes *decreases* as x increases (see Figure 6.1). The function $y = Ae^{ax}$ is a positive exponential. An example of a positive exponential relationship is bacterial cell growth – as time goes on, the number of bacteria increases exponentially. Compound interest relating to the growth of an investment with time is a further example of a positive exponential relationship.

After a single bolus, plasma concentration of drug falls at a rate that decreases with time and is dependent on the concentration itself. This describes a *negative* exponential relationship (Figure 6.1a). The simplest mathematical model that describes this is a single negative exponential function – it describes a single-compartment model:

$$C = C_0 e^{-kt}$$

In this relationship the independent variable is time (t) and the dependent variable drug concentration (C). C_0, the concentration at time $t = 0$, and k, **the rate constant for elimination**, represent the constants that define the exact equation for a given drug. This relationship is commonly referred to as a wash-out curve for the drug. The starting point on the concentration axis is C_0 and the 'steepness' of the curve depends on the rate constant, k.

Mathematically we talk about the **time constant** (τ) for an exponential process – this is the time it takes the concentration to fall by a factor of e and is the inverse of the rate constant for elimination ($\tau = 1/k$). A consequence of this is that concentration falls by the same proportion over equal time periods. In one time constant the process is approximately 63% complete (concentration has fallen from C to C/e) so after three time constants the process is virtually completed. Similarly it takes one **half-life** ($t_{1/2}$) for concentration to halve (concentration has fallen from C to C/2) and the process will be virtually complete in five half-lives. Note that the time constant is longer than the half-life (because *e* is greater than 2).

The way in which plasma concentration increases during a constant rate infusion, a wash-in curve, is also described by a *negative* exponential; although plasma concentration increases with time, the *rate* at which it approaches its maximum value is *decreasing* with time, making it a negative exponential (see Figure 6.1).

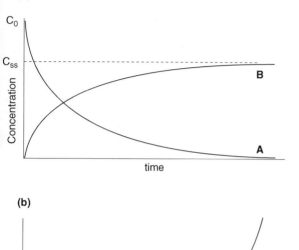

(a)

(b)

Figure 6.1 The exponential function. (a) Negative exponential function. Curve A is a simple wash-out curve for drug elimination, for example after a single bolus dose; the equation is $C = C_0 e^{-kt}$, the asymptote is zero and the starting point on the concentration-axis is defined as C_0. Curve B is a simple wash-in curve such as is seen when a constant rate infusion is used. The starting point on both axes is now zero and the asymptote is the concentration at steady-state C_{ss}. The equation is $C_{ss}(1 - e^{-kt})$. In both cases the rate constant for elimination is k. (b) Positive exponential function. This represents the exponential growth in a bacterial colony starting from a single organism. This organism divided; the two resultant organisms both divide and so on. There is a regular doubling of the number of bacteria so the equation is $N = 2^{t/d}$, where N is the number of organisms at time t and d is the time between consecutive cell divisions.

Logarithms

Any number can be expressed as a *power* of 10, for example 1000 can be written 10^3 and 5 as $10^{0.699}$. We call the power the *exponent* and 10 the *base*. Any number can be written in this way so that for any positive value of x:

$$x = 10^y$$

We define the value y as the *logarithm* to the base 10 of x, so the logarithmic function is (see Figure 6.2):

$$y = \log x$$

Thus any number can be written as:

$$x = 10^{\log x}$$

The exponent in 10^y is therefore equivalent to the logarithm (log) to the base 10 of x. Thus log1000 is 3 and log5 is 0.699. Similarly log10 is 1 ($10^1 = 10$) and log1 is 0 (because 10^0 is 1).

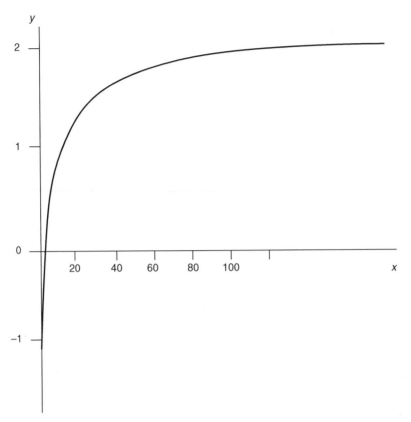

Figure 6.2 The logarithmic function. This shows the function y = log(x) for logarithms to the base 10. When x = 1 y = 0, which is a point common to all logarithmic relationships. Notice that unlike the exponential function, there is no asymptote corresponding to a maximum value for y. There is an asymptote on the x-axis, since the logarithm approaches negative infinity as x gets smaller and smaller and approaches 0; there is no such thing as a logarithm for a negative number.

So far we have described the familiar situation where the *base* is 10 and the exponent is the logarithm to the base 10. We can actually write a number in terms of *any* base, not just 10, with a corresponding exponent as the logarithm to that base.

In pharmacokinetics we are concerned with relationships involving the exponential function where the base is the natural number e, so we use e as the base for all logarithmic transformations.

By convention the logarithm of x to the base e is written as ln x, whereas log x is reserved for logarithms to base 10 and other logarithms to other bases are written as $\log_n$ x, where n is the base.

Logarithms to base e are known as *natural* logarithms, e.g. 2 can be written $e^{0.693}$, so the natural logarithm of 2, ln2, is 0.693 (this is a useful value to remember, as it is the factor that relates time constant to half-life).

Manipulating equations using logarithmic and exponential functions is described in more detail in the Appendix (page 62).

Calculus: Differentiation

Clinically we know that the rate of decline of plasma concentration with time in a wash-out curve is dependent on the plasma concentration. For a simple single-compartment model the constant of proportionality is k, the rate constant for elimination. Mathematically the rate at which concentration changes with time is expressed as the tangent to the curve. The tangent to any curve is described by its differential equation, so in the case of plasma concentration we can write:

$$dC/dt \propto C \text{ or } dC/dt = -kC$$

This simple expression describes a **first-order relationship** since the tangent depends on C raised to the power 1, also described as **linear kinetics**.

In mathematical terms we could start with the negative exponential describing the fall in plasma concentration and work out its differential:

$$d(C_0 e^{-kt})/dt$$

The exponential function differentiates to itself but we also need to take into account the factor $-k$ so:

$$d(C_0 e^{-kt})/dt = -C_0 e^{-kt}$$

Which gives us the relationship above, $dC/dt = -kC$

We also know clinically that for certain drugs, when elimination processes are saturated, drug concentration declines at a constant rate and the graph of concentration against time is a straight line rather than an exponential curve. When this happens the differential equation becomes:

$$dC/dt = -k$$

There is no dependence at all on concentration itself, so we describe this as **zero-order kinetics** since the tangent depends on C raised to the power zero ($C^0 = 1$).

Calculus: Integration

In differential calculus we use mathematics to calculate the gradient to a curve described by a mathematical function. In integral calculus mathematics is used to calculate the area under the curve of a function. It is possible to calculate the area between any two limits given by values on the x-axis. In pharmacokinetics we are interested in the entire area under the curve between time zero ($t = 0$) and infinity ($t = \infty$). Integration is the opposite of differentiation – if we integrate the function described by the differential equation given above, $dC/dt = -kC$, we can get back to the original equation, $C = C_0 e^{-kt}$, but only by knowing that at infinite time the plasma concentration must be zero.

This integral is written:

$$\int C_0 e^{-kt} dt, \ \text{with limits from 0 to } \infty$$

The 'dt' is used to show we are integrating with respect to time.
It is beyond the remit of this book to discuss integration in further detail.

Pharmacokinetic Models

Modelling involves fitting a mathematical equation to experimental observations of plasma concentration following drug administration to a group of volunteers or patients. These models can then be used to predict plasma concentration under a variety of conditions and, because for many drugs there is a close relationship between plasma concentration and drug activity, pharmacodynamic effects can also be predicted.

A number of models can be used:

- compartmental models
- physiological models
- non-compartmental models.

We will concentrate on compartmental models.

The Single-compartment Model

The simplest model is that of a single, well-stirred, homogenous compartment. If a single dose of drug is given, then the model assumes that it instantaneously disperses evenly throughout this compartment and is eliminated in an exponential fashion with a single rate constant for elimination (see Figure 6.3a). Although such a model rarely applies to drugs used in clinical practice, it is important to understand because it introduces the concepts that are further developed in more complex compartmental models. We have seen that this model is described by an equation with a single negative exponential term:

$$C = C_0 e^{-kt}$$

where C_0 is the concentration at time $t = 0$ and k is the rate constant for elimination. The volume of the single compartment is the volume of distribution, Vd. The rate constant for elimination, k, is the *fraction* of the volume of distribution from which drug is removed in unit time. The actual volume from which drug is removed in unit time is known as the **clearance** (Cl) of drug and has units of $ml.min^{-1}$ and is the product of volume of distribution and rate constant for elimination:

$$Cl = k.Vd$$

As described above, the time constant τ is the inverse of k so clearance also can be expressed as the ratio of the volume of distribution to the time constant:

$$Cl = Vd/\tau$$

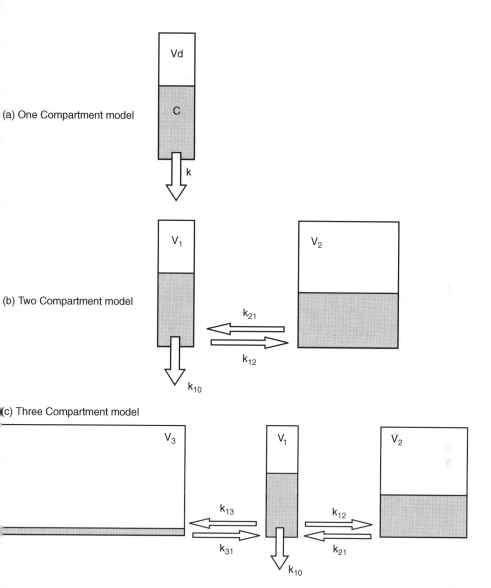

Figure 6.3 Compartmental models. (a) Single-compartment model, volume of distribution Vd, rate constant for elimination k. (b) Two-compartment model, central compartment has volume V_1 and peripheral compartment has volume V_2. Rate constants for transfer between compartments are described in the text. The rate constant for elimination is k_{10}. (c) Three-compartment model. This is similar to the two-compartment model but with the addition of a second peripheral compartment, volume V_3, with slower kinetics.

For any particular model k and Vd are constant, so clearance must also be constant. Because clearance is a ratio it is possible for drugs with very different values for Vd and τ to have the same clearance as long as the ratio of these two parameters is the same.

The values of the two parameters describing the relationship $C = C_0 e^{-kt}$ can be found by converting this equation to its logarithmic equivalent using natural logarithms (see Appendix (page 62) for the intermediate steps).

$$\ln C = \ln(C_0 e^{-kt})$$

$$\ln C = \ln C_0 - kt$$

This gives the equation of a straight line with a gradient $-k$ and $\ln C_0$ the intercept on the $\ln C$ axis (see Figure 6.4). Since we know the dose of drug given (X) and C_0, the concentration at time zero, the volume of distribution will be:

$$Vd = X/C_0$$

When a single bolus dose, X mg, of drug is given the concentration at time zero is C_0 or X/Vd mg.ml^{-1}. If we follow the amount of drug remaining in the body (X_t) it declines in a negative exponential manner towards zero in the same way as concentration:

$$X_t = Xe^{-kt}$$

The rate at which the drug is eliminated (in mg per minute) is the tangent to this curve, described by the differential expression:

$$dX_t/dt = -kX_t$$

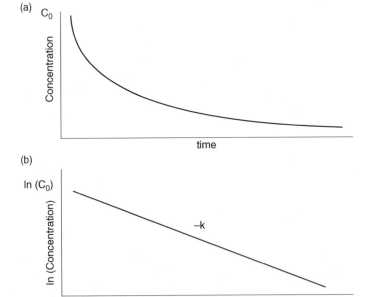

Figure 6.4 Semilogarithmic transformation of the exponential wash-out curve. (a) An exponential decrease in plasma concentration of drug against time after a bolus dose of a drug displaying single-compartment kinetics. (b) A natural logarithmic scale on the y-axis produces a straight line (C_0 is the plasma concentration at time, $t = 0$).

We know that clearance is the product of k and Vd, so k is the ratio of clearance (Cl) and Vd. If we put this into the expression above we can see that the **rate of elimination** is:

$$dX_t/dt = -(Cl/Vd)X_t = -Cl(X_t/Vd) = -Cl.C$$

At a plasma concentration C, the drug is eliminated at a rate determined by the product of clearance and the plasma concentration with units $mg.min^{-1}$, the negative sign indicating that the amount of drug falls with time. Note that this is the rate of elimination, quite different from the rate *constant* for elimination.

So far we have considered how the plasma concentration falls after a single bolus dose. If we give multiple doses, each one given before the concentration has fallen to zero, then the plasma concentration will build up in a saw-tooth fashion. The clearance of the drug determines how rapidly the required plasma level builds up. A smoother rise in plasma concentration will be achieved if a fixed-rate infusion is used. The curve of concentration against time is a negative exponential (see Figure 6.1b) with the steady-state concentration (Css) determined by clearance (Cl), the concentration of the solution infused (Ci) and infusion rate (I).

At steady-state the input of drug must be equal to output. This is a very important concept in kinetics. At steady state:

Input is the amount of drug given in unit time – the product of drug concentration in the syringe and infusion rate: Ci.I

Output is the rate of elimination of drug at steady state concentration, which is the product of steady-state concentration and clearance: Css.Cl

   Input = output

$$Ci.I = Css.Cl$$

Rearranging:

$$Css = Ci.I/Cl$$

The steady-state concentration can be determined by the amount of drug infused and clearance.

The time constant, τ, is the inverse of the rate constant for elimination and is commonly defined as the time it would have taken plasma concentration to fall to zero if the original rate of elimination had continued (see Figure 6.5). It represents the time it takes for the plasma concentration to fall by a factor of *e* – from C to C/*e*. Time constant is longer than the half-life:

$$t_{1/2} = 0.693\tau$$

It is easier to use time constants rather than half-lives when discussing models.

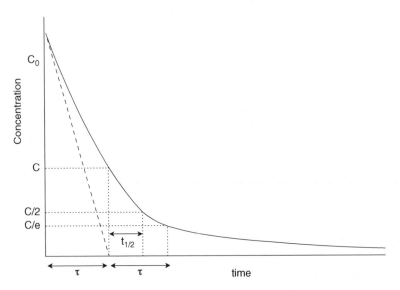

Figure 6.5 Time constant. The dashed line shows the tangent to the concentration–time curve at C_0; if this rate of decline had continued then the time it would have taken the concentration to reach zero is the time constant, τ. The time taken for the plasma concentration to fall from C to C/e, i.e. to 37% of C, is also one time constant.

Multi-compartment Models

Multi-compartment models make allowance for the uptake of drug by different tissues within the body, and for the different blood flow rates to these tissues. Different tissues that share pharmacokinetic properties form compartments. Convenient labels include 'vessel rich' and 'vessel poor' compartments. The number of theoretical compartments that may be included in any model is limitless, but more than three compartments become experimentally indistinguishable. In these models it is important to realise that elimination can occur *only* from the central compartment. Models for individual drugs differ in the volume of compartments and in transfer rates between compartments; the values for these pharmacokinetic parameters can vary enormously and depend on the physicochemical properties of a drug as well as the site and rate of drug metabolism.

Two Compartments

In the two-compartment model the central compartment connects with a second compartment; the volume of the central compartment is V_1 and that of the peripheral compartment V_2 (see Figure 6.3b). The total volume of distribution is the sum of these two volumes. Unlike the single-compartment model, there are now two pathways for drug elimination from plasma: an initial transfer from the central to peripheral compartment and removal from the central compartment. The latter removes the drug from the system, whereas after distribution to the second compartment, the drug can re-distribute to the central compartment when conditions allow. Inspection of the experimental concentration–time curve shows that the initial rate of decline in plasma concentration is much faster than would be expected from a single-compartment model; this represents the effect of the additional elimination pathway to the second compartment. A semi-logarithmic plot of lnC against

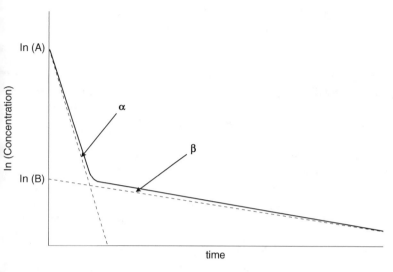

Figure 6.6 Bi-exponential decline. For a two-compartment model, plasma concentration declines with a rapid exponential phase that has time constant α, this is due largely to distribution. Once distribution has occurred plasma concentration falls at a slower exponential rate – terminal elimination – with a time constant β. Neither α nor β equate to any one particular rate constant for the model.

time is now a curve, rather than a straight line. It is actually the sum of two straight lines representing exponential processes with rate constants α and β (see Figure 6.6).

Transfer from one compartment to another occurs in an exponential fashion at a rate depending on the concentration difference between compartments and the rate constant for transfer. Rate constants for transfer in each direction are important: k_{12} is the rate constant for the transfer from the central to peripheral compartment and k_{21} is the rate constant for the transfer from the peripheral to central compartment. The rate constant for elimination from the central compartment is now referred to as k_{10}. The drug is given into the central compartment and there is a rapid initial decline in concentration due to distribution into the peripheral compartment in addition to elimination. Alongside this is a slower decline, the terminal elimination, which is influenced both by elimination from the body and re-distribution of the drug back to the central compartment from the second compartment.

Consider a dose X mg of drug given into the central compartment with X_1 and X_2 representing the amount of drug in the central and peripheral compartments respectively after time t. We know that movement of the drug is an exponential process depending on the rate constant and the amount of drug present so the rate at which the amount of drug in the central compartment changes with time depends on three processes: (1) removal of drug from the central compartment, determined by X_1 and k_{10}; (2) drug distribution to the second compartment determined by X_1 and k_{12}; (3) re-distribution from the second compartment determined by X_2 and k_{21}. We can therefore write a differential equation for the rate of change of the amount of drug in the central compartment:

$$dX_1/dt = -k_{10}X_1 - k_{12}X_1 + k_{21}X_2$$

This is much more complicated than the simple single-compartment model and requires a special form of integral calculus to solve (Laplace transforms). It can be shown that using the result from integral calculus for the amount of drug, and dividing X_1 by V_1 to give the concentration in the central compartment, C, we get the equation:

$$C = A\,e^{-\alpha t} + B\,e^{-\beta t}$$

The semi-logarithmic plot of lnC against time is the sum of two straight lines representing the two exponential processes in the relationship above (see Figure 6.6). The intercepts of these two straight lines on the lnC axis (i.e. when t = 0) allows the constants A and B to be found and C_0 is the sum of A and B.

The volume of the central compartment is found by dividing the dose given, X, by C_0. As in the simple model, the central and peripheral compartments do not correspond to actual anatomical or physiological tissues. Thus, the central compartment is often larger than just the plasma volume, representing all tissues that, in pharmacokinetic terms, behave like plasma.

The rate constants, α and β, are found from the gradients of these two straight lines and the reciprocals of these rate constants give the time constants τ_α and τ_β, which are related to the half-lives $t_{1/2\alpha}$ and $t_{1/2\beta}$, respectively (see above for relationship between time constant and half-life). Neither of these rate constants equates to any individual rate constant in the model, but each is a complex combination of all three.

The steepness of the initial decline is determined by the ratio k_{12}/k_{21}. If the ratio k_{12}/k_{21} is high then the initial phase will be very steep: the higher the value the more rapid the transfer into the second compartment compared with movement back into the central compartment. For example, after a bolus dose of fentanyl, where the ratio of k_{12}/k_{21} is about 4:1, the plasma concentration falls very rapidly.

Three Compartments

Modelling drug behaviour using three compartments requires three exponential processes. The equation for the plasma concentration (C) is now given by:

$$C = Ae^{-\alpha t} + Be^{-\beta t} + Ce^{-\gamma t}$$

This is similar to the relationship for the two-compartment model, but with the addition of a third exponential process resulting from the presence of an additional compartment; the kinetic constants G and γ describe that additional process. The model consists of a central compartment into which a drug is infused and from which excretion can occur, together with two peripheral compartments with which a drug can be exchanged (see Figure 6.7). These may typically represent well-perfused (the second compartment) and poorly perfused (the third compartment) tissues, respectively, with the central compartment representing plasma. Distribution into the second compartment is always faster than into the third compartment. This is a reasonable model for the majority of anaesthetic agents, where drug reaches the plasma and is distributed to muscle and fat. The volume of distribution at steady-state is the sum of the volumes of the three compartments. The mathematics is similar to that for two compartments, but more complicated as transfer into and out of the third compartment also must be taken into account.

As in the two-compartment model, there is a final phase that can be described by a single exponential and the half-life associated with this phase is known as the **terminal elimination half-life**, which reflects both elimination from the body and re-distribution from the peripheral compartments. The rate constant for elimination is therefore *not* the inverse of

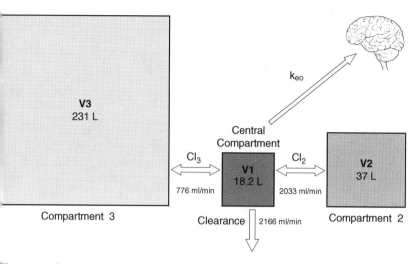

Figure 6.7 Three-compartment model for propofol including the effect compartment.

the terminal elimination time constant; it can be calculated once the model parameters have been found. Clearance of the drug out of the body is still defined as the product of V_1 and the rate constant for elimination.

Effect Compartment

Three-compartment models are used in clinical practice to target plasma or effect concentration. The effect compartment is considered to be in equilibrium with the central compartment but with a lag-time to account for blood–brain equilibration. There is no volume associated with the effect compartment but, to account for the lag-time, there is an associated elimination rate constant k_{eo}. The half-life for equilibration is known as the $t_{1/2k_{eo}}$.

Non-compartmental Models

Non-compartmental models make no assumptions about specific volumes but use information from the AUC, as this reflects the removal of the drug from plasma. The area under the concentration–time curve can be used to find clearance because AUC is the ratio of dose to clearance. Clearance (Cl) is therefore:

$$Cl = dose/AUC$$

If we plot the *product* of concentration and time on the y-axis against time, we produce what is known as the first moment curve. The area under this curve (AUMC) can be used to find a parameter known as mean residence time (MRT). Mean residence time is a measure of how long the drug stays in the body and is similar to a time constant in the compartmental models.

$$MRT = AUMC/AUC$$

The product of clearance and MRT is the steady-state volume of distribution (V_{ss}). So volume of distribution is:

$$Vss = Cl \times MRT$$

Measurement of Pharmacokinetic Parameters

The parameters described in the compartmental models are useful for comparing the persistence of different drugs in the body, namely: volume of distribution (Vd), clearance (Cl) and time constants (τ in the single compartment and α, β and γ in multi-compartment models). Half-lives ($t_{1/2}$) are related to their corresponding time constants by a factor of ln2 (0.693).

Volume of Distribution

Volume of distribution (Vd) is defined as the apparent volume into which a drug disperses in order to produce the observed plasma concentration. It does not correspond to any particular physiological volume and can be much larger than total body water.

Vd has units of volume (e.g. litres) but can be indexed to bodyweight and expressed as litres.kg^{-1}. The physicochemical properties of a drug including its molecular size, lipid solubility and charge characteristics all influence the volume of distribution. Propofol is a very lipid-soluble drug and has a large volume of distribution of about 250 litres; vecuronium and atracurium are charged molecules and have relatively small volumes of distribution of about 19 and 11 litres respectively. Tissue binding of drug, particularly intracellular sequestration, can account for extremely high volumes of distribution; the anti-malarial chloroquine has a volume of distribution in excess of 10,000 litres. Pathology also influences the kinetic parameters; in hepatic and renal disease volumes of distribution are increased as the relative volumes of body fluid compartments change.

In a simple kinetic model, Vd is the initial dose divided by the plasma concentration occurring immediately after administration:

$$Vd = dose/plasma\ concentration = X/C_0$$

In multi-compartment models, the central compartment volume is the initial volume into which the drug disperses ($V_{initial}$). The volume of this compartment depends partly on the degree of protein binding; a highly protein-bound drug will have a larger central compartment volume than a drug that is poorly bound. Propofol is 98% protein-bound and has a central compartment volume of about 16 litres, compared with an actual plasma volume of about 3 litres. The volume of this central compartment can be estimated from the rapid distribution phase; if the dose given was X and the intercept on the y-axis is A then:

$$V_{intial} = X/A$$

The total volume of distribution is the sum of all the volumes that comprise the model. There are several methods available that attempt to estimate this volume: V_{extrap}, V_{area} and V_{ss}. The first of these simply ignores the contribution made by any volume apart from that associated with the terminal phase of elimination. On a semi-logarithmic plot, the line representing terminal elimination is extrapolated back to its intercept on the ln-(concentration) axis, which gives a concentration M that can be used to give V_{extrap}:

$$V_{extrap} = X/M$$

It greatly overestimates the total volume of distribution for many drugs, particularly when the distribution phase contributes significantly to drug dispersion. The second method, V_{area}, is of more use because it is related both to clearance and the terminal elimination constant. This uses the non-compartmental method of calculating clearance from AUC and assumes that an 'average' rate constant for removal of drug from plasma can be approximated by the inverse of the terminal elimination time constant (β for the two-compartment model: substitute γ for the three-compartment model):

$$V_{area} = Clearance/\beta = X/(AUC. \beta)$$

This gives a better estimate of volume of distribution than V_{extrap}, but is still an over-estimate; using β as the 'average' rate constant is an underestimate, particularly if there is significant distribution and re-distribution to and from compartments. However, it has the advantage of being easily calculated from experimental data. The final method V_{ss} is entirely based on non-compartment models (see above) and is calculated from the product of clearance and mean residence time:

$$V_{ss} = (dose/AUC). (AUMC/AUC) = dose. AUMC/AUC^2$$

This gives an estimate of volume of distribution that is independent of elimination, which can be useful. The estimate of volume of distribution using this method is smaller than for either of the other methods, but is usually closer to the area method:

$$V_{extrap} > V_{area} > V_{ss}$$

Clearance

Clearance is defined as that volume of plasma from which a drug is completely removed per unit of time – the usual units are $ml.min^{-1}$. For the single-compartment model we saw that clearance is the product of the rate constant for elimination and the volume of distribution. In the multi-compartment model, there are inter-compartmental clearances as well as clearance responsible for drug loss from the system. Clearance describing the removal of drug from the body is the product of the rate constant for elimination k_{10} and V_1, the volume of distribution of the central compartment. For example, propofol has a k_{10} of approximately 0.12, so about 1/8 of the plasma-equivalent volume has the drug removed by elimination in unit time. For propofol, V_1 is about 16 litres and k_{10} is approximately 0.12, so the clearance of propofol is 16×0.12, which is about 2 litres per minute. Remifentanil has a much smaller central compartment volume but a higher k_{10}, so the clearance of remifentanil is 5.1×0.5, which is 2.5 litres, quite similar to that of propofol.

In general, clearance is usually calculated using a non-compartmental method (see above):

Clearance = Dose/AUC

Inter-compartmental clearance relates to the movement of the drug between compartments; C_{12} and C_{13} define drug transfer between compartments one and two and one and three, respectively. For drugs with comparable compartmental volumes, the higher the inter-compartmental clearance the more rapidly distribution and re-distribution takes place.

Non-linear Kinetics

So far we have considered models in which first-order kinetics determines elimination of the drug from the body. Metabolic processes are usually first order, as there is a relative excess of enzyme over substrate, so enzyme activity is not rate limiting. However, in certain situations, some metabolic enzymes become saturated and obey zero-order kinetics, in which the rate of change of plasma drug concentration is constant rather than being dependent upon the concentration of drug. This is also known as saturation kinetics and indicates that enzyme activity is maximal, so cannot be influenced by increasing substrate concentration. An example is the metabolism of ethanol, which proceeds at a relatively constant rate after the ingestion of a moderate amount of alcohol. This is because the rate-limiting step in its metabolism by alcohol dehydrogenase is the presence of a co-factor for the reaction, which is present only in small quantities.

Certain processes obey first-order kinetics at low dose, but zero-order at higher doses. For example, the metabolism of phenytoin becomes saturable within the upper limit of the normal range, and the pharmacokinetics of thiopental obeys zero-order kinetics when used by infusion for prolonged periods, such as in the treatment of status epilepticus. There are two important implications of a process obeying zero-order kinetics within a normal dose range.

First, during zero-order kinetics, a small increase in dose may cause a large increase in plasma level. If this occurs at a level near the upper limit of the therapeutic range, toxicity may be experienced after a modest dose increase. Checking plasma concentration is essential to avoid toxic levels when prescribing drugs where this is a problem, such as occurs with phenytoin.

Second, during zero-order kinetics there is no steady state. If the rate of drug delivery exceeds the rate of drug excretion, plasma levels will continue to rise inexorably until ingestion stops or toxicity leads to death (see Figure 6.8).

Appendix

Examples of Using Logarithms

Multiplication

Let $w = 10^x$ and $z = 10^y$

Then $\log w = x$ and $\log z = y$

To multiply w by z we add their logarithms to find the exponent of the product

$w.\ z = 10^x.10^y = 10^{(x+y)}$

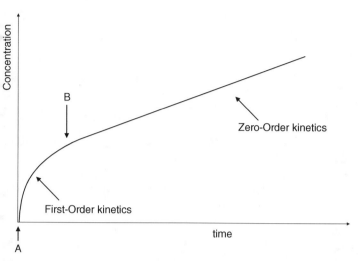

Figure 6.8 Transition to non-linear (zero-order) kinetics. If an infusion is started at a constant rate at point A, initially plasma concentration rises in a negative exponential fashion according to first-order kinetics. At point B the elimination process is overwhelmed and the plasma concentration continues to rise in a linear fashion, according to zero-order kinetics. This usually occurs because hepatic enzymes become saturated and work at maximum capacity.

An example: multiply 13 by 257 using their logarithms. There are tables containing logarithms for numbers between 1 and 9.999 (with values between 0 and 0.999) but these days we can use a calculator:

log 13 = 1.1139, log 257 = 2.4100

We add their logarithms to give the exponent of the product

1.1139 + 2.4100 = 3.5239

The answer is therefore $10^{3.5239}$

To convert back to a numerical value we need to find the antilog of 3.5239 either using a calculator or looking up in log tables. To use log tables we have to split the exponent into an integer part and a positive decimal part; for the example we used this gives $10^3 \times 10^{0.5239}$. We know this is 1000 × antilog(0.5239); we can look up 0.5239 in the body of the logarithm tables and find it corresponds to 3.341.

So the result of multiplying 13 by 257 is 1000 × 3.341, which is 3341.

Division

To divide w by z we subtract their logarithms to find the exponent of the result.

$$w/z = 10^x/10^y = 10^{(x-y)}$$

An example: divide 13 by 257 using their logarithms:

log 13 = 1.1139, log 257 = 2.4100

We subtract their logarithms to give the exponent of the result:

$$1.1139 - 2.4100 = -1.2961$$

The answer is therefore $10^{-1.2961}$. We can use a calculator to find the antilog or we can use log tables. If we use tables we need to split the exponent into an integer part and a positive decimal part because there are no values for negative logarithms so we actually need $10^{-2} \times 10^{0.7039}$ ($-2 + 0.7039 = -1.2961$).

We now have $0.01 \times$ antilog(0.7039) and the antilog of 0.7039 is 5.057, so the result of dividing 13 by 257 is 0.01×5.057, which is 0.05057.

Of course, this is a very old-fashioned way of multiplying and dividing numbers – a calculator can do both with much greater accuracy. However, it has introduced us to the idea of logarithms and shown that the logarithm to the base 10 of a number is the same as its exponent when it is written as a power of 10.

Adding and Subtracting Logarithms

When adding logarithms together, it is important to remember that this is equivalent to multiplication:

$$\log (w.z) = \log w + \log z$$

When subtracting logarithms, this is equivalent to division

$$\log (w/z) = \log w - \log z$$

Logarithms of Numbers with Exponential Terms

We are used to finding the logarithms to the base 10 of numbers such as 10^{-3}, 10^2, 10^4, 10^x – their logarithms are –3.0, 2.0, 4.0 and x respectively. The same is true for natural logarithms where the base is e.

The natural logarithms of e^{-2}, e^4, e^7, e^t are –2.0, 4.0, 7.0 and t respectively.

In our pharmacokinetic models we come across the exponential function involving e^{-kt}.

The natural logarithm of this is simply –kt.

Sometimes we want to take the logarithm to base 10 of a number with an exponent raised to a different base. For example we want

$$\log e^4$$

This is the same as:

$$\log (e.e.e.e)$$

Since we add logarithms of numbers multiplied together:

$$\log (e.e.e.e) = \log e + \log e + \log e + \log e$$

So

$$\log e^4 = 4 \log e$$

In a similar manner:

$$\ln 10^y = y \ln 10$$

Conversion of Logarithms from One Base to Another

There is a simple relationship between logarithms to the base 10 and natural logarithms. For example, we can express plasma concentration, C, either as a natural logarithm or as a logarithm to base 10:

$$C = e^{\ln C} \text{ or } C = 10^{\log C}$$

so $e^{\ln C} = 10^{\log C}$

If we take the natural logarithms of both sides

$$\ln C = \ln 10^{\log C}$$

We saw above how to deal with logarithms for numbers that have an exponent raised to a different base:

$$\ln 10^{\log C} = \log C . \ln 10$$

So

$$\ln C = \log C . \ln 10$$

We know that $\ln 10$ is 2.302

$$\ln C = 2.302 \log C$$

$$\log C = \ln C / 2.302 = 0.434 \ln C$$

So, if we know the natural logarithm of a number we can find its logarithm to base 10 simply by dividing by the natural logarithm of 10.
We can do this the other way around:

$$10^{\log C} = e^{\ln C}$$

Taking logarithms to base 10 of both sides:

$$\log C = \log e^{\ln C}$$

$$\log C = \ln C. \log e$$

$$\ln C = \log C / \log e \text{ and we know log } e \text{ is } 0.434$$

So, if we know the logarithm to base 10 we find its natural logarithm by dividing by log e.

A Semi-logarithmic Plot of Concentration against Time

To find values for k and C_0 in a single-compartment model we need a semi-logarithmic plot of our exponential relationship. It is easier to use natural logarithms for the concentration axis, since our equation involves the base e:

$$C = C_0 e^{-kt}$$

Taking natural logarithms of both sides:

$$\ln C = \ln(C_0 e^{-kt})$$

The logarithm of two numbers multiplied together is the same as the sum of their individual logarithms so:

$$\ln C = \ln C_0 + \ln e^{-kt}$$

We have seen that $\ln e^n$ is simply n so:

$$\ln C = \ln C_0 + (-kt) \text{ or more simply, } \ln C = \ln C_0 - kt$$

This is the equation of a straight line with $\ln C$ on the y-axis and t on the x-axis, with a slope of $-k$.

If logarithms to the base 10 are taken the slope will be different, by a factor of log e (0.434):

$$\log C = \log (C_0 e^{-kt})$$

$$\log C = \log C_0 + \log e^{-kt}$$

The second term is more tricky, but from the relationships shown above, $\log x = (\ln x)/2.302$ and since $\ln e^{-kt}$ is simply $-kt$ we can substitute:

$$\log C = \log C_0 - kt/2.302 \text{ or } \log C = \log C_0 - 0.434kt$$

Relationship between Half-life and Time Constant

We have seen that $\ln C = \ln C_0 - kt$ and rearranging this equation gives

$$t = (\ln C_0 - \ln C)/k$$

If C is the concentration at time t_1 and C/2 is the concentration later at time t_2, the half-life ($t_{1/2}$) is the difference between these two times.

$$t_2 - t_1 = t_{1/2} = (\ln C_0 - \ln(C/2))/k - (\ln C_0 - \ln C)/k$$

Rearranging and eliminating the term $\ln C_0$ this gives

$k.t_{1/2} = \ln C - \ln(C/2)$ Since subtracting logarithms represents division (see above)

$$k.t_{1/2} = \ln (C \div C/2)$$

$$k.t_{1/2} = \ln 2 = 0.693$$

since $k = 1/\tau$, substituting and rearranging gives

$$t_{1/2} = 0.693\tau$$

This clearly shows that half-life is shorter than time constant, the factor relating them being $\ln 2$.

Applied Pharmacokinetic Models

In the previous chapter we explored the mathematical principles and models that can be used to predict plasma concentrations of drugs, particularly compartment models. This chapter will discuss the use of drugs for which commercial infusion devices are available that are programmed with kinetic models, in particular propofol and remifentanil.

Ideal Drugs for Intravenous Use in Anaesthesia

Total intravenous anaesthesia (TIVA) describes the provision of anaesthesia by intravenous infusions alone. Anaesthesia may be induced and maintained either by an infusion of a hypnotic alone or by a combination of hypnotic and analgesic. An ideal drug for induction and maintenance of anaesthesia should have the following properties:

- predictable plasma concentrations according to a known pharmacokinetic model
- predictable link between pharmacokinetic and pharmacodynamic effects
- no active metabolites
- a rapid onset of action
- a rapid offset of action
- stable in a plastic syringe.

The delivery of TIVA has been improved by pumps that contain algorithms specific to the anaesthetic agents with the most favourable kinetic profiles. These pumps deliver infusions to maintain a constant (plasma or effect site) concentration – target-controlled infusions (TCIs). Propofol and remifentanil are the commonest combination of hypnotic and analgesic, each being delivered by a separate pump so that either can be altered independently of the other. A mixture of propofol and alfentanil has been used via a single pump for shorter cases, although the target concentration of alfentanil is impossible to control directly with this technique.

Propofol

The intravenous anaesthetic propofol can be used both for induction and maintenance of anaesthesia, largely due to its favourable 'wake up' profile. Although it is possible to give a bolus dose of propofol without understanding its pharmacokinetics, to use it sensibly by infusion requires some understanding of kinetics.

Propofol is a sterically hindered phenol: the potentially active hydroxyl (-OH) group is shielded by the electron clouds surrounding the attached isopropyl ($(CH_3)_2CH-$) groups, which reduces its reactivity. So, unlike phenol, propofol is insoluble in water but highly soluble in fat hence its preparation as a lipid emulsion. The phenolic hydroxyl group makes propofol a weak acid, but significant ionisation occurs only at a pH greater than 10. High lipid solubility means that after long infusions there is the risk of accumulation in fatty tissues. There are no active metabolites of propofol. The combination of high lipid solubility and insignificant ionisation means that once propofol distributes into fat it will redistribute back into plasma relatively slowly. The extremely large volume of distribution of propofol is accounted for mainly by the third compartment and although a relatively large amount of drug, in terms of milligrams, may distribute into this volume, the concentration rises only very slowly.

An induction dose of propofol is extensively bound to plasma proteins (98% bound to albumin) following intravenous injection. After the initial bolus dose there is rapid loss of consciousness as the lipid tissue of the central nervous system (CNS) takes up the highly lipophilic drug. Over the next few minutes propofol then distributes to peripheral tissues and the concentration in the CNS falls (see Figure 7.1), such that in the absence of further doses or another anaesthetic agent the patient will wake up. Its distribution half-life is 1–2 minutes and accounts for the rapid fall in plasma levels with a short duration of action. The very rapid elimination of propofol by hepatic and extra-hepatic metabolism also contributes significantly to this rapid reduction in plasma concentration. The terminal elimination half-life is very much longer (5–12 hours) reflecting relatively slow redistribution from the fatty tissues and plays an insignificant role in offset of clinical action following a bolus dose.

The pharmacodynamic profile of propofol lags behind plasma concentration due to the short delay in access to and from the CNS. Time-to-peak effect of a bolus dose of propofol is in the order of a few minutes ('t', Figure 7.1) and has been described by different models as 1.7–3.9 minutes, so the brain concentration of propofol is lower than that of plasma on induction but higher during the elimination phase. There is a relationship between plasma concentration and effect when equilibrium is reached between brain and plasma, but the lag-time before equilibrium is reached must be accounted for in a kinetic model. Modelling

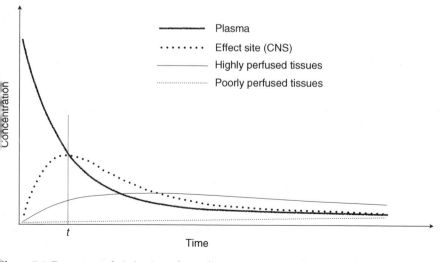

Figure 7.1 Time course of a bolus dose of propofol.

this lag-time requires use of depth of anaesthesia monitoring, usually the bispectral monitor (BIS), as a surrogate measure of brain (effect compartment) concentration.

Anaesthesia with propofol can be induced and maintained by its delivery according to a three-compartment model with an effect compartment that equilibrates with the central compartment. The lag-time referred to above between plasma and effect compartments is included by considering the effect compartment as one with no volume but a rate constant of elimination, k_{eo}. The half-life for equilibration is known as the $t_{1/2keo}$.

Remifentanil

Remifentanil is a fentanyl derivative that is a pure μ agonist. It has an ester linkage, which is very rapidly broken down by plasma and non-specific tissue esterases, particularly in muscle. The metabolites have minimal pharmacodynamic activity. With increasing age, muscle bulk decreases and this significantly influences the rate of remifentanil metabolism. The offset of clinical activity is rapid and not greatly affected by duration of infusion; as discussed below remifentanil has a relatively constant context-sensitive half-time between 3 and 8 minutes. Therefore, a patient may be maintained on a remifentanil infusion for a long period, without significant drug accumulation as seen with other opioids. The advantage of this pharmacokinetic profile is that a patient may be given prolonged infusions of remifentanil for analgesia during surgery, with rapid offset of action when this is no longer required. The potential disadvantage is that its analgesic effect wears off so rapidly that pain may be a significant problem immediately post-operatively. Inadequate provision of analgesia before discontinuing remifentanil may be associated with hyperalgesia in the recovery area that can be difficult to treat without using high doses of other opiates, which may lead to adverse consequences. Post-operative pain must therefore be anticipated, either by using a regional technique or by the administration of a longer-acting opioid before the end of surgery.

Total Intravenous Anaesthesia

A strict definition of total intravenous anaesthesia (TIVA) refers to the induction and maintenance of anaesthesia using intravenous agents and an oxygen/air mix. Nitrous oxide has been used as an adjunct, but now this is much less common as the familiarity of TIVA increases and the environmental impact of nitrous oxide is better understood. The intravenous agent(s) may be given by manual infusion or by an infusion device programmed with pharmacokinetic model(s) to target either plasma (TCI plasma) or brain (TCI effect) concentration of drug. When using an infusion of propofol or remifentanil there is no 'point-of-delivery' measure of the target concentration comparable to the end-tidal monitoring of inhalational agents. A TCI will display a *calculated* value for plasma concentration based on the software model used and the information it has been given, which may include some or all of the patient's weight, height, age and sex.

Manual Total Intravenous Anaesthesia: The Bristol Model

The Bristol algorithm provides a simple manual infusion scheme for propofol to achieve a target blood concentration of about 3 $\mu g.ml^{-1}$ within 2 minutes and to maintain this level for the duration of surgery (see Figure 7.2). This is based on plasma concentrations obtained from healthy patients premedicated with temazepam and induced with fentanyl 3 $\mu g.kg^{-1}$

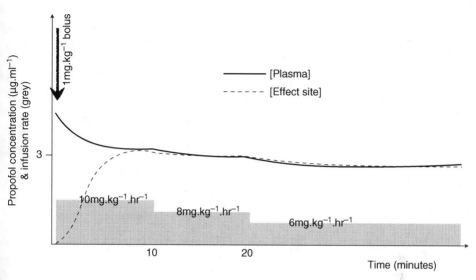

Figure 7.2 The Bristol Model, '10–8–6'.

followed by a propofol bolus of 1 mg.kg^{-1}. Induction is followed by a variable-rate infusion of propofol at 10 mg.kg^{-1}.h^{-1} for 10 minutes, 8 mg.kg^{-1}.h^{-1} for 10 minutes then 6 mg.kg^{-1}. h^{-1} thereafter. This '10–8–6' infusion scheme was supplemented with nitrous oxide and patients were ventilated. Clearly, if higher plasma concentrations of propofol are needed to maintain adequate anaesthesia, then the 10–8–6 algorithm should be adjusted appropriately or an additional intravenous supplement used, such as a remifentanil infusion.

Although anaesthesia can be delivered using a manual infusion, studies have shown that using a TCI provides anaesthesia using a lower total dose of propofol with the associated benefits of more haemodynamic stability and a more rapid awakening.

Target-controlled Infusion

Target-controlled infusion is a technique that uses a microprocessor-controlled infusion pump programmed with a three-compartment model of drug pharmacokinetics. It is possible to target either plasma or effect site concentration (see Figure 7.3). The pump uses the pharmacokinetic model, the concentration of the drug being infused and the type of syringe, to calculate a variable rate infusion in order to achieve the targeted drug concentration. In adults there are two commonly used models for propofol TCI, Marsh and Schnider. Due to different kinetics in children, specific paediatric models are required, for example Paedfusor. The Minto model is used exclusively for remifentanil TCI.

The recently published pharmacokinetic-pharmacodynamic algorithm by Eleveld et al. characterises propofol for the broadest range of patients yet, from neonates to the elderly and in the morbidly obese. Its complex underpinning mathematics may simplify the process of TCI in practice by reducing the number of target adjustments at induction and over time, although ultimately for the individual patient, all anaesthetic drugs will still need to be titrated carefully to effect. Much of the discussion below, as models and targeting options are compared and contrasted, is predicated on a single identical target value. This is not to

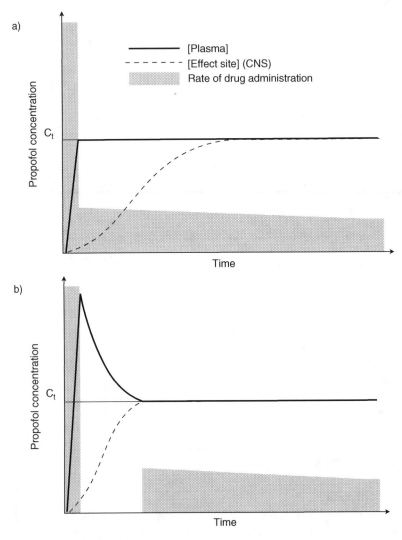

Figure 7.3 TCI targeting options. a) Plasma Site targeting, the TCI pump delivers a bolus dose to reach the set plasma target, and then continues the infusion to maintain the target. The rate at which the effect site is projected to reach the target is determined by the kinetic model and the k_{eo}. b) Effect Site targeting, the TCI pump administers a bolus dose and then pauses. As the plasma concentration falls it meets the rising effect site concentration at exactly the target concentration, at which point the TCI pump restarts at a rate to maintain the target. Importantly, there is no overshoot in the effect site concentration.

suggest that administering drugs by TCI is done in this fashion, rather it is simply a means of illuminating differences.

It is obvious that different algorithms do not change the nature of propofol and as such are only an attempt to reflect how it is handled by and affects the body, rather than actually determining how it is handled. In other words, propofol does not induce anaesthesia more rapidly when the Modified Marsh model is used compared to the Marsh model in plasma targeting mode (see Figure 7.4a), despite the model calculating (due to a larger K_{eo}) the effect site concentration reaching its target more rapidly. This becomes even more obvious as the dose / time profiles are the same – both models giving the same initial bolus dose in plasma targeting mode (see Figure 7.5).

However, when the Modified Marsh model is used in effect site targeting mode (Figure 7.4b) induction may be more rapid but only by virtue of a slightly larger initial bolus dose (Figure 7.5). It is also worth noting that the high initial (induction) plasma concentration generated when using Schnider in the effect site mode does not imply a larger (induction) dose compared with that seen when the Modified Marsh model is used in effect targeted mode. This is due to the fundamentally different 'build' of the two

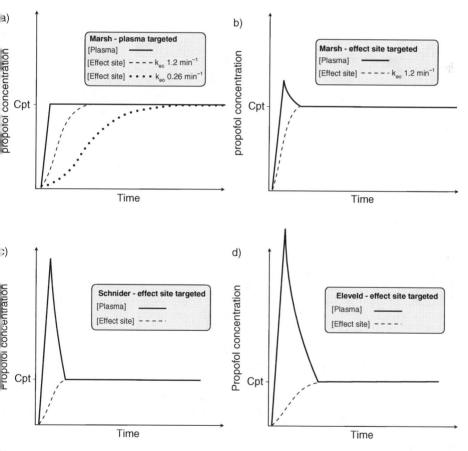

Figure 7.4 Comparison of different kinetic models and targeting options, for an average adult assuming a single identical target value. a) The Marsh model in plasma targeting mode. The rate at which the effect site reaches the target depends on the k_{eo}. Typically this is 0.26 min^{-1} and equilibration is slow, but with a k_{eo} of 1.2 min^{-1} it is faster. b) The Modified Marsh model (k_{eo} =1.2 min^{-1}) in effect site mode. A slightly larger initial bolus is given compared to a)) followed by a characteristic 'infusion pause'. The peak plasma concentration is only slightly above the target concentration because of the relatively large k_{eo}. c) The Schnider model in effect site mode. The combination of a small V1 and k_{eo} of 0.45 min^{-1} drives the plasma concentration to high levels despite a similar initial dose to that seen with Marsh. d) The k_{eo} of 0.146 min^{-1} used in the Eleveld model means a large initial dose is required, leading to a high plasma concentration which is only partly offset by its modest V1 of 6.28 litres.

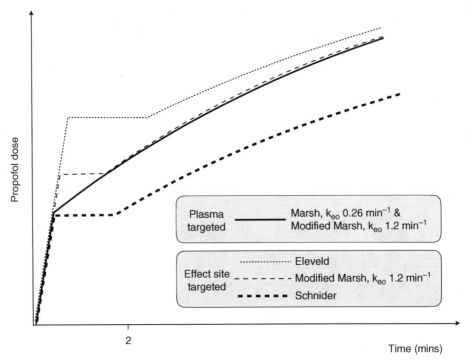

Figure 7.5 The dose / time profiles for propofol with various models and targeting options for an average adult, assuming a single identical target value.

algorithms, but especially the smaller V1. In practice, the anaesthetist chooses plasma or effect site targets of their chosen algorithm, considering the patient and clinical scenario, to deliver an appropriate dose that results in induction of anaesthesia over an appropriate time scale. Maintenance target concentrations will be lower and typical values are described below.

The Marsh model for propofol was originally developed to target the *plasma* concentration whereas the Schnider model was specifically designed for targeting the *effect site*, and ordinarily this is how they are used. The Modified Marsh model differs from the Marsh model by using a k_{eo} of 1.21 min^{-1}, which facilitates effect site targeting. The differences between the Marsh and Schnider algorithms can be considered by comparing their key parameters (Table 7.1), and also by comparing the amount of propofol infused for a given target concentration (Figure 7.5).

The Marsh model describes V1 as 0.228 L.kg^{-1}. A doubling in weight leads to a doubling in V1 (70 kg, V1 = 15.96 litres; 140 kg, V1 = 31.92 litres). Consequently, as weight (and V1) increases, so does the amount of propofol calculated to achieve an initial target concentration. Conversely, lighter patients will have a smaller V1 and will receive a reduced amount of propofol to achieve the same target concentration. For normally proportioned patients this is logical, but specifically where the amount of adipose tissue is disproportionately large, V1 becomes an overestimate resulting in an overdose of propofol if typical target

Table 7.1 Parameters affecting TCI algorithms

	Marsh	Modified Marsh	Schnider
V1	weight	weight	fixed at 4.27 L
V2	weight	weight	age
V3	weight	weight	fixed
k12 & k21	fixed	fixed	age
k13 & k31	fixed	fixed	fixed
k_{eo} (min^{-1})	0.26	1.21	0.456
clearance	weight	weight	weight, height

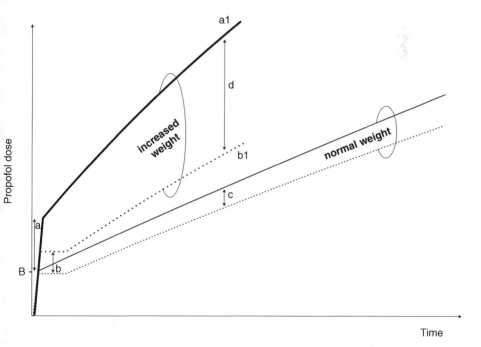

Figure 7.6 The effect of weight on propofol TCI administration against time, for Marsh and Schnider with the same target concentration. Similar bolus doses are given (B), but for normal weight 'c' describes the difference over time between plasma targeted Marsh (solid line) and effect site targeted Schnider (dotted line). As weight increases, Marsh delivers a greater initial bolus than Schnider 'a' vs 'b', and then a greater subsequent infusion rate 'a1' vs 'b1'. Consequently the difference between Marsh and Schnider increases over time, 'd'.

concentrations are used. These differences are most profound at the start of a TCI infusion but continue during the maintenance phase (Figure 7.6).

In complete contrast, V1 in the Schnider model is fixed at 4.27 litres (Table 7.1), nearly four times smaller (for a 70 kg patient) compared to Marsh. Were V1 the only factor, the amount of propofol delivered at the start of a TCI would not change between patients of different weights, and would be much less than delivered by the Marsh model, assuming identical targets. Indeed, if target values typically used at the start of an effect site targeted Schnider infusion were used in a plasma targeted Schnider infusion, the dose of propofol delivered would be too small to reliably induce anaesthesia. However, when Schnider is used in an effect site targeted manner, the bolus dose of propofol is larger and approximates to that given in the initial rapid infusion phase of a plasma targeted Marsh infusion (see Figure 7.5). The rapid infusion phase is by default 1200 ml.hr^{-1} and is represented by the steepest part of the curves in Figure 7.5. The horizontal part of the curve is characteristic of effect site targeting, as the pump is paused (administered dose remains static as time passes), while the plasma concentration falls following the initial bolus, to meet the rising effect site concentration at the target concentration (see Figure 7.3b).

The rate of drug infusion for a typical 70 kg patient during the maintenance phase (Figure 7.6) is similar for both plasma targeted Marsh and effect site targeted Schnider, assuming the same target concentration. This is to be expected given that both are used to maintain anaesthesia with the same drug, but the situation becomes more complicated as weight increases. In both algorithms the initial dose increases with weight, but more so with Marsh. The increase is amplified during the maintenance phase with a greater increase seen with Marsh so that the curves (representing dose against time), diverge. In practice this is often compensated for by entering a value that is below the actual weight. A number of different methods based on weight scalars and proportions of excess weight have been proposed in search of this optimal value. Depth of anaesthesia monitoring is especially useful in these situations.

Total Intravenous Anaesthesia in Practice

There are a number of obstacles to navigate in order for TIVA to be delivered successfully. Many of these do not relate to pharmacology, but rather obtaining equipment (TCI pumps, appropriate giving sets, depth of anaesthesia monitors) and standardising the setup. Assuming these are in place the delivery of TIVA need not be complicated and for decades the vast majority of anaesthesia has been induced using only intravenous drugs! The analogy of volatile induction / maintenance is helpful in that the induction phase typically involves a high concentration (albeit sometimes with a steady increase to customise the patient to the smell), followed by a lower maintenance concentration, at approximately 1MAC. The same is true for TIVA, where an initial higher target concentration, delivering an induction bolus, is followed by a lower target concentration delivering a maintenance infusion.

The values selected for induction will depend on the model chosen, effect of other drugs, patient factors and the clinical scenario. Induction strategies are no different compared to a 'non-pump' intravenous anaesthetic, where larger initial amounts result in a faster induction but risk cardiovascular instability, while smaller amounts offer the converse. Maintenance targets are typically, 2.5–4 mcg.ml^{-1} for propofol and 3–6 ng.ml^{-1} for remifentanil when used together. However, as the isobologram suggests (see Figure 7.7), if the remifentanil target concentration is increased, the propofol target concentration may be reduced for the same clinical effect (and vice versa). Of course, a higher target concentration risks side effects and offers less synergy. Where TIVA is used for long operations, priority may be given to keeping the propofol target concentration low while using a higher remifentanil target concentration as its context-sensitive half-time is small and fixed (see below). In many cases, using a combination of the two drugs near the most concave part of the isobologram (greatest synergy) will be most effective in terms of minimising drug use;

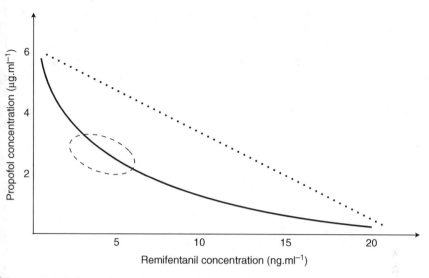

Figure 7.7 Isobologram for combining propofol and remifentanil. The concave shape indicates synergy which is maximal within the dashed area.

however, the exact combination chosen depends on whether analgesic requirements exceed hypnotic requirements or vice versa.

It is important to realise that the actual blood level achieved by TCI in any individual patient is not necessarily the exact target level due to pharmacokinetic variations between patients. Studies suggest that displayed plasma concentration will generally be within 25% of the actual concentration. In addition, the target level may or may not be appropriate for the stage of surgery. While a convenient aid to the anaesthetist, the infusion must be adjusted to effect, just as the vaporiser setting is adjusted during volatile anaesthesia.

Some TCI pumps have a **decrement time** displayed for the drug in use. This is the predicted time for the plasma level to fall to a lower value (often set at 1.2 $\mu g.ml^{-1}$ for propofol) at which the patient is expected to awaken. However, there are a number of reasons why this time may be longer, particularly with the use of other drugs with hypnotic or analgesic effects (especially opioids).

Safety of Total Intravenous Anaesthesia and Target-controlled Infusion in Clinical Practice

The setup of TIVA is arguably more complicated than that of an inhalational anaesthetic. Additional equipment needs checking and unlike the 'key index' system used to ensure that the correct volatile agent is used to refill the appropriate vaporiser, no such equivalent system exists for TIVA, so that it is possible to incorrectly programme the current generation of TCI pumps with the wrong drug, or wrong concentration of the correct drug.

Delivering volatile anaesthesia allows analysis of exhaled gas, providing a real-time proxy measure of depth of anaesthesia. By contrast, there is no equivalent mechanism for TIVA to assure the anaesthetist that adequate drug has reached the patient. Consequently, failure to deliver volatile agent to the patient, due to, for example, a breathing circuit failure will be detected unlike a disconnected propofol infusion. Depth of anaesthesia monitors have been recommended where TIVA is used in conjunction with muscle relaxants.

Using the same anaesthetic agent for induction and maintenance of anaesthesia is useful to prevent 'the gap', where the effects of the induction agent have worn off before the effects of the second agent have taken effect. Single agent induction/maintenance, be it either propofol or a volatile, negate this risk. TIVA has the additional advantage of being able to maintain anaesthesia independently of ventilation.

Context-sensitive Half-time

The terminal elimination half-life is a value often cited for comparing the duration of action of different drugs, but this has little clinical relevance. It is clear that the time course for the decline in plasma concentration at the end of an infusion depends on the duration of the infusion. The term context-sensitive half-time (CSHT) has been introduced to describe this variability; where 'context' refers to the duration of infusion. Context-sensitive half-time is defined as the time taken for the plasma concentration to fall by half, when an infusion (designed to maintain a constant plasma concentration) is stopped. The longest possible context-sensitive half-time is seen when the infusion has reached steady state, when there is no net transfer between compartments and input rate is the same as elimination rate. In general

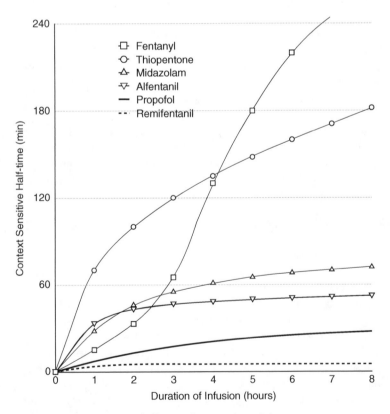

Figure 7.8 Context-sensitive half-times of commonly used drugs.

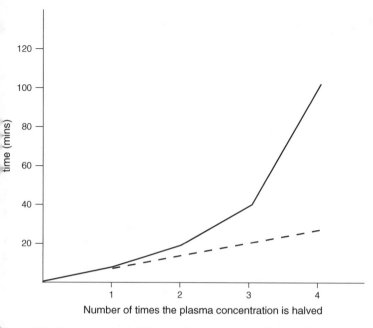

Figure 7.9 Context-sensitive half-times and times to repeated halving of plasma concentration of propofol. The dotted line shows what would have been seen if CSHT were *constant*.

terms, the higher the ratio of distribution clearance to clearance due to elimination, the greater the range for context-sensitive half-time. Fentanyl re-distributes much more rapidly than propofol; in addition, its clearance due to elimination is about one-fifth that for distribution. As a consequence, the CSHT for fentanyl increases rapidly with increasing duration of infusion. For propofol the clearance due to elimination is similar to that for distribution into the second compartment, so plasma concentration falls rapidly after a propofol infusion, mainly due to rapid elimination with a smaller contribution from distribution.

The maximum possible CSHT for propofol is about 25 minutes, compared with 300 minutes for fentanyl, based on current pharmacokinetic models. For remifentanil the longest possible CSHT is only 8 minutes since the ratio of distribution clearance to elimination clearance is less than one (the opposite of the situation with fentanyl) and as a result, elimination always dominates and there is very little variation in CSHT.

The variation of context-sensitive half-time with duration of infusion for different intravenous agents is shown in Figure 7.8. It must be remembered that after one CSHT, the next period of time required for plasma concentration to halve again will not be the same as the CSHT and is likely to be much longer (see Figure 7.9). This reflects the increasing importance of the slower redistribution and metabolism phases that predominate after initial drug distribution has taken place. This explains the emphasis on half-*time* rather than half-*life*: half-lives are constant whereas half-times are not.

Although the CSHT for propofol has a maximum value of about 25 minutes, during long, stimulating surgery infusion rates will have been high and the plasma concentration when wake-up is required may be much less than half the plasma concentration at the end of the infusion. Thus, time to awakening using propofol alone may be much longer than the CSHT. This is why the TCI pumps display a decrement time rather than a CSHT.

Chapter

8

Medicinal Chemistry

Structure–activity relationships (SAR) describe how the structure of related drugs influences their behaviour, for example whether they are agonists or antagonists. In order to understand how differences in drug structure can affect activity it is necessary to appreciate drug development methods and some basic organic chemistry. Once the properties of the contributing groups are understood, then it becomes easier to predict the likely behaviour of a drug molecule compared with the parent drug. In addition, knowledge of the structural properties of a drug may help us appreciate some of their physicochemical properties, such as their solubility in oil and water, their pK_a values and whether they are weak acids or bases. These in turn help us understand the pharmacokinetic behaviour of a drug.

Drug design starts with a lead compound that has the required action in an animal model, but is not necessarily ideal; for example, the drug may resemble a neurotransmitter or be an enzyme inhibitor. By adding various functional groups to this compound it is possible to develop a more specific drug to target the required system. Once a compound with the most favourable pharmacodynamic effects is found, further modifications may be made to make the drug's pharmacokinetic behaviour more desirable.

In this chapter we will introduce some basic organic chemistry and identify the structures associated with drugs commonly used in anaesthesia. Those basic structures that should be readily identified are mentioned briefly below, together with diagrams of their structures and examples relevant to anaesthesia. These should be used in conjunction with a description of drug activity in Sections II–IV.

Organic chemistry is the study of carbon-based compounds. The position of carbon in the middle of the periodic table (Group IV) gives it an atomic structure that can form covalent bonds with elements from either end of the table. This contrasts with inorganic chemistry, where ionic bonds are most common. Covalent bonds are stronger than ionic bonds and do not interact readily with water, making many organic molecules insoluble in water. By the addition of functional groups (such as hydroxyl, –OH or amine, –NH$_2$) these organic compounds can become water-soluble. Organic molecules are the basis of life, from DNA to structural proteins and chemical messengers. Knowledge of these basic building blocks and signalling systems is crucial to an understanding of how therapeutic agents modify existing physiological processes at the molecular level.

Building Blocks: Amino Acids, Nucleic Acids and Sugars

Amino Acids

The basic structure of an α-amino acid is a hydrocarbon group with both a carboxyl and amine group attached to the end carbon (the α-carbon). There are 20 commonly occurring α-amino acids that form the building blocks for protein synthesis (of which five cannot be synthesised – the essential amino acids). Not all amino acids form peptides and proteins; some amino acids are important precursors in neurotransmitter synthesis. For example, phenylalanine can be metabolised to tyrosine which then enters adrenergic neurones as the substrate for catecholamine synthesis (see Chapter 13). Other α-amino acids are central neurotransmitters in their own right, for example, glycine and glutamate. Not all amino acids of importance are α-amino acids. GABA (γ-amino butyric acid), as its name suggests, is a γ-amino acid that has the carboxyl and amine groups on opposite ends of a butyl backbone; GABA is an important inhibitory neurotransmitter.

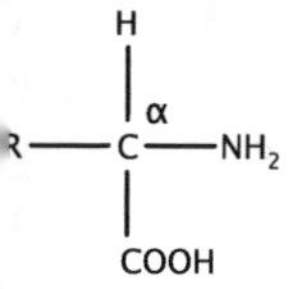

An α–amino acid

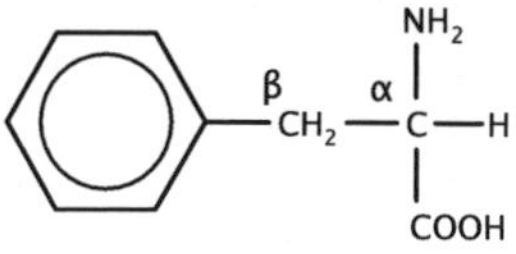

Phenylalanine

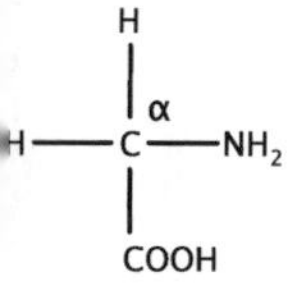

Glycine

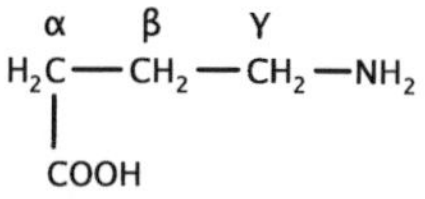

GABA, γ–amino buteric acid

Nucleic Acids, Nucleosides and Nucleotides

Nucleosides are formed from the combination of a nucleic acid with a sugar, usually ribose (e.g. adenosine, guanosine). Nucleotides are the building blocks of DNA/RNA and are formed from nucleosides linked to a phosphate group. The nucleic acids are either purines (adenine or guanine) or pyrimidines (cytosine, uracil or thymine). Many anti-cancer drugs are analogues of nucleic acids or nucleotides. Nucleosides are important intermediates in metabolic processes as they can combine with high-energy phosphate groups to act as co-factors in metabolic and catabolic processes within the cell.

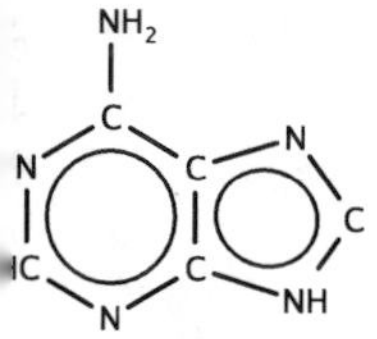

Adenine

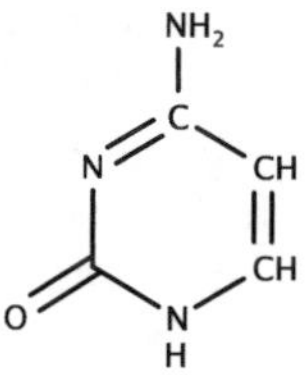

Cytosine (4–amino 2 oxopyrimidine)

Sugars

These are carbohydrates with a chemical formula $(CH_2O)_n$, where n can be 3 (a triose, e.g. glyceraldehyde), 4 (a tetrose), 5 (a pentose, e.g. ribose) or 6 (a hexose, e.g. glucose). They are naturally occurring compounds and glucose is metabolised to carbon dioxide and water through oxidative tissue respiration. The pentoses and hexoses exist in cyclic forms in vivo.

Glyceraldehyde (a triose)

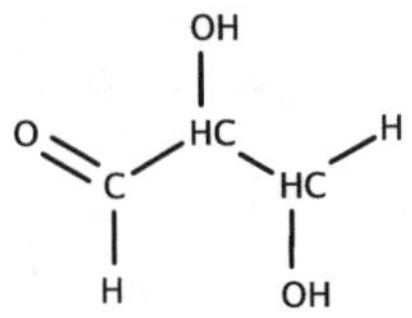

Ribose (a pentose)

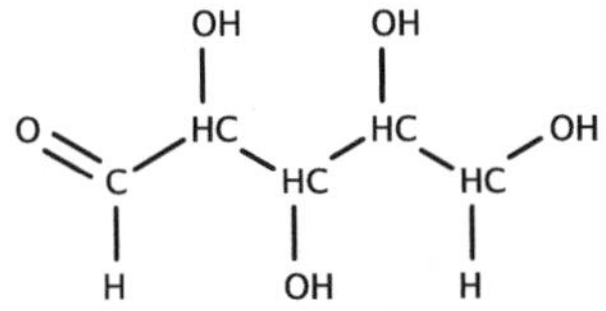

Glucose (a hexose)

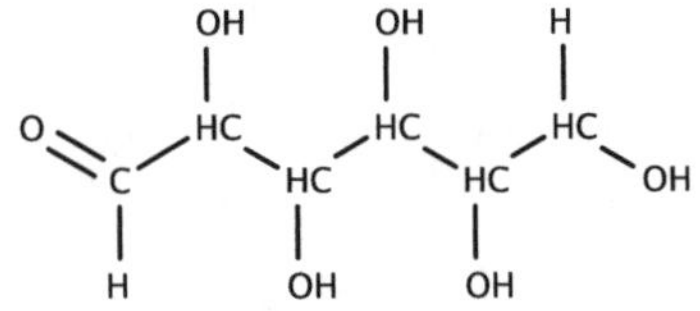

Drugs and their Structures

Many drugs are organic molecules and often derived from plant material. It is not possible here to describe all the molecular structures of groups of anaesthetically important drugs. In this section the following selected structures will be described: catecholamines, barbiturates, benzodiazepines, non-depolarising muscle relaxants (bis-benzylisoquinoliniums and aminosteroids) and opioids.

Catecholamines and Derivatives

These are derived from the amino acid tyrosine (see also Figure 13.3), which is hydroxylated (addition of an –OH group) and decarboxylated (removal of a –COOH group). The side chain (ethylamine) consists of two carbons attached to an amine group. The α-carbon is bound to the amine group and the β-carbon is covalently linked to the catechol ring. The size and nature of the functional groups on the terminal amine and the α-carbon determine whether an agent is active at either α- or β-adrenoceptors or is an agonist or antagonist. In addition, only catechols (two adjacent –OH groups on the benzene ring) are metabolised by catechol-O-methyl transferase (COMT); derivatives without this feature may have a longer duration of action. Similarly, monoamine oxidase (MAO) will metabolise only drugs with a single amine group, preferably a primary amine, although adrenaline, a secondary amine (see mini-dictionary below), is a substrate (see Chapter 13).

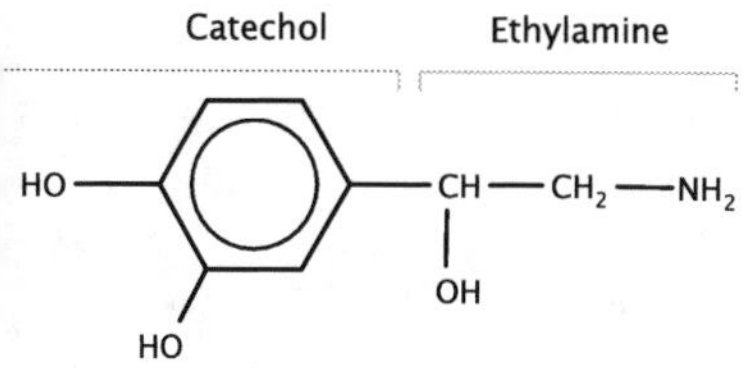

Catechol   Ethylamine

HO — [benzene ring] — CH — CH$_2$ — NH$_2$
              |
              OH
HO

Noradrenaline

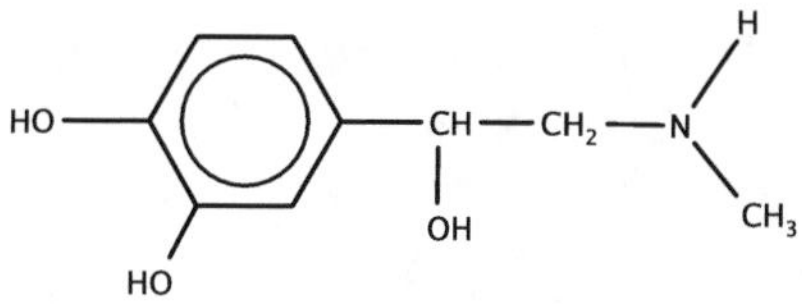

HO — [benzene ring] — CH — CH$_2$ — N — H
              | \
              OH   CH$_3$
HO

Adrenaline

HO — [benzene ring] — CH — CH$_2$ — N — H
              | \
              OH   CH
                                    / \
                              H$_3$C   CH$_3$
HO

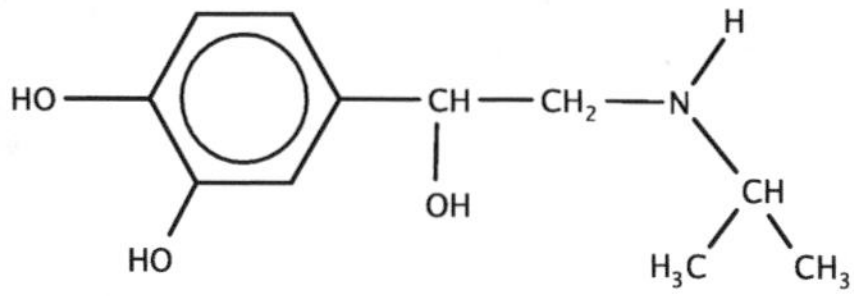

Isoprenaline
A β–selective agonist;
not a substrate for MAO,
a substrate for COMT

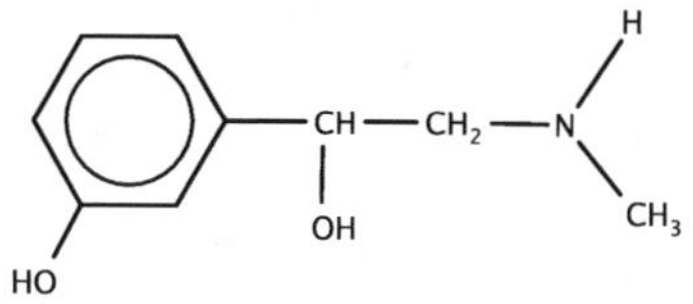

[benzene ring] — CH — CH$_2$ — N — H
                   | \
                   OH   CH$_3$
HO

Phenylephrine
An α–selective agonist;
a substrate for MAO,
not a substrate for COMT

Barbiturates

Barbiturates are derivatives of barbituric acid, which is formed by a condensation reaction (i.e. water is also formed) between malonic acid and urea. Barbiturates are weak acids, but also have imino groups present (see Figure 9.3). Thio barbiturates have, as their name suggests, a thio (=S) substitution for the keto group (=O). The types of hydrocarbon groups on the 5-carbon determine the duration of pharmacological action. Oxybarbiturates undergo less hepatic metabolism than the corresponding thiobarbiturate.

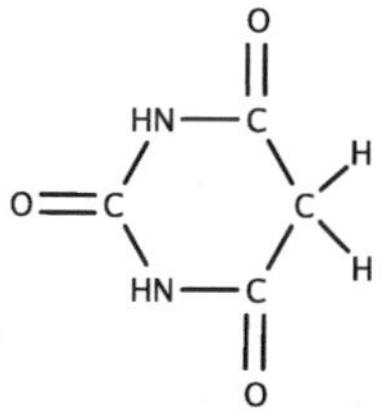

Barbituric acid

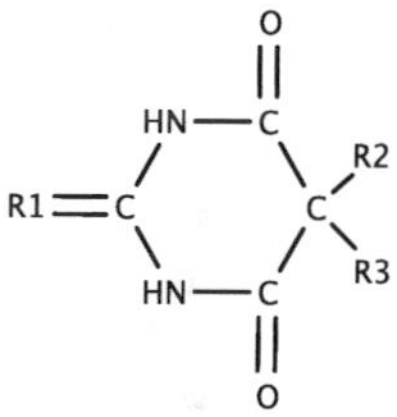

Barbiturates:

	R$_1$	R$_2$	R$_3$
Long acting Phenobarbitone	O	— CH$_2$CH$_3$	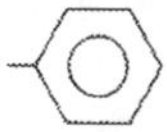 [benzene ring]
Intermediate acting Pentobarbitone	O	— CH$_2$CH$_3$	— CH CH$_2$ CH$_2$ CH$_3$ with CH$_3$
Short acting Thiopentone	S	— CH$_2$CH$_3$	— CH CH$_2$ CH$_2$ CH$_3$ with CH$_3$

Benzodiazepines

Members of this group of heterocyclic compounds are interesting in that structurally they have both six- and seven-membered rings, and some also have a five-membered ring. Their C-containing ring structures make benzodiazepines (BDZs) poorly water-soluble and diazepam requires a special lipid emulsion preparation (diazemuls) to be used intravenously. However, by altering the hydrocarbon groups and pH, an alternative tautomeric form without a closed seven-membered ring can be formed. Thus midazolam is presented in the ampoule as a water-soluble drug, but when it reaches the plasma it returns to the more lipid-soluble ring form (see Figure 18.1). There are three groups of BDZs: 1,4-BDZs (diazepam, temazepam, lorazepam), heterocyclic BDZs (midazolam) and 1,5-BDZs (clobazam). Some of the 1,4-BDZs are metabolically related; diazepam is metabolised to oxazepam and temazepam.

Diazepam,
a 1,4–benzodiazepine

Clobazam,
a 1,5–benzodiazepine

Midazolam
(closed ring form)

Non-depolarising Muscle Relaxants

Bis-benzylisoquinoliniums

Bis-benzylisoquinoliniums are one of the two groups into which the non-depolarising muscle relaxants can be divided, the other being the aminosteroids (see below). These are based on the structure of the naturally occurring drug tubocurarine. They are so named from their underlying structure of two (hence the bis-) isoquinolinium structures, linked through a carbon chain containing two ester linkages. The isoquinolinium structure is related to papaverine, which is a smooth muscle relaxant. Features of the molecular structure of atracurium are: the distance between quaternary nitrogens (approximately 1 nm); the heterocyclic, bulky ring structures and the reverse orientation of the ester linkages that favours Hofmann degradation. In mivacurium the ester linkages are oriented the opposite way, which does not allow Hofmann degradation to occur. The nitrogen atom in each isoquinolinium group is quaternary, so the molecules are permanently charged and are presented as a salt. Multiple isomers exist, with differing activity (see Chapter 5).

Aminosteroids

The steroid nucleus is a complex polycyclic hydrocarbon structure. It is important to recognise that many hormones have this basic structure as well as many drugs. It has been popular as a drug skeleton because it is relatively inflexible. The aminosteroid non-depolarising muscle relaxants are steroids, as was the intravenous agent althesin and the corticosteroid hormones. It is worth recognising the numbering of the carbon atoms, since this will help identify metabolites and substitutions especially for muscle relaxants. Importantly, the steroid nucleus is not readily water-soluble; this requires hydrophilic substitution. In the aminosteroid family, not all are readily water-soluble and vecuronium has to be presented as a lyophilised preparation to ensure its stability (rapid freezing and dehydration of the frozen product under a high vacuum). Important features are: the distance between nitrogen atoms; the acetyl groups ester-linked to the 3 and 17 positions and the bis-quaternary structure of pancuronium but the monoquaternary structure of vecuronium and rocuronium with the N- in the 2 position protonated at pH 7.4.

Atracurium

Vecuronium
The two acetylcholine moieties are highlighted; loss of the 3- or 17-acetyl groups reduces potency

Opioids

The parent compound is morphine, which has a complex ring structure. The important features include the phenolic hydroxyl (-OH) group in the 3 position, which is different from the cyclohexanol -OH group in the 6 position. The former is essential for activity in morphine-like opioids, but the latter is not; the 6-glucuronide metabolite of morphine is active, the 3-glucuronide is not. Modifications include acetylation at both the 3 and 6 positions to the pro-drug diamorphine; this increases lipid solubility and reduces onset time as only de-acetylation at the 3 position is essential for activity. Codeine is methylated through the 3 hydroxyl group increasing lipid solubility but reducing activity. The 6-keto derivatives are more active. The second important feature is the amine group, which is also necessary for receptor binding. Substitutions here can result in antagonists, such as naloxone. Not all rings are necessary for activity, with the phenolic ring being most important. Loss of various rings results in drugs such as fentanyl and its derivatives.

Morphine   Naloxone   Fentanyl

Medicinal Chemistry Mini-Dictionary

The following is not meant to be an exhaustive list of every possible chemical group or underlying drug structure. However, it covers terms encountered most commonly. It is designed as a quick reference to features of drug molecules.

Acetyl: Acetyl group CH_3COO-R (where R is a C-based group), acetic acid (= ethanoic acid) is CH_3COOH. A proton (H^+) donor group therefore acidic and hydrophilic. Aspirin is *acetyl*salicylic acid and some NSAIDs are phenyl*acetic acid* derivatives (e.g. diclofenac, ketorolac and indomethacin); present in the neurotransmitter *acetyl*choline.

$H_3C - C - O - CH_2 - CH_2 - N^+(CH_3)_3$ Acetylcholine

Acetyl

Alkane: A compound containing just carbon and hydrogen atoms (a hydrocarbon) forming a chain of carbon atoms with fully saturated bonds. The *normal* alkanes are unbranched and form a series starting with methane (CH_4), ethane (CH_3CH_3), propane ($CH_3CH_2CH_3$) and butane ($CH_3CH_2CH_2CH_3$). Lipid-soluble, short-chain alkanes are miscible with water.

Alkanol: Alkanes with one or more –OH substitutions. If one such substitution occurs on a terminal C, then this is an n-alkanol (or normal alkanol). If the substitution occurs on an inner C then this is an iso-alkanol. Presence of an –OH increases water solubility.

Alkyl: Indicates the presence of an alkane group. Naming depends on length of chain: 1 = methyl; 2 = ethyl; 3 = propyl; 4 = butyl; 5 = pentyl; 6 = hexyl; 7 = heptyl; 8 = octyl; 9 = nonyl; 10 = decyl; 11 = undecyl; 12 = duodecyl. The longer the chain, the less water-soluble and more lipid-soluble. Compare the butyl- (bupivacaine) and propyl- (ropivacaine) substitutions in the mepivacaine local anaesthetic series.

Amide: This has an R-CO · NH_2 conformation. It is found in the chain linking the xylidine ring with the substituted amine in amide local anaesthetics (e.g. lidocaine).

Amine: A primary amine group is $R–NH_2$. A secondary amine is R–NH-R′; a tertiary amine has all three H groups replaced. A monoamine contains just one amine group in its structure. Each amino acid has one terminal with an amine group, the other with a carboxyl group; some amino acids are monoamines, others are diamines. Amine groups are proton acceptors and at a pH above their pK_a will become protonated and therefore carry a (+) charge. This can then increase water solubility. Conversely, below their pK_a they are more lipid soluble. A quaternary nitrogen (sometimes misnamed a quaternary amine) is one where the N has four bonds and so is permanently charged. The non-depolarising muscle relaxants have quaternary nitrogens (e.g. vecuronium, atracurium).

Benzyl: This group has an unsaturated (i.e. contains some double C=C bonds) 6-carbon ring structure; benzene has the formula C_6H_6. It has a planar ring structure and is a solvent for lipids but is not water-soluble. It is a common group in drug molecules, for example, etomidate, and often substituted with a halogen as in ketamine (chlorine) and some BDZs (chlorine).

Carbamyl: The group $-CONH_2$. The dimethyl derivative of this group is present and ester-linked in some of the anticholinesterase inhibitors, such as neostigmine (hence a carbamate ester). As a result of enzyme interaction the enzyme becomes carbamylated instead of acetylated with slower recovery of the esteratic site.

Neostigmine

Dimethylcarbamyl

Carboxylic acid: Generic term for acids derived from alkanols. The first two members of the series have special names: formic acid and acetic acid from methanol and ethanol. The others are named according to the alkanol, for example, propionic acid from n-propanol. As acids, they are proton donors and water soluble.

Formic acid   Acetic acid   Proprionic acid

Catechol: 1, 2-hydroxybenzene. Both $-OH$ groups are required before a compound can be metabolised by COMT (catechol O-methyltransferase) when the $-OH$ group is methylated to $-OCH_3$. In noradrenaline, the main substituent on the benzyl ring is the ethylamine group, which is therefore numbered 1, so the two $-OH$ groups are renumbered as 3 and 4.

Catechol   Noradrenaline

Choline: $CH_3 N(CH_3)_3$, a precursor in acetylcholine (ACh) synthesis.

Cyclohexanol: A cyclic alkanol with formula $C_6H_{11}OH$. It has very different properties from phenol, the cyclic alcohol with a benzene ring structure. Tramadol is based on cyclohexanol.

Enol: The enol form in organic cyclic molecules is an –OH (hydroxyl) group adjacent to a C=C double bond, so allowing for tautomeric interconversion to the keto form =O with a single C–C bond. Seen in barbiturates.

Ester: A link formed by the interaction of a carboxylic acid with an alcohol, resulting in an ester and water, R–O–CO–R'. It is susceptible to hydrolysis, either by plasma or hepatic esterases. Many examples: aspirin, remifentanil, esmolol, mivacurium.

Ether: A link between two carbon-containing groups, R–O–R'. Important in the structure of currently available volatile agents, all but halothane are ethers. Halothane is a halogen-substituted ethane (see **Alkane**). Not water-soluble, but lipid-soluble.

Glucuronide: A polar glucose group added during phase II hepatic metabolism, often through a hydroxy group (–OH). For example, BDZs are glucuronidated after phase I metabolism, morphine is glucuronidated to an active (-6) and inactive (-3) glucuronide, propofol and its quinol derivative are also glucuronidated.

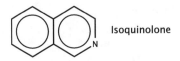

Glucuronidation of propofol

Halogen: A member of group VII of the periodic table. Includes fluorine, chlorine and bromine. Halogens are important substitutions on lead compounds in development of volatile anaesthetics. Fluorine is the most electronegative element and stabilises the ethers, reducing the likelihood of metabolism.

Heterocyclic: A ring structure with at least one member of the ring *not* carbon.

Imidazole: Heterocyclic ring containing two N atoms and three C atoms. Part of the structures of etomidate, enoximone and phentolamine. These are weak bases, proton acceptors, so that pH will determine the degree of ionisation and hence water solubility.

Imidazole (1,3 diazole)

Isoquinoline: A heterocyclic ring system, part of bis-benzylisoquinolinium structure of certain non-depolarising blockers and found in papaverine.

Isoquinolone

Keto: A keto group is the equivalent of an aldehyde group (=O) but in a ring structure. Under certain circumstances it exists in equilibrium with its enol form.

Laudanosine: One of the products of atracurium and cis-atracurium breakdown by Hofmann degradation. It is neurotoxic in certain non-primate species. The other product is an acrylate (CH_2CH-R).

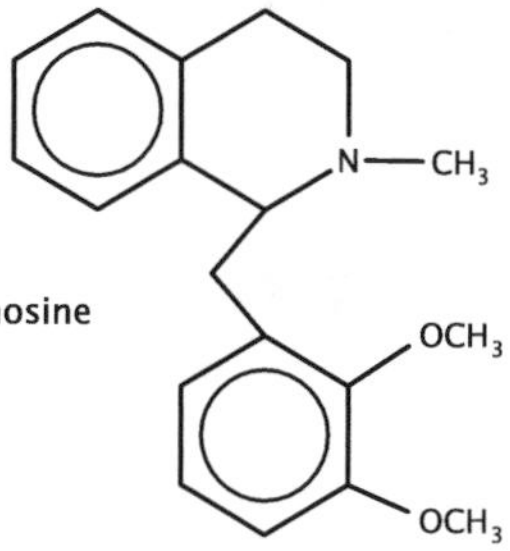

Laudanosine

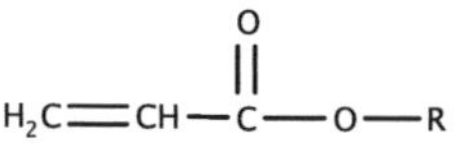

Acrylate

Mandelic acid: Derivatives of mandelic acid are formed as a result of adrenaline and noradrenaline metabolism by MAO and COMT, e.g. 3-methoxy-4-hydroxymandelic acid.

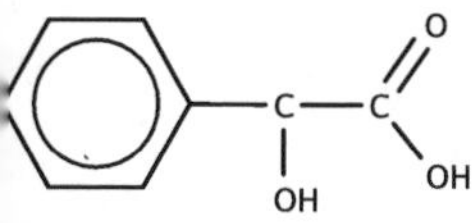

Mandelic acid

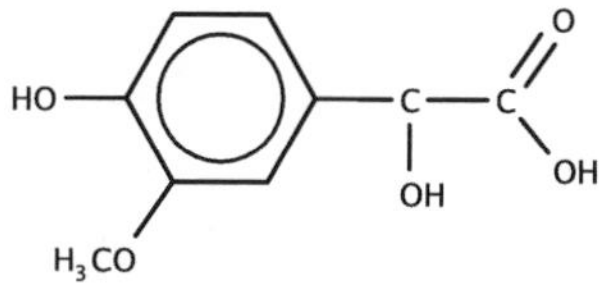

3–methoxy–4–hydroxy mandelic acid

Methoxy: $-OCH_3$ group, this has better lipid solubility than $-OH$. Codeine is 3-methoxymorphine. There are several methoxy- group substitutions in the benzylisoquinolinium non-depolarising muscle relaxants which make them water-soluble.

Methyl: $-CH_3$ group (see **Alkyl**). Methylation and demethylation are important routes of metabolism for many drugs, both in the liver and in other tissues. Noradrenaline is methylated to adrenaline in adrenal medullary cells whereas diazepam is demethylated to nordiazepam and ketamine demethylated to norketamine in the liver. Note that the prefix nor- and the prefix desmethyl- can both imply the removal of a methyl group from a parent structure.

Oxicam: Piroxicam and meloxicam are two examples of the NSAIDs with this underlying structure.

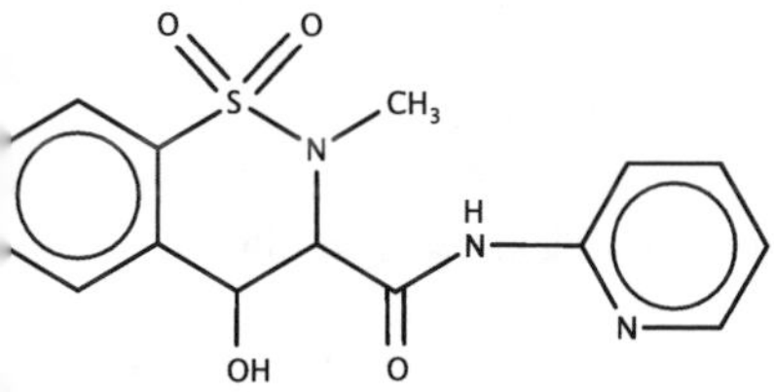

Piroxicam

Papaverine: Heterocyclic ring structure related to opioids and found with morphine in opium. Two papaverine-like ring structures are found in bis-benzylisoquinoliniums. Papaverine is a smooth muscle relaxant.

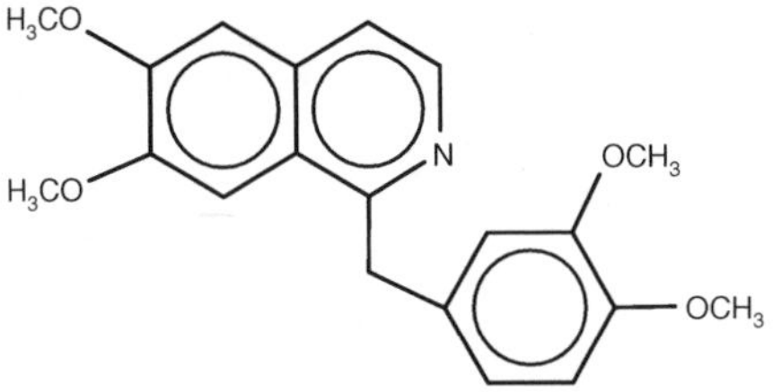

Papaverine

Phenanthrene: A polycyclic carbon ring structure related to morphine.

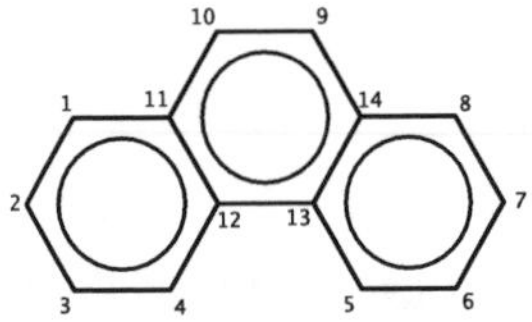

Phencyclidine: A cyclic hexacarbon with a phenolic substituent group. The underlying structure of ketamine.

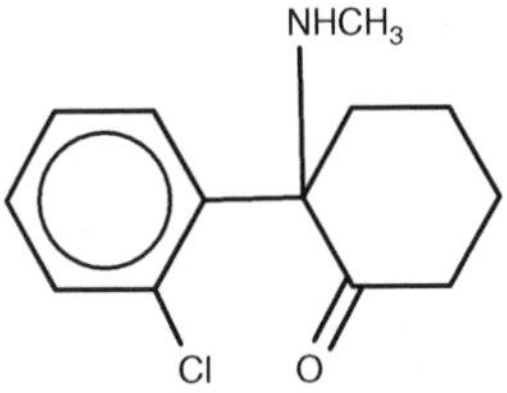

Ketamine

Phenyl: Phenol is hydroxylated benzene, C_6H_5OH. A phenyl group is $-C_6H_4OH$. Commonly part of drug structures, for example, paracetamol, propofol and edrophonium, and as a substituent, for example, in phentolamine and fentanyl. Phenol is water-soluble.

Piperazine: Heterocyclic ring containing two N atoms and four C atoms, $C_4H_{10}N_2$. The N atoms are in opposition, that is, in the 1 and 4 positions. The $-NH$ groups are bases, proton acceptors, so that pH and pK_a will determine degree of ionisation and hence water solubility.

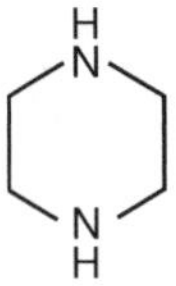

Piperazine

Piperidine: Heterocyclic ring containing one N atom and five C atoms, $C_5H_{11}N$. The NH group is a proton acceptor; pH and pK_a determine degree of ionisation. Piperidine rings are found in many drugs including fentanyl, alfentanil, remifentanil, bupivacaine and ropivacaine.

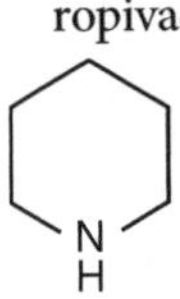

Piperidine

Propionic acid: Another of the chemical groups upon which NSAIDs are based, the underlying structure is the carboxylic acid of propanol, for example, ibuprofen.

Pyrazalones: Keto-modified pyrazole ring on which phenylbutazone and related NSAIDs are based.

Pyrazolone   Phenylbutazone

Pyrazole: A five-membered ring with two N and three C atoms, $C_3H_3 \cdot N \cdot NH$. Celecoxib and rofecoxib are based on the pyrazole nucleus.

Pyrazole

Quinol: 1,4-dihydroxybenzene, also known as hydroquinone. One metabolite of propofol is the 4-glucuronide of 2,6-diisopropylquinol. The quinols are responsible for the green colour of urine in patients receiving propofol infusions.

Quinol   2,6,diisopropylquinol

Salicylate: Aspirin is acetyl salicylate and is metabolised to salicylic acid.

Aspirin   Salicylic acid

Thiazide: Sulfur-containing heterocyclic ring, the core structure of thiazide diuretics.

Xanthene: Methylxanthenes are important phosphodiesterase inhibitors, e.g. aminophylline.

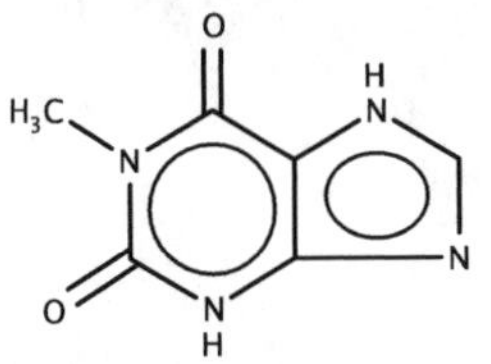

Methylxanthene

Xylidine: 2,6-bismethylaminobenzene. Xylides are metabolites of many amide anaesthetics. Lidocaine is metabolised to MEGX, monoethylglycine-xylide.

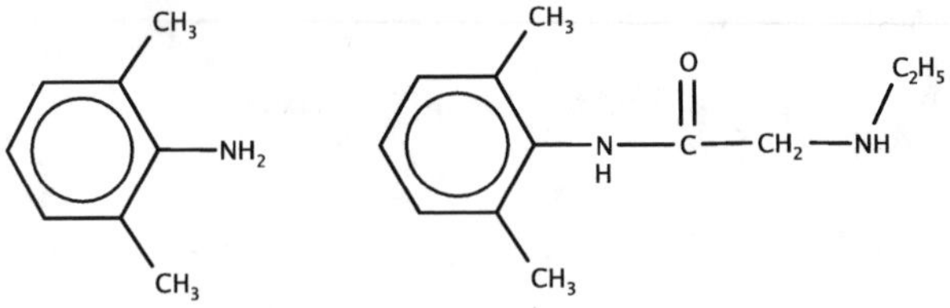

Xylidine

MEGX

General Anaesthetic Agents

Our understanding of the mechanisms involved in the action of general anaesthetics has increased considerably in recent times and is discussed below. This is followed by sections discussing intravenous and inhaled anaesthetic agents.

Mechanisms of General Anaesthetic Action

Any mechanism of general anaesthetic action must be able to explain: loss of conscious awareness; loss of response to noxious stimuli (anti-nociceptive effect); and, perhaps most important of all, reversibility.

Anatomical Sites of Action

General anaesthetic agents affect both brain and spinal cord to account for physiological responses to nociception, loss of consciousness and inhibition of explicit memory. Auditory and sensory evoked potential data implicate the thalamus as the most likely primary target, but secondary sites such as the limbic system (associated with memory) and certain cortical areas are also important. Halogenated volatile anaesthetics appear to have a greater influence on the spinal cord than do the intravenous agents.

Molecular Theories

At the beginning of the twentieth century, Overton and Meyer independently described the linear correlation between the lipid solubility of anaesthetic agents and their potency (see Figure 9.1). This correlation was so impressive, given the great variation in structure of these agents, that it suggested a non-specific mechanism of action based on this physicochemical property. Later interpretation pointed out that any highly lipophilic area was a potential site of action, with cell membranes being the most likely contender, given the high concentration of lipids. There are problems with a unified theory based on lipid interactions: some general anaesthetics, such as ketamine, are extreme outliers, and the stereoisomers R-etomidate and S-etomidate have identical lipid solubility but only R-etomidate has anaesthetic properties.

Membrane Lipids

There are several potential lipophilic sites in cell membranes, including the lipid bilayer itself and the annular lipids surrounding ionic channels.

Initially it was suggested that anaesthetic agents could penetrate the bilayer and alter the molecular arrangement of the phospholipids, which led to expansion of the membrane and disruption of the function of membrane-spanning ionic channels. Calculations identifying

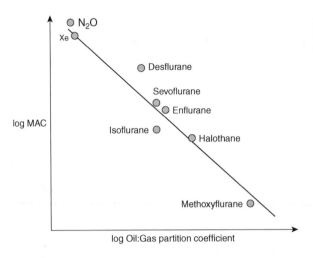

Figure 9.1 Straight line relationship between MAC and an index of lipid solubility (note: logarithmic scales).

the volume of anaesthetic agent required to expand membranes led to a 'critical volume hypothesis'. Against such a theory, a 1°C rise in temperature increases membrane thickness to a similar extent as that seen with volatile agents, yet increased temperature does not enhance anaesthesia – the opposite is true.

A further theory suggested anaesthetic agents act at specific lipid site(s). The composition of phospholipids in the immediate vicinity of ion channels is different from that of the general lipid bilayer. This proposed disruption of annular lipids associated with specific ion channels led to the perturbation theory.

A rapid advance in receptor protein identification within the central nervous system (CNS) has led to newer theories based on interactions with specific proteins. It now seems likely that the correlation between potency and lipid solubility reflects the lipophilic nature of specific protein-based binding site(s).

Protein Site(s) of Action

Ligand-gated ionic channels are more sensitive to the action of general anaesthetics than are voltage-gated channels. The interaction at inhibitory (GABA$_A$ and glycine) and excitatory (neuronal nicotinic and NMDA) channels have all been studied. Table 9.1 summarises the relative activity of a number of agents at these receptors.

GABA$_A$ Receptor

The GABA$_A$ receptor, like the nicotinic acetylcholine receptor, belongs to the pentameric family of ligand-gated ion-channel receptors. It has binding sites for GABA associated with α subunits and modulatory sites at the α/γ interface for benzodiazepines and on the β subunit for etomidate, barbiturates, propofol and volatile agents (see Figure 9.2). The stereospecificity of the action of etomidate, presented as an enantiopure preparation of the R(+) isomer, supports the protein-based action of anaesthetics. The S(−) form of etomidate is clinically inactive and at the GABA$_A$ receptor there is a 30-fold difference in activity.

Anaesthetics increase channel opening time, so allowing for increased chloride entry resulting in hyperpolarisation. The effect is seen for etomidate, propofol and barbiturates, as well as halogenated volatiles. Etomidate is selective for the $GABA_A$ receptor but propofol will also increase glycine channel opening time and is inhibitory at neuronal nicotinic and $5HT_3$ receptors. The site(s) on the $GABA_A$ receptor associated with anaesthetic action are associated with the β subunit and are distinct from the benzodiazepine receptor site. There are at least 30 types of $GABA_A$ receptor, each with different subunit composition; $β_2$ and $β_3$ subunits are more sensitive to the effects of etomidate than is the $β_1$ subunit.

Glycine Receptor

The major inhibitory transmitter in the spinal cord and brain stem is glycine, which is associated with a chloride channel similar to the $GABA_A$ receptor. The volatile anaesthetics all markedly potentiate the action of glycine, although there is no evidence of stereoselectivity. It has been suggested that the spinal cord is an important site of action for volatile rather than intravenous anaesthetic agents. Efficacy here correlates more with immobility than awareness.

Table 9.1 General anaesthetic effects at central receptors

	Inhibitory neurotransmitters		Excitatory neurotransmitters	
	GABA_A	Glycine	NMDA	Neuronal nACh
Propofol	++++	+	0	–
Thiopental	+++++	++	0	–
R-etomidate	+++++	0	0	0
S-etomidate	0	0	0	0
Ketamine	0	0	–	0
Isoflurane	++++	+++	0	–
Nitrous oxide	0	0	–	0
Xenon	0	0	–	0

+: enhances effect of neurotransmitter; –: reduces effect of neurotransmitter; 0: no effect on neurotransmitter. nACh: central nicotinic acetylcholine receptor.

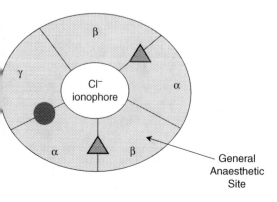

Figure 9.2 The $GABA_A$ receptor complex, from above. The grey triangles show the two agonist sites for gamma amino butyric acid (GABA). Diazepam, temazepam and midazolam are agonists and flumazenil is an antagonist at the benzodiazepine site (grey circle). Propofol, etomidate, barbiturates and halogenated volatile agents are agonists at the general anaesthetic site. Both sites produce positive allosteric modulation.

NMDA Receptor

Neuronal signalling may also be reduced by inhibition of excitatory pathways. The NMDA receptor is involved in long-term signal potentiation associated with learning and memory; it is activated by glutamate, modulated by magnesium and inhibited in a non-competitive manner by ketamine, nitrous oxide and xenon. This glutamate-mediated mechanism represents an additional pathway for anaesthesia. Other anaesthetic agents, such as barbiturates, can reduce the effectiveness of glutamate but at a lower potency than for inhibition of $GABA_A$ receptor function.

Intravenous Anaesthetic Agents

Intravenous anaesthetics have been defined as agents that will induce loss of consciousness in one arm–brain circulation time.

The introduction of barbiturates in the 1930s was a significant advance in anaesthesia. Their rapid onset and relatively short duration of action made them different from previously used agents. Hexobarbitone was introduced first, followed by thiopental and subsequently methohexitone. Phencyclidine (angel dust) was withdrawn due to serious psychotomimetic reactions, but the chemically related compound ketamine is still used. The imidazole ester, etomidate, is useful due to its cardiovascular stability but side effects limit its use. The phenolic derivative propofol has become the most popular agent in recent years due to its ready-to-use formulation, favourable recovery profile and use in target-controlled infusions (TCIs). Steroidal compounds have also been used; however, poor solubility (pregnalolone) together with an association with anaphylactic reactions (due to cremophor EL – used to solubilise the steroid althesin) has led to their demise.

The Ideal Intravenous Anaesthetic Agent

Were an ideal intravenous anaesthetic agent to exist, it should have the following properties:

- rapid onset (mainly unionised at physiological pH)
- high lipid solubility
- rapid recovery, no accumulation during prolonged infusion
- analgesic at sub-anaesthetic concentrations
- minimal cardiovascular and respiratory depression
- no emetic effects
- no pain on injection
- no excitation or emergence phenomena
- no interaction with other agents
- safe following inadvertent intra-arterial injection
- no toxic effects
- no histamine release
- no hypersensitivity reactions
- water-soluble formulation
- long shelf-life at room temperature
- minimal environmental impact.

The currently used agents are discussed below under the following headings:

- **Barbiturates (thiopental)**
- **Non-barbiturates (propofol, ketamine, etomidate).**

Barbiturates

All barbiturates are derived from barbituric acid, which is the condensation product of urea and malonic acid (see Figure 9.3). When oxygen is exchanged for sulfur at the C2 position, oxybarbiturates become thiobarbiturates.

Barbiturates are not readily soluble in water at neutral pH. Their solubility depends on transformation from the keto to the enol form (tautomerism), which occurs most readily in alkaline solutions (see Figure 9.4). In general, thiobarbiturates are very lipid-soluble, highly protein-bound and completely metabolised in the liver. In contrast, the oxybarbiturates are less lipid-soluble, less protein-bound, and some are excreted almost entirely unchanged in the urine.

Thiopental

Thiopental is the sulfur analogue of the oxybarbiturate pentobarbital.

Presentation

Thiopental is formulated as the sodium salt and presented as a pale yellow powder. The vial contains sodium carbonate (Na_2CO_3, 6% by weight) and nitrogen in place of air. These two measures are designed to improve solubility of the solution by the following mechanisms:

1. Sodium carbonate reacts with water in the following manner:

   $$Na_2CO_3 + H_2O \rightarrow NaHCO_3 + Na^+ + OH^-$$

   The result is a strongly alkaline solution (pH 10.5) favouring the water-soluble enol form which is more desirable as a preparation.

2. Air contains small amounts of carbon dioxide. Were this to be present and react with water it would tend to release bicarbonate and hydrogen ions which in turn would result in a less alkaline solution. As a result, more thiopental would be in the less water-soluble keto form. Nitrogen is used in place of air to prevent this.

   The 2.5% solution is stable for many days and should be bacteriostatic due to its alkaline pH.

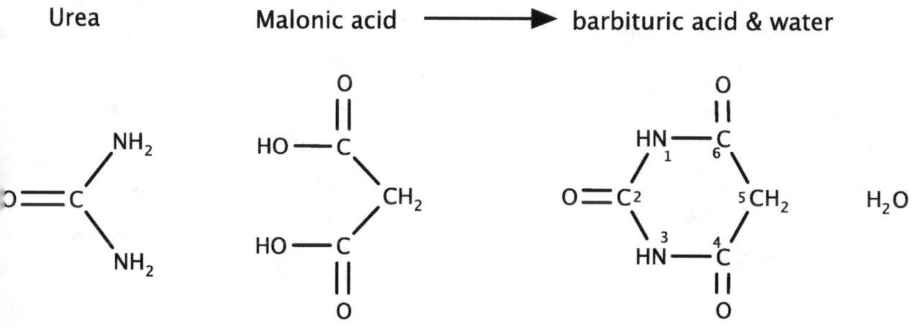

Urea   Malonic acid   ⟶   barbituric acid & water

Figure 9.3
Formation of barbituric acid.

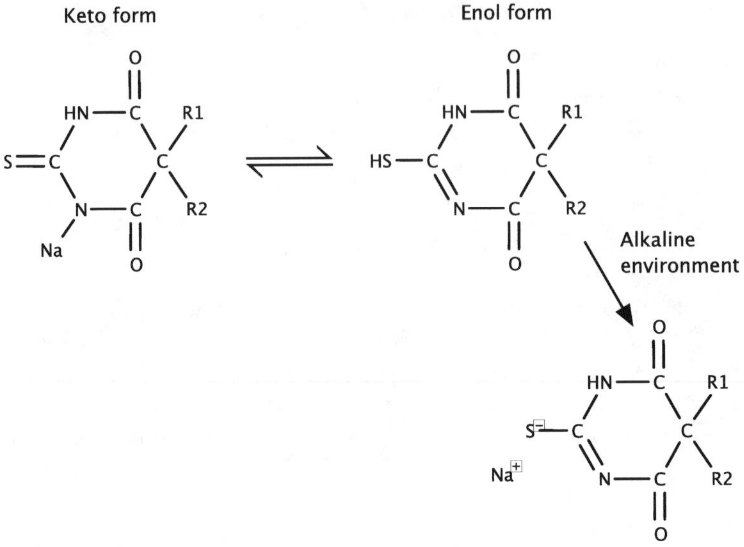

Figure 9.4 Keto-enol transformation of barbiturates – tautomerism. Alkaline solutions favour the water-soluble enol form.

Uses

Apart from induction of anaesthesia (3–7 mg.kg^{-1} intravenously) thiopental is occasionally used in status epilepticus. At sufficient plasma concentrations (most easily maintained by continuous infusion) thiopental produces an isoelectric EEG, confirming maximal reduction of cerebral oxygen requirements. Inotropic support may be required to maintain adequate cerebral perfusion at these doses. It has previously been used rectally, although it has a slow onset via this route.

Effects

- *Cardiovascular* – there is a dose-dependent reduction in cardiac output, stroke volume and systemic vascular resistance that may provoke a compensatory tachycardia. These effects are more common in patients that are hypovolaemic, acidotic and have reduced plasma protein binding.
- *Respiratory* – respiratory depression is dose-dependent. It may produce a degree of laryngospasm and bronchospasm.
- *Central nervous system* – a single dose will rapidly induce general anaesthesia with a duration of about 5–10 minutes. There is a reduction in cerebral oxygen consumption, blood flow, blood volume and cerebrospinal fluid pressure. When used in very low doses it is antanalgesic.
- *Renal* – urine output may fall, not only as a result of increased antidiuretic hormone release secondary to CNS depression, but also as a result of a reduced cardiac output.
- *Severe anaphylactic reactions* – these are seen in approximately 1 in 20,000 administrations of thiopental.
- *Porphyria* – thiopental may precipitate an acute porphyric crisis and is therefore absolutely contraindicated in patients with porphyria. The following drugs may also precipitate an acute porphyric crisis:
  - other barbiturates
  - etomidate

- halothane
- cocaine
- lidocaine and prilocaine (bupivacaine is safe)
- clonidine
- metoclopramide
- hyoscine
- diclofenac
- ranitidine.

Kinetics

Thiopental is predominantly bound by plasma proteins with only 20% free and unbound within the plasma. Its pK_a of 7.6 means that 60% of the free form is unionised (i.e. 12% of the total drug in the plasma). This relatively small fraction is *immediately* available to achieve its effects. Despite this it has a rapid onset due to its high lipid solubility and the large cardiac output that the brain receives. In addition, a dynamic equilibrium exists between protein-bound and free drug. Critically ill patients tend to be acidotic and have reduced plasma protein binding, resulting in a greater fraction of drug in the unionised form and fewer plasma protein binding sites, so that a smaller administered dose of thiopental is required to induce anaesthesia. Non-steroidal anti-inflammatory drugs may also reduce available protein binding sites and increase the fraction of free drug.

Rapid emergence from a single bolus dose is due to rapid initial distribution into tissues, not metabolism. A tri-exponential decline is seen representing distribution to well-perfused regions (brain, liver) followed by muscle and skin. The final decline is due to hepatic oxidation mainly to inactive metabolites (although pentobarbital is also a metabolite). When given as an infusion its metabolism may become linear (zero-order, see p. 62) due to saturation of hepatic enzymes. The hepatic mixed-function oxidase system (cytochrome P450) is induced after a single dose.

Intra-arterial Injection

If 2.5% thiopental at pH 10.5 is injected into arterial blood with a pH of 7.4 the tautomeric equilibrium swings away from the enol towards the keto form, resulting in a less water-soluble solution. This in turn leads to the precipitation of thiopental crystals which become wedged into small blood vessels leading to ischaemia and pain. Treatment should begin immediately and may include intra-arterial injection of papaverine or procaine, analgesia, sympathetic block of the limb and anticoagulation.

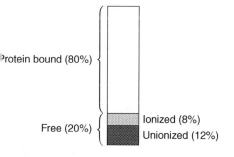

Figure 9.5 Thiopental in plasma. Only 12% is immediately available as non-protein-bound and unionised drug.

Protein bound (80%)

Free (20%)

Ionized (8%)

Unionized (12%)

Thiopental does not precipitate when injected intravenously as it is continually diluted by more venous blood. Peri-vascular injection is painful and may cause serious tissue necrosis if large doses extravasate.

Non-barbiturates

Propofol

Presentation

This phenolic derivative (2,6 diisopropylphenol, see Figure 9.6) is highly lipid-soluble and is presented as a 1% or 2% lipid–water emulsion due to poor solubility in water. There are a number of generic formulations which differ in their excipients although all contain soya bean oil, egg lecithin and glycerol. The addition of medium chain triglycerides has been used to reduce the proportion of free propofol and the incidence of pain during administration. It is a weak organic acid with a pK_a of 11 so that it is almost entirely unionised at pH 7.4.

Uses

Propofol is used for the induction and maintenance of general anaesthesia and for sedation of ventilated patients in intensive care. The induction dose is 1–2 $mg.kg^{-1}$ while a plasma concentration of 4–8 $\mu g.ml^{-1}$ will maintain anaesthesia.

Effects

- *Cardiovascular* – the systemic vascular resistance falls, resulting in a drop in blood pressure. A reflex tachycardia is rare and propofol is usually associated with a bradycardia, especially if administered with an opioid. Sympathetic activity and myocardial contractility are also reduced.

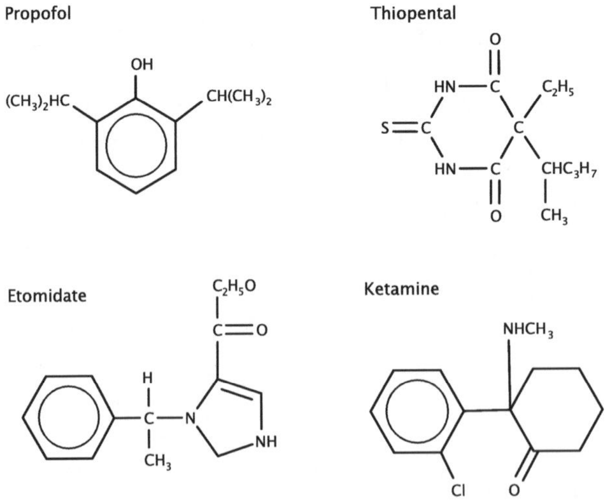

Propofol

Thiopental

Etomidate

Ketamine

Figure 9.6 Chemical structure of some intravenous anaesthetics.

- *Respiratory* – respiratory depression leading to apnoea is common. It is rare to observe cough or laryngospasm following its use and so it is often used to facilitate placement of a supraglottic airway.
- *Central nervous system* – excitatory effects have been associated with propofol in up to 10% of patients. They probably do not represent true cortical seizure activity; rather they are the manifestation of subcortical excitatory–inhibitory centre imbalance. The movements observed are dystonic with choreiform elements and opisthotonos. Propofol has been used to control status epilepticus.
- *Gut* – limited evidence exists to suggest that propofol possesses antiemetic properties following its use for induction, maintenance or in subhypnotic doses post-operatively. Antagonism of the dopamine D_2 receptor is a possible mechanism.
- *Pain* – injection into small veins is painful but may be reduced if lidocaine is mixed with propofol or if the affected limb is raised to facilitate venous drainage.
- *Metabolic* – a fat overload syndrome, with hyperlipidaemia, and fatty infiltration of heart, liver, kidneys and lungs can follow prolonged infusion, see below, 'Toxicity'.
- *Miscellaneous* – propofol may turn urine and hair green.

Kinetics

Propofol is extensively bound to both plasma proteins (mainly albumin) and erythrocytes, with only 1–2% remaining free in the plasma. It readily crosses the blood–brain barrier leaving the cardiac output and speed of administration as keys to the speed of induction. Following bolus administration, its duration of action is short due to the rapid decrease in plasma levels as it is distributed to well-perfused tissues. It has the largest volume of distribution of all the induction agents at 4 l.kg^{-1} (see Table 9.2) due to it's high lipid solubility. Even after long durations of administration its offset is still relatively fast as redistribution from these fat stores is slow compared with the rates of metabolism and excretion (*cf.* context-sensitive half-time, p. 78).

Metabolism is mainly hepatic, with approximately 70% being conjugated to propofol glucuronide while 30% undergoes a Phase 1 reaction to 4-hydroxypropofol within CYP2B6 (and CYP2C9). From here it is conjugated to form 4-hydroxypropofol-sulphate, 4-hydroxypropofol-glucuronide and 1-hydroxypropofol-glucuronide. All the conjugated forms are then excreted in the urine, alongside a tiny fraction (less than 1%) of unchanged propofol. None of the major metabolites (Figure 9.7) have hypnotic activity. The liver is very efficient at propofol metabolism with a blood extraction ratio of 90% so that reductions in hepatic blood flow lead to reductions in its metabolism. Its clearance (of about 2.2 l.min^{-1}) exceeds hepatic blood flow, indicating some extra-hepatic metabolism, which may reach up to 40%. In addition, the kidneys are responsible for up to 30% of its metabolism. Owing to this high clearance, plasma levels fall more rapidly than those of thiopental following the initial distribution phase. Its terminal elimination half-life is 5–12 hours although it has been suggested that when sampling is performed for longer than 24 hours the figure approaches 60 hours and may reflect the slow release of propofol from fat. During prolonged infusion its context-sensitive half-time increases, although where the infusion has been titrated carefully, waking may still be relatively rapid.

Table 9.2 Pharmacokinetics of some intravenous anaesthetics

	Dose (mg.kg^{-1})	Volume of distribution (l.kg^{-1})	Clearance (ml.kg^{-1}.min^{-1})	Elimination half-life (h)	Protein binding (%)	Metabolites
Thiopental	3–7	2.5	3.5	6–15	80	active
Propofol	1–2	4.0	30–60	5–12	98	inactive
Ketamine	1–2	3.0	17	2	25	active
Etomidate	0.3	3.0	10–20	1–4	75	inactive

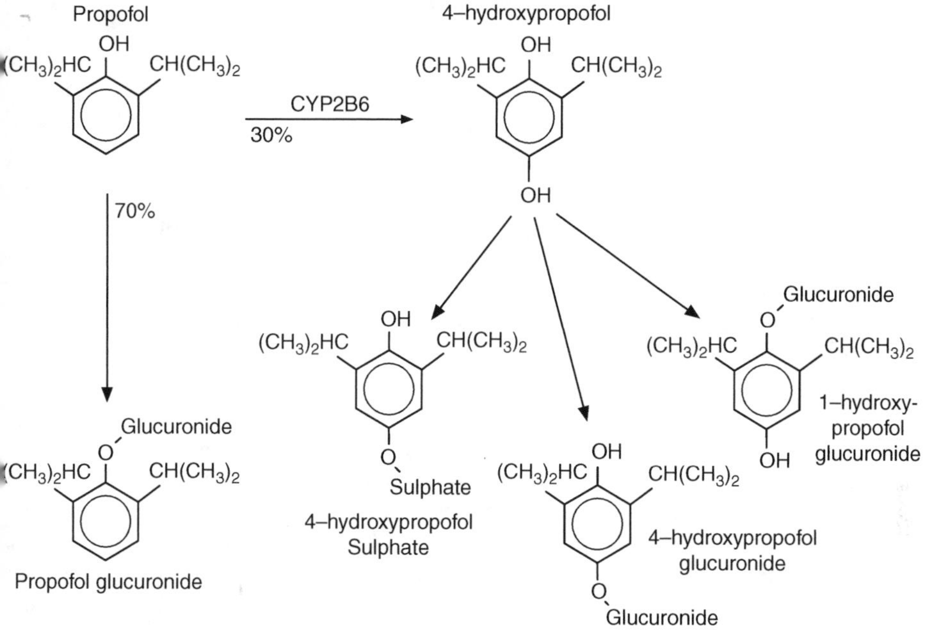

Figure 9.7 The metabolic pathway of propofol

Toxicity

The term Propofol Infusion Syndrome (PRIS) has been used to describe an acute refractory bradycardia, leading to asystole, in the presence of at least one of the following features: metabolic acidosis (BE > –10 mmol.l^{-1}), rhabdomyolysis or myoglobinuria, lipaemic plasma or an enlarged/fatty liver. It was originally described in children but has also been reported in adults during periods of sedation in Intensive Care Units (ICUs).

It typically occurs after 3 days of propofol-based sedation, and is associated with an increased mortality compared with patients being sedated with other drugs. It presents most commonly with new onset metabolic acidosis and cardiac dysfunction which is pre-empted by ECG changes which are similar (but not limited) to those seen in Brugada syndrome. Direct muscle necrosis with creatine kinase (CK) levels of > 10,000 units.l^{-1} may occur. Animal and human models have demonstrated that propofol interferes with oxidative phosphorylation, mitochondrial energy production and electron transfer in myocytes. This leads to a mismatch between energy demand and utilisation and ultimately to muscle necrosis.

Where propofol sedation is used it should not exceed 4 mg.kg^{-1}.hr^{-1} for more than 48 hours and should be done with regular CK, lactate and triglyceride monitoring. Patients with sepsis, burns, trauma, pancreatitis and neurological injuries are at high risk. It is contraindicated in patients of 16 years and younger for sedation in ICU.

Following a single case of pruritis in a patient with egg allergy, and a subsequent report of two patients who developed bronchospasm after propofol administration, it was suggested that soybean oil and egg yolk lecithin might have been responsible, despite an absence of allergy testing. A further case of hypotension and bronchospasm in a child, known to be allergic to egg and peanut (but not soy), gave further credence to this narrative, also in the absence of allergy testing. A more thorough analysis of much larger patient cohorts allergic to egg, soy and peanut has concluded that propofol is safe in this group. However, the picture is more complicated in children where there is no persuasive evidence that propofol is unsafe in those allergic to soy or peanut, but for children allergic to egg it is advised that more evidence is required for propofol to be used with confidence.

Propofol does not appear to cause any adverse effects when given intra-arterially, although onset of anaesthesia is delayed. Caution is required when using a peripheral intravenous cannula whose tip does not lie in a superficial vein. If its lumen is not intravascular, deep subcutaneous injection of propofol is not especially painful and may only be recognised when induction fails. Erythema, pain and swelling over the subsequent 24 hours appears to be dose-dependent.

Environmental Impact

Unlike the inhaled agents, propofol has no direct global warming potential. Its environmental footprint relates to production, transport and the electricity used when delivered via a syringe pump. Consequently, its global warming potential is four orders of magnitude less when compared to the inhaled agents. It is said to have 'moderate persistence' in the environment where it is toxic to aquatic organisms, but the overall risk is low. In order to prevent environmental contamination, unused propofol should not be discarded down the sink, but disposed of in containers destined for incineration.

Ketamine

Ketamine is a phencyclidine derivative.

Presentation and Uses

Ketamine is presented as a racemic mixture or as the single S(+) enantiomer, which is two to three times as potent as the R(−) enantiomer. It is soluble in water forming an acidic solution (pH 3.5–5.5). Three concentrations are available: 10, 50 and 100 mg.ml^{-1}, and it may be given intravenously (1–2 mg.kg^{-1}) or intramuscularly (5–10 mg.kg^{-1}) for induction of anaesthesia. Intravenous doses of 0.2–0.5 mg.kg^{-1} may be used to facilitate the positioning of patients with fractures before regional anaesthetic techniques are performed. It has been used via the oral and rectal route for sedation and also by intrathecal and epidural routes for analgesia. Historically, its use has been limited by unpleasant side effects. It has gained popularity at low doses in combination with other analgesics and may be particularly useful in those with an element of chronic pain.

Effects

- *Cardiovascular* – ketamine is unlike other induction agents in that it produces sympathetic nervous system stimulation, increasing circulating levels of adrenaline and noradrenaline. Consequently heart rate, cardiac output, blood pressure and myocardial oxygen requirements are all increased (see Table 9.3). However, it does not appear to precipitate arrhythmias. This indirect stimulation masks the mild direct myocardial depressant effects that racemic ketamine would otherwise exert on the heart. S(+) ketamine produces less direct cardiac depression in vitro compared with R(−) ketamine. In addition, while racemic ketamine has been shown to block ATP-sensitive potassium channels (the key

Table 9.3 Pharmacological properties of some intravenous anaesthetics

	Thiopental	Propofol	Ketamine	Etomidate
BP	↓	↓↓	↑	→
CO	↓	↓↓	↑	→
HR	↑	↓→	↑	→
SVR	↑↓	↓↓	→	→
RR	↓	↓	↑	↓
ICP	↓	↓	↑	→
IOP	↓	↓	↑	→
Pain on injection	no	yes	no	yes
Nausea and vomiting	no	? reduced	yes	yes

mechanism of ischaemic myocardial preconditioning), S(+) ketamine does not, which therefore must be considered advantageous for patients with ischaemic heart disease.

Respiratory – the respiratory rate may be increased and the laryngeal reflexes relatively preserved. A patent airway is often, but not always, maintained, and increased muscle tone associated with the jaw may precipitate airway obstruction. It causes bronchodilation and may be useful for patients with asthma.

Central nervous system – ketamine produces a state of dissociative anaesthesia that is demonstrated on EEG by dissociation between the thalamocortical and limbic systems. In addition, intense analgesia and amnesia are produced. The α rhythm is replaced by θ and δ wave activity. Ketamine is different from other intravenous anaesthetics as it does not induce anaesthesia in one arm–brain circulation time – central effects becoming evident 90 seconds after an intravenous dose. Vivid and unpleasant dreams, hallucinations and delirium may follow its use. These emergence phenomena may be reduced by the concurrent use of benzodiazepines or opioids. S(+) ketamine produces less intense although no less frequent emergence phenomena. They are less common in the young and elderly and also in those left to recover undisturbed. Cerebral blood flow, oxygen consumption and intracranial pressure are all increased. Muscle tone is increased and there may be jerking movements of the limbs. A nasal spray of S(+) ketamine has been approved by the FDA for the treatment of resistant depression.

Analgesia – when given by infusion at doses low enough to avoid side effects ketamine may still retain useful analgesic effects and reduce morphine consumption.

Gut – nausea and vomiting occur more frequently than after propofol or thiopental. Salivation is increased requiring anticholinergic premedication.

Bladder – non-prescription, high-dose use has been associated with severe interstitial cystitis that may require cystectomy.

Kinetics

Following an intravenous dose the plasma concentration falls in a bi-exponential fashion. The initial fall is due to distribution across lipid membranes while the slower phase is due to hepatic metabolism. Ketamine is the least protein-bound (about 25%) of the intravenous anaesthetics and is demethylated to the active metabolite norketamine by hepatic P450 enzymes. Norketamine (which is 30% as potent as ketamine) is further metabolised to inactive glucuronide metabolites. The conjugated metabolites are excreted in the urine.

Etomidate

Etomidate is an imidazole derivative and an ester. While it continues to be used infrequently in the UK it has been withdrawn in North America and Australia.

Presentation

Etomidate is prepared as a 0.2% solution at a pH of 4.1 and contains 35% v/v propylene glycol to improve stability and reduce its irritant properties on injection. A lipid formulation is now also available.

Uses

Etomidate is used for the induction of general anaesthesia at a dose of 0.3 mg.kg^{-1}.

Effects

At first glance etomidate would appear to have some desirable properties, but due to its side effects its place in anaesthesia has remained limited.

- *Cardiovascular* – of the commonly used intravenous anaesthetics, etomidate produces the least cardiovascular disturbance. The peripheral vascular resistance may fall slightly (but less so than with other induction agents), while myocardial oxygen supply, contractility and blood pressure remain largely unchanged. Hypersensitivity reactions are less common following etomidate and histamine release is rare.
- *Metabolic* – it suppresses adrenocortical function by inhibition of the enzymes 11β-hydroxylase and 17α-hydroxylase, resulting in inhibition of cortisol and aldosterone synthesis. It was associated with an increase in mortality when used as an infusion to sedate septic patients in the ICU. Single doses can influence adrenocortical function but are probably of little clinical significance in otherwise fit patients. However it is unlikely to be used to induce elective patients. In other words the situation in which it has the best cardiovascular profile is the unwell patient in whom the consequences of steroid inhibition are likely to be the most detrimental.
- *Miscellaneous* – unpleasant side effects relate to pain on injection in up to 25% of patients, excitatory movements and nausea and vomiting. It may also precipitate a porphyric crisis.

Kinetics

Etomidate is 75% bound to albumin. Its actions are terminated by rapid distribution into tissues, while its elimination from the body depends on hepatic metabolism and renal excretion. Non-specific hepatic esterases, and possibly plasma cholinesterase, hydrolyse etomidate to ethyl alcohol and its carboxylic acid metabolite. It may also inhibit plasma cholinesterase.

Inhaled Anaesthetic Agents

Inhaled anaesthetic agents in current use include nitrous oxide (N_2O) and the volatile liquids isoflurane, sevoflurane, desflurane, halothane and enflurane. Xenon has useful properties but is expensive to extract from the atmosphere, which limits its clinical use.

Minimum Alveolar Concentration

Minimum alveolar concentration (MAC) is a measure of potency and is defined as the MAC at steady state that prevents reaction to a standard surgical stimulus (skin incision) in 50% of subjects at one atmosphere. Because the majority of anaesthetics involving inhaled agents are given at approximately one atmosphere the indexing of MAC to atmospheric pressure may be forgotten and lead the unwary to conclude that concentration is the key measure. However, the key measure is the *partial pressure* of the agent. When measured using kPa, the concentration and partial pressure are virtually the same as atmospheric pressure which approximates to 100 kPa.

MAC is altered by many physiological and pharmacological factors (see Table 9.4) and is additive when agents are administered simultaneously.

The Ideal Inhaled Anaesthetic Agent

While the agents in use today demonstrate many favourable characteristics, no single agent has all the desirable properties listed below. 'Negative' characteristics (e.g. not epileptogenic) are simply a reflection of a currently used agent's side effect.

Table 9.4 Factors altering minimum alveolar concentration

Factors increasing MAC	Factors decreasing MAC
Infancy	During the neonatal period
	Increasing age
	Pregnancy
	Hypotension
Hyperthermia	Hypothermia
Hyperthyroidism	Hypothyroidism
Catecholamines and sympathomimetics	α_2-agonists
	Sedatives
Chronic opioid use	Acute opioid use
Chronic alcohol intake	Acute alcohol intake
Acute amphetamine intake	Chronic amphetamine intake
Hypernatraemia	Lithium

Physical Properties

- Stable to light and heat
- Inert when in contact with metal, rubber and soda lime
- Preservative-free
- Not flammable or explosive
- Pleasant odour
- Not a greenhouse gas
- Cheap.

Biochemical Properties

- High oil:gas partition coefficient; low MAC
- Low blood:gas partition coefficient
- Not metabolised
- Non-toxic
- Only affects the CNS
- Not epileptogenic
- Some analgesic properties.

Environmental Impact

Despite the increasing use of intravenous agents, it is the inhaled agents that are used most commonly for the maintenance of general anaesthesia. Determining their total environmental impact requires a life cycle assessment (LCA) of resource extraction, production, transport, delivery and disposal, which is complex.

However, of particular note is their ability to absorb infrared radiation that would otherwise leave the earth's lower atmosphere. It is this property that defines them as greenhouse gases (GHGs) and can be quantified in the following ways.

- *Global warming potential* (GWP). This is a measure of how much heat is trapped in the atmosphere and may be quoted for 20 years (GWP_{20}) in an anaesthetic context due to the relatively short lifespans of the inhaled agents (with the exception of N_2O), but is more widely quoted over 100 years (GWP_{100}). The values are indexed to CO_2, which by convention has a GWP_{100} of 1 (see Table 9.5).

Table 9.5 Environmental impact of some inhaled anaesthetic agents

	Nitrous oxide	Isoflurane	Sevoflurane	Desflurane
Atmospheric lifetime (yrs)	114	3.2	1.1	14
Radiative efficiency (W.m^{-2}.ppb^{-1})	0.00303	0.453	0.351	0.469
GWP_{100}	298	510	130	2,540

• *Carbon dioxide equivalency* (CO_2e). For a given amount of gas, this is the amount of CO_2 that would have the same GWP when measured over a specified time span, usually 100 years. The CO_2e for a gas is its mass multiplied by its GWP.

The commonly used volatile agents all absorb infrared light with a wavelength between 7–10 μm. Their specific absorption profile determines their Radiative Efficiency (RE) which is a measure of the influence a substance has on incoming and outgoing atmospheric energy. When weighted by their atmospheric lifespan this determines the GWP_{100}. The RE for isoflurane and desflurane are similar but due to its five-fold atmospheric lifespan, desflurane has a much larger GWP_{100}. In addition, desflurane is the least potent volatile agent so that more is needed for anaesthesia, further worsening its profile. Globally, desflurane makes up approximately 80% of the CO_2e of all the volatile agents despite being vented in roughly equal quantities, by mass. However, N_2O has the largest CO_2e, due to its even higher MAC, longer atmospheric lifespan and high volume use during labour. But in the wider context, less than 4% of N_2O emissions are due to medical use, the majority being agricultural in origin, although natural sources may be twice anthropogenic ones.

While GHGs retain infrared radiation, the ozone layer forms an important part of the earth's ability to deflect harmful ultraviolet radiation. Many man-made compounds have the ability to break down the ozone layer. This ability is determined primarily by the presence of chlorine within the molecular structure. As a result only isoflurane has ozone depleting potential, but this is minimal due to its short atmospheric lifetime. By a contrasting mechanism, N_2O releases its oxygen atom by a photolytical process high in the stratosphere, breaking down ozone (O_3) and forming O_2. New work suggests that N_2O is currently the dominant ozone depleting substance and is expected to remain so throughout the twenty-first century.

Kinetics of Inhaled Anaesthetic Agents

At steady state, the partial pressure of inhaled anaesthetic within the alveoli (P_A) is in equilibrium with that in the arterial blood (P_a) and subsequently the brain (P_B). Therefore, P_A gives an indirect measure of P_B. However, for most inhaled anaesthetics, steady state is rarely achieved in the clinical setting as the process may take many hours (see Figure 9.8).

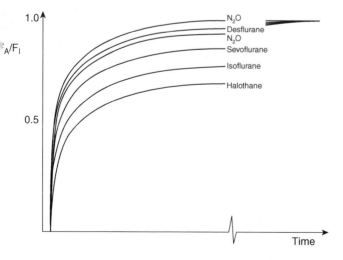

Figure 9.8 Different agents approach a F_A/F_I ratio of 1 at different rates. Agents with a low blood:gas partition coefficient reach equilibrium more rapidly. (F_A/F_I represents the ratio of alveolar concentration to inspired concentration.) For an explanation of the two N_2O curves see Figure 9.9.

Physiological and agent-specific factors influence the speed at which inhaled anaesthetics approach equilibrium.

Alveolar Ventilation

Increased alveolar ventilation results in a faster rise in P_A. Consequently, P_B increases more rapidly and so the onset of anaesthesia is faster. A large functional residual capacity (FRC) will effectively dilute the inspired concentration and so the onset of anaesthesia will be slow. Conversely, those patients with a small FRC have only a small volume with which to dilute the inspired gas and so P_A rises rapidly, resulting in a fast onset of anaesthesia.

Inspired Concentration

A high inspired concentration leads to a rapid rise in P_A and so onset of anaesthesia is also rapid.

Cardiac Output

A high cardiac output will tend to maintain a concentration gradient between the alveolus and the pulmonary blood so that P_A rises slowly. Conversely, a low cardiac output favours a more rapid equilibration and so onset of anaesthesia will also be more rapid. However, modern anaesthetic agents, which are relatively insoluble in blood, are affected to a much lesser extent by cardiac output when compared with agents of greater blood solubility.

Blood:Gas Partition Coefficient

The blood:gas partition coefficient is defined as the ratio of the amount of anaesthetic in blood and gas when the two phases are of equal volume and pressure and in equilibrium at 37°C.

Although it might be expected that agents with a high blood:gas partition coefficient (i.e. high solubility) would have a rapid onset, this is not the case because these agents only exert a low partial pressure in blood, even when present in large amounts. It is the partial pressure of the agent in the blood and subsequently the brain that gives rise to anaesthesia and not the total amount present. Agents with a low blood:gas partition coefficient exert a high partial pressure and will, therefore, produce a more rapid onset and offset of action. Although a low blood:gas partition coefficient is important, MAC and respiratory irritability can also alter the speed of induction.

Concentration and Second Gas Effect

These are described in the section on nitrous oxide.

Metabolism

Hepatic cytochrome P450 (CYP2E1) metabolises the C-(halogen) bond to release halogen ions (F^-, Cl^- Br^-), which may cause hepatic or renal damage. The C–F bond is a stable one and is only minimally metabolised, unlike C–Cl, C–Br and C–I which become progressively easy to metabolise (see Table 9.6).

Table 9.6 Metabolism of inhaled anaesthetic agents

Agent	Percentage metabolised	Metabolites
N_2O	< 0.01	(N_2)
Halothane	20	Trifluoroacetic acid, Cl^-, Br^-
Sevoflurane	3.5	Inorganic and organic fluorides
		Compound A in the presence of soda lime and heat (Compound B, C, D and E)
Enflurane	2	Inorganic and organic fluorides
Isoflurane	0.2	Trifluoroacetic acid and F^-
Desflurane	0.02	Trifluoroacetic acid

Pharmacology of Inhaled Anaesthetic Agents

Nitrous Oxide

Nitrous oxide (N_2O) may be used alongside the volatile agents and in combination with oxygen (O_2) as entonox. Apart from a high MAC, it has favourable physical properties. However, its use in theatre is decreasing due to its potential to cause nausea and vomiting and concerns over its environmental impact (see above, p. 108).

Manufacture

Nitrous oxide is manufactured by heating ammonium nitrate to 250°C.

$$NH_4NO_3 \rightarrow N_2O + 2H_2O$$

Unless the temperature is carefully controlled N_2O may contain the following contaminants: NH_3, N_2, NO, NO_2 and HNO_3. These impurities are actively removed by passage through scrubbers, water and caustic soda.

Storage

Nitrous oxide is stored as a liquid in French blue cylinders (C = 450 litres up to G = 9,000 litres) with a gauge pressure of 51 bar at 20°C, which therefore bears no correlation to cylinder content until all remaining N_2O is in the gaseous phase. The filling ratio (mass of N_2O in cylinder/mass of water that the cylinder could hold) is 0.75 in temperate regions, but it needs to be reduced to 0.67 in tropical regions to avoid cylinder explosions. Its critical temperature is 36.5°C; its critical pressure is 72 bar.

Effects

- *Respiratory* – it causes a small fall in tidal volume that is offset by an increased respiratory rate so that minute volume and $PaCO_2$ remain unchanged.

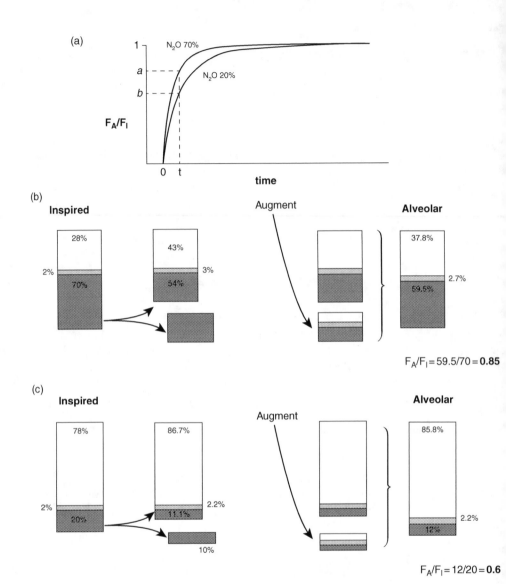

Figure 9.9 The concentration effect. See text for details.

- *Cardiovascular* – although N_2O has mild direct myocardial depressant effects, it also increases sympathetic activity by its central effects. Therefore, in health the circulatory system is changed very little. However, for patients with cardiac failure who are unable to increase their sympathetic drive, the direct myocardial depressant effects may significantly reduce cardiac output. It does not sensitise the heart to catecholamines.

- *Central nervous system* – N_2O increases cerebral blood flow and is sometimes avoided in patients with a raised intracranial pressure. Despite a MAC of 105%, its potential to cause anaesthesia in certain patients (the old), should not be ignored.

- *Gut* – N_2O probably increases the risk of post-operative nausea and vomiting (PONV), especially in those with risk factors.

Concentration Effect, Second Gas Effect and Diffusion Hypoxia

The Concentration Effect

The concentration effect is an observed phenomenon that describes the disproportionate rate of rise of the alveolar fraction compared with the inspired fraction when high concentrations of N_2O are inspired (see Figure 9.9a). The rate of rise is disproportionate when compared with the situation where low concentrations of N_2O are inspired. The concentration effect only applies to N_2O because N_2O is the only agent used at sufficiently high concentration. Various models have been used to explain the phenomenon; all have limitations.

However, the fundamental driving force for the process is the large gradient which the high concentrations of N_2O generate. As a result large amounts of N_2O (50% is assumed in the model shown in Figure 9.9b) are absorbed into the pulmonary capillaries despite the fact that it is usually considered an insoluble agent (blood:gas solubility coefficient 0.47). In order for the alveolar volume to remain constant, gas that was in the conducting airways is drawn down into the alveoli so that the various alveolar concentrations change.

In the final analysis, when comparing two separate scenarios, the first using high concentrations of N_2O (Figure 9.9b) and the second using low concentrations of N_2O (Figure 9.9c), the F_A/F_I ratio is disproportionately high (point a at time t, see Figure 9.9a) where large concentrations of N_2O are used, compared to the F_A/F_I ratio when lower concentrations of N_2O are used (point b at time t, see Figure 9.9a).

The model described in Figure 9.9 is limited in numerous ways (N_2O is not the only gas absorbed and the effects of N_2 leaving the body are not included), but it does serve to illustrate the mechanism by which the concentration effect is thought to occur. In addition, it illustrates the second gas effect. It assumes that half the N_2O in the alveoli is absorbed into the pulmonary capillaries, the volume deficit being made good by augmented ventilation which has the same fractional composition as the initial alveolar gas.

The Second Gas Effect

The second gas effect is a direct result of the concentration effect. Oxygen plus or minus volatile agents used alongside high concentrations of N_2O will be concentrated by the rapid uptake of N_2O and augmented alveolar ventilation. This leads to increased concentrations of oxygen and volatile agents, resulting in a reduced induction time.

Diffusion Hypoxia

At the end of anaesthesia when N_2O/O_2 is replaced by air (N_2/O_2) the reverse of the second gas effect is seen. The volume of N_2O entering the alveolus will be greater than the volume of N_2 entering the pulmonary capillaries, resulting in a dilution of all alveolar gases. Most volatile anaesthetics end by changing N_2O/O_2 to 100% O_2 which prevents diffusion hypoxia.

In addition to the effects seen across the alveolar membrane, N_2O will cause a rapid expansion of any air-filled space (pneumothorax, vascular air embolus and intestinal lumen).

Toxicity

The cobalt ion present in vitamin B_{12} is oxidised by N_2O so that it is unable to act as the co-factor for methionine synthetase (Figure 9.10). The result is reduced synthesis of

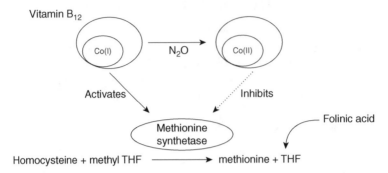

Figure 9.10 N_2O inhibits methionine synthetase by oxidising cobalt (Co(I)). THF, tetrahydrofolate.

methionine, thymidine, tetrahydrofolate and DNA. Methionine synthetase also appears to be directly inhibited by N_2O. Exposure of only a few hours may result in megaloblastic changes in bone marrow but more prolonged exposure (i.e. days) may result in agranulocytosis. Recovery is governed by synthesis (taking a few days) of new methionine synthetase, but may be helped by the administration of folinic acid, which provides a different source of tetrahydrofolate.

In a properly scavenged environment where N_2O concentrations are less than 50 ppm there is no effect on DNA synthesis. However, in unscavenged dental surgeries where large amounts were used, chronic exposure resulted in neurological syndromes that resembled subacute combined degeneration of the cord, as a result of chronic vitamin B_{12} inactivation.

In experimental conditions N_2O has been shown to be teratogenic to rats but this effect is prevented by folinic acid. While this has never been unequivocally demonstrated in humans, N_2O is often not used in the first trimester when anaesthesia is required.

Entonox

Entonox is a 50:50 mixture of N_2O and O_2. The two gases effectively dissolve into each other and do not behave in a way that would be predicted from their individual properties. This phenomenon is called the Poynting effect.

Uses

Entonox is used commonly for analgesia during labour and other painful procedures.

Storage

Entonox is stored as a gas in French blue cylinders (G = 3,200 litres; J = 6,400 litres) with white and blue checked shoulders, at 137 bar. It separates into its constituent parts below its pseudo-critical temperature, which is about −7°C, and is most likely to occur at 117 bar. Higher or lower pressures reduce the likelihood of separation. When delivered via pipeline at 4.1 bar the pseudo-critical temperature is less than −30°C. If a cylinder is used following separation, the inspired gas will initially produce little analgesia as it contains mainly O_2, but as the cylinder empties the mixture will become progressively potent and hypoxic as it approaches 100% N_2O.

Isoflurane

This halogenated ethyl methyl ether is a structural isomer of enflurane (see Figure 9.11). It is used widely to maintain anaesthesia. Its physical properties are summarised in Table 9.7.

Effects

- *Respiratory* (see Table 9.8) – isoflurane depresses ventilation more than halothane but less than enflurane. Minute volume is decreased while respiratory rate and $PaCO_2$ are increased. It is rarely used to induce anaesthesia due to its pungent smell, which may cause upper airway irritability, coughing and breath-holding. However, despite its pungent smell it causes some bronchodilation.
- *Cardiovascular* (see Table 9.9) – its main effect is to reduce systemic vascular resistance. The resulting reflex tachycardia suggests that the carotid sinus reflex is preserved. It causes only a small decrease in myocardial contractility and cardiac output. It has been suggested that isoflurane may cause coronary steal whereby normally responsive coronary arterioles are dilated and divert blood away from areas supplied by

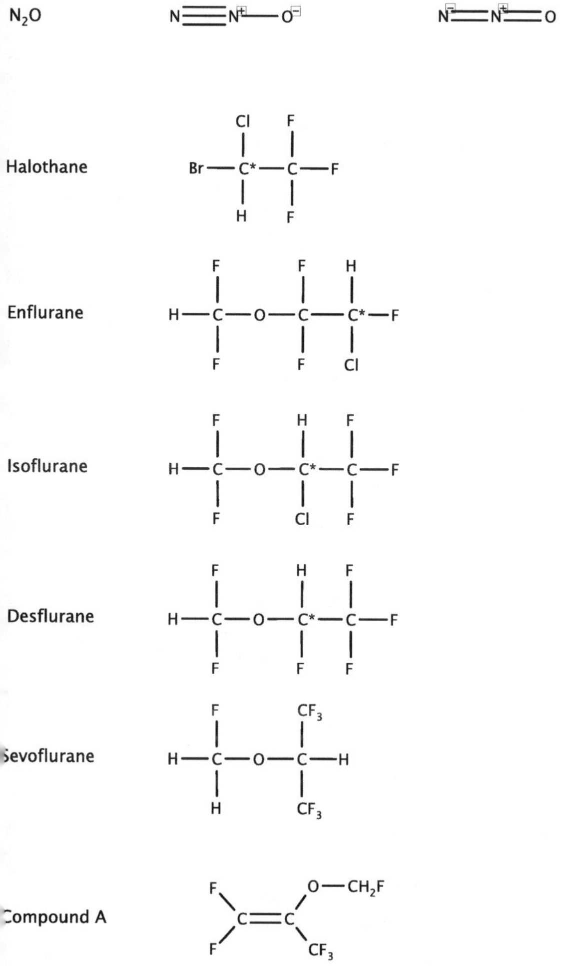

Figure 9.11 Structure of some inhaled anaesthetics and Compound A. An asterisk represents a chiral centre.

Table 9.7 Physiochemical properties of inhaled anaesthetics

	Halothane	Isoflurane	Enflurane	Desflurane	Sevoflurane	N$_2$O	Xenon
MW	197.0	184.5	184.5	168.0	200.1	44.0	131.0
BP (°C)	50.2	48.5	56.5	23.5	58.5	−88.0	−108
SVP at 20°C (kPa)	32.3	33.2	23.3	89.2	22.7	5200	
MAC (%)	0.75	1.17	1.68	6.60	1.80	105	71.0
Blood:gas partition coefficient	2.40	1.40	1.80	0.42	0.70	0.47	0.14
Oil:gas partition coefficient	224	98	98	29	80	1.4	1.9
Odour	non-irritant, sweet	irritant	non-irritant	pungent	non-irritant	odourless	odourless

Table 9.8 Respiratory effects of inhaled anaesthetics

	Halothane	Isoflurane	Enflurane	Desflurane	Sevoflurane
Respiratory rate	↑	↑↑	↑↑	↑↑	↑↑
Tidal volume	↓	↓↓	↓↓↓	↓↓	↓
$PaCO_2$	unchanged	↑↑	↑↑↑	↑↑	↑

unresponsive diseased vessels, resulting in ischaemia. However more recent work has suggested that as long as coronary perfusion is maintained, coronary steal does not occur. In addition isoflurane may have myocardial protective properties via its effects on ATP-dependent potassium channels.

- *Central nervous system* (see Table 9.10) – of all the volatile agents isoflurane produces the best balance of reduced cerebral oxygen requirement and minimal increase in cerebral blood flow. At concentrations up to 1 MAC cerebral autoregulation is preserved. Stimulation of the area postrema at the base of the fourth ventricle in the medulla is the likely mechanism leading to nausea and vomiting. This effect may be dose-related, the longer the anaesthetic duration the more likely it is to occur, although prolonged surgery is likely to be associated with greater opioid use. However, any effect is limited to the early post-operative period.

Metabolism

Only 0.2% is metabolised and none of the products has been linked to toxicity.

Toxicity

Owing to the presence of a $-CHF_2$ group in its structure it may react with dry soda lime (or baralyme), producing carbon monoxide. Reports of this relate to circle systems that have been left with dry gas circulating over a weekend so that subsequent use of isoflurane causes release of carbon monoxide. Enflurane and desflurane also possess $-CHF_2$ groups and may react in a similar manner.

Sevoflurane

Sevoflurane is a polyfluorinated isopropyl methyl ether and has the favourable combination of a relatively low blood:gas partition coefficient (0.7), pleasant odour and relatively low MAC (1.8). However, during storage where the concentration of added water is below 100 ppm it is susceptible to attack by Lewis acids at its ether and halogen bonds, releasing the highly toxic hydrofluoric acid (HF). (A Lewis acid is defined as any substance that can accept an electron pair and includes many metal oxides but also H^+; glass is a source of Lewis acids.) Hydrofluoric acid corrodes glass, exposing sevoflurane to further Lewis acids. As a result sevoflurane is formulated with 300 ppm of water, which acts as a Lewis acid inhibitor. In addition it is stored in polyethylene napthalate bottles rather than glass. A dry formulation containing less than 130 ppm water is now available and is presented in an aluminium bottle lined with an epoxyphenolic resin lacquer. Unlike the other volatile agents sevoflurane is achiral.

Table 9.9 Cardiovascular effects of inhaled anaesthetics

	Halothane	Isoflurane	Enflurane	Desflurane	Sevoflurane
Contractility	↓↓↓	↓	↓↓	minimal	→
Heart rate	↓↓	↑↑	↑	↑(↑↑ > 1.5 MAC)	nil
Systemic vascular resistance	→	↓↓	→	↓↓	→
Blood pressure	↓↓	↓↓	↓↓	↓↓	→
Coronary steal syndrome	no	possibly	no	no	no
Splanchnic blood flow	→	unchanged	→	unchanged	unchanged
Sensitisation to catecholamines	↑↑↑	nil	↑	nil	nil

Table 9.10 Other effects of inhaled anaesthetics

	Halothane	Isoflurane	Enflurane	Desflurane	Sevoflurane
Cerebral blood flow	↑↑↑	↑ (nil if < 1 MAC)	↑	↑	↑
Cerebral O_2 requirement	→	→	→	→	→
EEG	burst suppression	burst suppression	epileptiform activity (3 Hz spike and wave)	burst suppression	burst suppression
Effect on uterus	some relaxation	some relaxation	some relaxation	some relaxation	some relaxation
Potentiation of muscle relaxation	some	significant	significant	significant	significant
Analgesia	none	some	some	some	some

Manufacture

- The one pot method – all the ingredients are added together to produce sevoflurane and then water is added to 300 ppm.
- The chloro-fluoro method – here the basic molecular architecture is manufactured but with chlorine attached. This is then substituted with fluorine to produce sevoflurane.

Effects

- *Respiratory* (see Table 9.8) – sevoflurane is a useful agent for induction of anaesthesia due to its pleasant odour and favourable physical properties. It does, however, depress ventilation in a predictable fashion with a reduction in minute volume and a rise in $PaCO_2$.
- *Cardiovascular* (see Table 9.9) – the systemic vascular resistance falls and, due to an unchanged heart rate, the blood pressure falls. Cardiac contractility is unaffected and the heart is not sensitised to catecholamines. Vascular resistance to both cerebral and coronary circulations is decreased.
- *Central nervous system* (see Table 9.10) – compared with halothane, there is evidence that children exhibit a higher incidence of post-operative agitation and delirium, which may extend beyond the initial recovery period. In common with other volatile agents sevoflurane causes nausea and vomiting by a similar mechanism.

Metabolism

Sevoflurane undergoes hepatic metabolism by cytochrome P450 (isoform 2E1) to a greater extent than all the other commonly used volatile agents except halothane (see Table 9.6) to produce hexafluoroisopropanol and inorganic F^- (known to cause renal toxicity).

Toxicity

Compounds A, B, C, D and E have all been identified when sevoflurane is used in the presence of carbon dioxide absorbents. Only compounds A and B (which is less toxic) are present in sufficient amount to make analysis feasible. Their formation is favoured in the presence of potassium hydroxide rather than sodium-hydroxide-based absorbents, particularly when dry. The reaction releases heat and consumes sevoflurane, both of which are readily detectible.

The lethal concentration of compound A in 50% of rats is 300–400 ppm after 3 hours exposure. Extrapolation of these and other animal studies suggest a human nephrotoxic threshold of 150–200 ppm. Recent work suggests that even with flow rates of 0.25 l.min^{-1} for 5 hours the level of compound A peaks at less than 20 ppm and is not associated with abnormal tests of renal function.

Halothane

This halogenated hydrocarbon is unstable when exposed to light, and corrodes certain metals. It is stored with 0.01% thymol to prevent the liberation of free bromine. It dissolves into rubber and may leach out into breathing circuits after the vaporiser is turned off. Its physical properties are summarised in Table 9.7. It retains niche use but has largely been superseded by sevoflurane.

Effects

- *Respiratory* (see Table 9.8) – owing to its sweet non-irritant odour it may be used to induce anaesthesia. Higher concentrations significantly reduce minute ventilation. It has significant bronchodilator properties that are useful in asthmatic patients.

- *Cardiovascular* (see Table 9.9) – halothane has a number of significant effects on the heart. Cardiac output is reduced indirectly by an increased vagal tone and directly by a myocardial depressant effect. Despite this the myocardium is sensitised to endogenous and exogenous catecholamines and local anaesthetic/adrenaline preparations should be used with caution.
- *Central nervous system* (see Table 9.10) – halothane increases cerebral blood flow more than any other volatile agent, leading to significant increases in intracranial pressure above 0.6 MAC. Cerebral oxygen requirements are reduced.

Metabolism

Up to 25% of inhaled halothane undergoes oxidative metabolism by hepatic cytochrome P450 to produce trifluoroacetic acid, Br^- and Cl^-. However, reductive metabolism producing F^- and other reduced metabolites predominate when the liver becomes hypoxic. While these reduced metabolites are toxic it is thought that they are not involved in halothane hepatitis.

Toxicity

Hepatic damage may take one of two forms:

- A reversible form that is often subclinical and associated with a rise in hepatic transaminases. This is probably due to hepatic hypoxia.
- Fulminant hepatic necrosis (halothane hepatitis). Trifluoroacetyl chloride (an oxidative metabolite of halothane) may behave as a hapten, binding covalently with hepatic proteins, inducing antibody formation. The diagnosis of halothane hepatitis is based on the exclusion of all other forms of liver damage. The incidence in children is between 1 in 80,000–200,000 while in the adult it is 1 in 2,500–35,000. The following are risk factors: multiple exposures, obesity, middle age and female sex. The mortality rate is 50–75%. Halothane should be avoided if administered within the previous 3 months, there is a history of a previous adverse reaction to halothane or pre-existing liver disease. Enflurane has also been reported to cause hepatic necrosis. Its incidence is much lower due to its lower rate of metabolism. In theory the other volatile agents may cause a similar reaction but due to their even lower rates of metabolism this becomes increasingly unlikely.

Enflurane

This halogenated ethyl methyl ether is a structural isomer of isoflurane that has been superseded by other agents. At high concentrations it produces a 3 Hz spike and wave pattern on EEG, consistent with grand mal activity. It is avoided in patients with renal impairment as its metabolism produces F^- ions (known to produce reversible nephropathy).

Desflurane

Desflurane (a fluorinated ethyl methyl ether) was slow to be introduced into anaesthetic practice due to difficulties in preparation and administration. It has a boiling point of 23.5°C, which renders it extremely volatile and, therefore, dangerous to administer via a conventional vaporiser. It is, therefore, administered via the electronic Tec 6 vaporiser that heats desflurane to 39°C at 2 atmospheres. Its low blood:gas partition coefficient (0.42) ensures a rapid onset and offset, which has made it the volatile agent of choice for prolonged surgery or bariatric surgery.

Its effects as a GHG are significantly worse than those of sevoflurane and isoflurane.

Effects

- *Respiratory* (see Table 9.8) – desflurane shows similar respiratory effects to the other agents, being more potent than halothane but less potent than isoflurane and enflurane. $PaCO_2$ rises and minute ventilation falls with increasing concentrations. Desflurane has a pungent odour that causes coughing and breath-holding. It is not suitable for induction of anaesthesia.
- *Cardiovascular* (see Table 9.9) – these may be thought of as similar to isoflurane. However, in patients with ischaemic heart disease particular care is required as concentrations above 1 MAC may produce cardiovascular stimulation (tachycardia and hypertension). It does not sensitise the heart to catecholamines. Vascular resistance to both cerebral and coronary circulations is decreased.

Metabolism

Only 0.02% is metabolised and so its potential to produce toxic effects is minimal.

Xenon

Xenon is an inert, odourless gas with no occupational or environmental hazards and makes up 0.0000087% of the atmosphere. It has a MAC of 71% and a very low blood:gas partition coefficient (0.14). Consequently, its onset and offset of action are faster than both desflurane and N_2O.

Manufacture

Xenon is produced by the fractional distillation of air, at about 2,000 times the cost of producing N_2O.

Effects

- *Respiratory* – in contrast to other inhaled anaesthetic agents xenon slows the respiratory rate, while the tidal volume is increased so that the minute volume remains constant. Compared with N_2O, xenon has a higher density ($\times 3$) and viscosity ($\times 1.5$), which might be expected to increase airway resistance when used in high concentrations. However, its clinical significance is probably minimal. Despite its use at high concentrations it does not appear to result in diffusion hypoxia in a manner similar to that seen with N_2O.
- *Cardiovascular* – xenon does not alter myocardial contractility but may result in a small decrease in heart rate.
- *Central nervous system* – xenon may be used to enhance CT images of the brain while [133]xenon may be used to measure cerebral blood flow. However, in humans it appears to increase the cerebral blood flow in a variable manner, and its use in anaesthesia for neurosurgery is not recommended.
- *Analgesia* – it has significant analgesic properties.

Elimination

Xenon is not metabolised in the body, rather it is eliminated via the lungs.

Non-Anaesthetic Medical Gases

Oxygen

Manufacture and Storage

Oxygen (O_2) is manufactured by the fractional distillation of air or by means of an oxygen concentrator in which a zeolite mesh adsorbs N_2 so that the remaining gas is about 97% O_2. It is stored as a gas in black cylinders with white shoulders at 137 bar and as a liquid in a vacuum insulated evaporator (VIE) at 10 bar and $-180°C$, which must be located outside. The VIE rests on three legs; two are hinged while the third serves as a weighing device, enabling its contents to be displayed on a dial.

Physiochemical Properties

- Boiling point $-182°C$
- Critical temperature $-119°C$
  Critical pressure 50 bar.

Uses

It is used to prevent hypoxaemia, and should be prescribed like other therapeutic interventions.

Measurement

Depending on the sample type, various means are used to measure O_2. In a mixture of gases a mass spectrometer, paramagnetic analyser or fuel cell may be used; when dissolved in blood a Clarke electrode, transcutaneous electrode or pulse oximetry may be used; in vitro blood samples may be analysed by bench or co-oximetry.

Effects

Cardiovascular – if O_2 is being used to correct hypoxaemia then an improvement in all cardiovascular parameters will be seen. However, prolonged administration of 100% O_2 will directly reduce cardiac output slightly and cause coronary artery vasoconstriction. It causes a fall in pulmonary vascular resistance and pulmonary artery pressure.

Respiratory – in healthy subjects, a high concentration causes mild respiratory depression. However, in those patients who are truly dependent on a hypoxic drive to maintain respiration, even a modest concentration of O_2 may prove fatal.

Toxicity

O_2 toxicity is caused by free radicals. They affect the CNS resulting in anxiety, nausea and seizures when the partial pressure exceeds 200 kPa. The alveolar capillary membrane undergoes lipid peroxidation and regions of lung may collapse. Neonates are susceptible to retrolental fibroplasia, which may be a result of vasoconstriction of developing retinal vessels during development.

Nitric Oxide

Nitric oxide (NO) is an endogenous molecule but it is potentially a contaminant in nitrous oxide cylinders. It was formerly known as endothelium-derived relaxing factor (EDRF).

Synthesis

It is manufactured as a by-product in nitric acid synthesis. In vivo it is synthesised from one of the terminal guanidino nitrogen atoms of L-arginine in a process catalysed by nitric oxide synthase (NOS), which is present in two forms:

- Constitutive – which is normally present in endothelial, neuronal, skeletal muscle, cardiac tissue and platelets. Here NOS is Ca^{2+}/calmodulin-dependent and is stimulated by cGMP.
- Inducible – which is seen only after exposure to endotoxin or certain cytokines in endothelium, vascular smooth muscle, myocytes, macrophages and neutrophils. Following induction large quantities of NO are produced, which may be cytotoxic. In addition, it may form radicals leading to cellular damage and capillary leakage.

Effects

- *Cardiovascular* – vasodilator tone in small arteries and arterioles is dependent on a continuous supply of locally synthesised NO. Shear stresses in these vessels increase NO production and may account for flow-dependent vasodilatation. Nitric oxide derived from the endothelium inhibits platelet aggregation. In septic shock there is overproduction of NO resulting in hypotension and capillary leakage.
- *Respiratory* – endogenous NO provides an important basal vasodilator tone in pulmonary and bronchial vessels, which may be reversed in hypoxia. When inhaled in concentrations of up to 40 ppm it may reduce V/Q mismatching in acute respiratory distress syndrome (ARDS) and reduce pulmonary hypertension in neonates. Inhaled NO has no effect on the systemic circulation due to its rapid inactivation within red blood cells. Its affinity for haemoglobin is 1,500 times that of CO. It has no bronchodilator properties.
- *Immune* – NO synthesised in macrophages and neutrophils can be toxic to certain pathogens and may be an important host defence mechanism.
- *Haematological* – NO inhibits platelet aggregation.
- *Neuronal* – nerves containing NO are widely distributed throughout the CNS. Proposed roles include modulation of the state of arousal, pain perception, programmed cell death and long-term neuronal depression and excitation whereby neurones may 'remember' previous signals. Peripheral neurones containing NO control regional blood flow in the corpus cavernosum.

N-monomethyl-L-arginine (L-NMMA) is a guanidino substituted analogue of L-arginine, which inhibits NOS. While L-NMMA has been used to antagonise NOS, resulting in an increased blood pressure in septic shock, it does not alter the course of the underlying pathology and has not been shown to alter survival.

Sodium nitroprusside and the organic nitrates (e.g. glyceryl trinitrate) exert their effect by the spontaneous release of NO or metabolism to NO in smooth muscle cells.

UK Guidelines for the Use of Inhaled Nitric Oxide in Adult Intensive Care Units

An expert group of physicians and representatives from the Departments of Health and Industry issued the following guidelines in 1997:

Indications: severe ARDS (optimally ventilated, $PaO_2 < 12$ kPa with $F_IO_2 = 1$), or right-sided cardiac failure.

Dose: maximum = 40 ppm, but use minimum effective dose.

Equipment: a synchronised inspiratory injection system is considered optimal. If a continuous delivery system is used it must be through a calibrated flowmeter. Stainless steel pressure regulators and connectors should be used.

Monitoring: chemiluminescence or electrochemical analysers should be used and are accurate to 1 ppm. Methaemoglobinaemia is only very rarely significant and is more likely in paediatric patients or those with methaemoglobin reductase deficiency, but levels should be checked before and after starting NO, and daily thereafter.

Exposure: environmental NO levels should not exceed 25 ppm for 8 hours (time-weighted average). Scavenging is not required in a well-ventilated unit.

Contraindications: methaemoglobinaemia (bleeding diathesis, intracranial haemorrhage, severe left ventricular failure).

Helium

Helium (He) is an inert gas presented as either Heliox (79% He, 21% O_2) in brown cylinders with white shoulders or as 100% helium in brown cylinders at 137 bar. It does not support combustion.

Its key physical characteristic is its lower density (and hence specific gravity) than both air and oxygen.

	Helium	Heliox	Oxygen	Air
Specific gravity	0.178	0.337	1.091	1

Therefore, during turbulent flow the velocity will be higher when Heliox is used. This will reduce the work of breathing and improve oxygenation in patients with an upper airway obstruction such as a tumour. Helium/oxygen mixtures are also used for deep water diving to avoid nitrogen narcosis. The lower density of helium/oxygen mixtures produces higher frequency vocal sounds, giving the typical squeaky voice.

Carbon Dioxide

Carbon dioxide (CO_2) is a colourless gas with a pungent odour at high concentrations. It is stored as a liquid at 51 bar at 20°C in grey cylinders (C = 450 litres up to E = 1,800 litres).

Physiochemical Properties

- Boiling point −78.5°C
- Critical temperature 31°C
- Critical pressure 73.8 bar.

Uses

It is used as the insufflating gas during laparoscopic procedures and occasionally to stimulate respiration following general anaesthesia. It is also used in cryotherapy.

Effects

- *Cardiovascular* – by sympathetic stimulation it increases heart rate, blood pressure, cardiac output and dilates the coronary arteries. Arrhythmias are more likely in the presence of a raised $PaCO_2$.
- *Respiratory* – the respiratory centre and peripheral chemoreceptors respond to a raised $PaCO_2$ resulting in an increased minute volume and bronchodilation. However, a $PaCO_2$ above 10 kPa may result in respiratory depression.
- *Central nervous system* – as $PaCO_2$ rises so does cerebral blood flow and intracranial pressure. Beyond 10 kPa narcosis may ensue.

Carbon Dioxide Absorbents

Absorbents consume CO_2 to prevent rebreathing in a circle system. In the UK they are mainly sodium-hydroxide- (sodalime) based while in the US they are potassium-hydroxide-based (baralyme). There are three steps in the chemical reaction:

$$H_2O + CO_2 \rightarrow H_2CO_3$$

$$H_2CO_3 + 2NaOH \rightarrow Na_2CO_3 + 2H_2O$$

$$Na_2CO_3 + Ca(OH)_2 \rightarrow CaCO_3 + 2NaOH.$$

Chapter 10

Analgesics

Pain is defined as an unpleasant sensory and emotional experience associated with actual or potential tissue damage. Since pain is so highly subjective, it may also be described as being what the patient says it is.

Pain may be classified according to its presumed aetiology. Nociceptive pain is the result of the stimulation of nociceptors by noxious stimuli, whilst neuropathic pain is the result of dysfunction of the nervous system. These may exist together as mixed pain. There is also visceral pain, the clearest example being that associated with gallstones.

An alternative classification is based on chronicity. The point at which acute pain becomes chronic has been suggested at about 12 weeks or when the pain is no longer thought to be due to the initial insult.

Physiology

Nociceptive impulses are triggered by the stimulation of nociceptors that respond to chemical, mechanical or thermal damage. The chemical mediators that initiate (H^+, K^+, acetylcholine, histamine, serotonin (5-HT), bradykinin) and sensitise (prostaglandins, leukotrienes, substance P, neurokinin A, calcitonin gene-related peptide) the nociceptors are legion. Two types of primary afferent fibres exist:

- small myelinated Aδ fibres (diameter 2–5 μm) that conduct sharp pain rapidly (40 m.s^{-1})
- unmyelinated C fibres (diameter < 2 μm) that conduct dull pain slowly (2 m.s^{-1}). These fibres enter the dorsal horn of the spinal cord and synapse at different sites (Aδ at Rexed laminae II and V; C at Rexed laminae II). The substantia gelatinosa (lamina II) integrates these inputs, from where second-order neurones form the ascending spinothalamic and spinoreticular pathways on the contralateral side. Descending pathways and the larger Aβ fibres conducting 'touch' stimulate inhibitory interneurones within the substantia gelatinosa and inhibit C fibre nociceptive inputs. This forms the basis of the 'gate theory' of pain (Figure 10.1).

Pain may be modified by altering the neural pathway from its origin at the nociceptor to its interpretation within the central nervous system (CNS). The commonly used agents are discussed below under the following headings:

- **Opioids and related drugs**
- **Non-steroidal anti-inflammatory drugs (NSAIDs)**
- **Other analgesics.**

Table 10.1 Classification of opioid receptors

Receptor	Effects
MOP, μ, mu	analgesia, miosis, euphoria, respiratory depression, bradycardia, inhibition of gut motility
KOP, κ, kappa	analgesia, sedation, miosis
DOP, δ, delta	analgesia, respiratory depression
NOP	anxiety, depression, appetite modulation

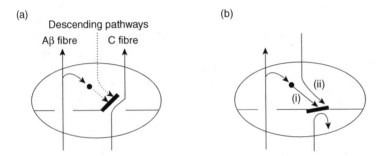

(a)

Descending pathways

Aβ fibre   C fibre

(b)

(ii)
(i)

Figure 10.1 Principle of the gate theory of pain within the dorsal horn of the spinal cord. (a) Pain mediated via C fibres passes through the gate centrally; (b) the gate is shut as Aβ fibres stimulate inhibitory interneurones (i) and by descending pathways, preventing the central passage of pain (ii).

Opioids and Related Drugs

The term 'opiate' refers to all naturally occurring substances with morphine-like properties, while 'opioid' is a more general term that includes synthetic substances that have an affinity for opioid receptors. Opioids are basic amines.

Receptor Classification

Classical receptor classification, that is, kappa and delta, was based on either the name of the agonist that acted at that receptor, *mu* (μ) – *morphine*, *kappa* (κ) – *ketcyclazocine* or the location of the receptor, *delta* (δ) – *vas deferens*. The latest reclassification is listed in Table 10.1 and includes an additional non-classical receptor, NOP, which was discovered at the time of receptor cloning. It is known as the nociceptin/orphanin FQ peptide receptor.

Both receptor types are serpentine (i.e. span the membrane seven times) and are linked to inhibitory G-proteins so that when stimulated by an appropriate opioid agonist (e.g. morphine to μ) the following sequence occurs: voltage-sensitive Ca^{2+} channels are closed, hyperpolarisation by K^+ efflux and adenylase cyclase inhibition lead to reduced cAMP. These processes result in inhibition of transmitter release between nerve cells.

MOP or μ-Receptor

The μ-receptor is located throughout the CNS including the cerebral cortex, the basal ganglia, the spinal cord (presynaptically on primary afferent neurones within the dorsal horn) and the periaqueductal grey (as the origin of the descending inhibitory control pathway). Apart from analgesia, μ-receptor stimulation produces wide-ranging effects including respiratory depression (by reducing chemoreceptor sensitivity to carbon dioxide), constipation (reduced secretions and peristalsis) and cardiovascular depression.

KOP or κ-Receptor

The original κ-receptor agonist was ketocyclazocine, which demonstrated a different set of effects when compared with μ-receptor stimulation. The main advantage of κ-receptor stimulation relates to a lack of respiratory depression, although κ-agonists do seem to have μ-antagonist effects thus limiting their use.

DOP or δ-Receptor

The δ-receptor was the first to be cloned and is less widely spread throughout the CNS. Like μ-receptors, when stimulated they inhibit neurotransmitter release. It may also be involved in regulating mood and movement.

NOP-Receptor

When stimulated by nociceptin/orphanin FQ the NOP receptor produces effects similar to μ-receptor stimulation. It acts at both spinal and supraspinal levels to produce hyperalgesia at low doses but analgesia at high doses. NOP-receptor antagonists produce long-lasting analgesia and prevent morphine tolerance, and may be useful in the future.

Morphine

Morphine is a naturally occurring phenanthrene derivative. It has a complex structure (Figure 10.2) and is the reference opioid with which all others are compared. It is a μ-receptor agonist (see Table 10.2).

Presentation and Uses

Morphine is formulated as tablets, suspensions and suppositories, and as slow-release capsules and granules in a wide range of strengths. The oral dose of morphine is 10–20 mg 4-hourly. The parenteral preparation contains 10–30 $mg.ml^{-1}$ and may be given intravenously or intramuscularly. The intramuscular dose is 0.1–0.2 $mg.kg^{-1}$ 4-hourly. Intravenous morphine should be titrated to effect, but the total dose is similar. It should be noted that these doses are only guidelines and the frequency of administration and/or the dose may have to be increased. The subcutaneous route is usually avoided due to its relatively low lipid solubility and therefore slow absorption. Delayed respiratory depression following intrathecal or epidural administration may occur and is again due to its relatively low lipid solubility.

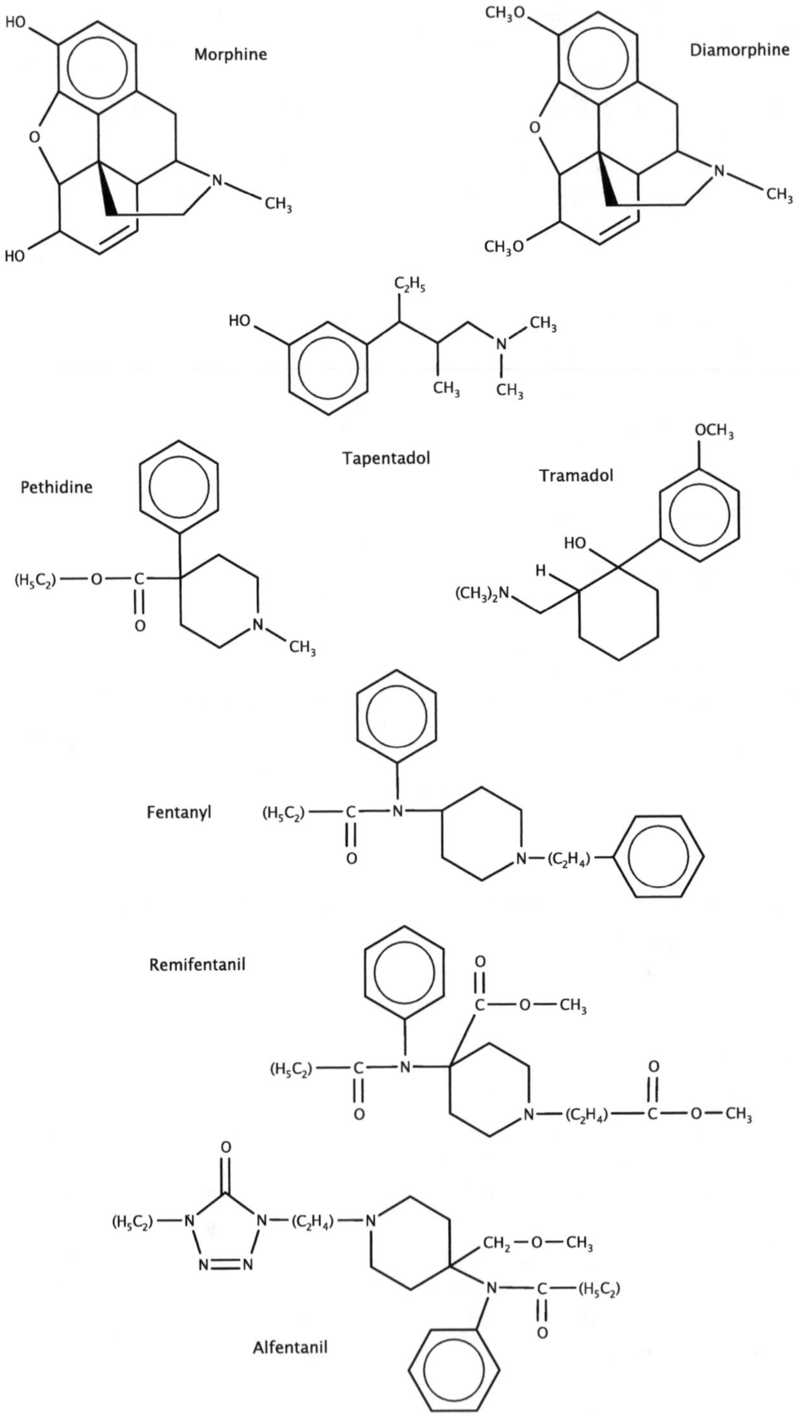

Figure 10.2 Structure of some opioids.

Table 10.2 Opioid receptor subtypes and their ligands

Ligand	μ	κ	δ	NOP
Endorphins	+++	+++	+++	
Enkephalins	+		+++	
Dynorphins	+	+++		
N/OFQ				+++
Morphine	+++	+	+	
Fentanyl	+++	+		
Naloxone	+++	++	++	

Note: + represents receptor affinity, blank represents no receptor affinity.

Effects

- *Analgesia* – particularly effective for visceral pain while less effective for sharp or superficial pain. Occasionally increased doses may be required but this is usually due to a change in pathophysiology rather than dependence.
- *Respiratory depression* – the sensitivity of the brain stem to carbon dioxide is reduced following morphine while its response to hypoxia is less affected. However, if the hypoxic stimulus is removed by supplementary oxygen then respiratory depression may be potentiated. The respiratory rate falls more than the tidal volume. Morphine is anti-tussive. It may precipitate histamine release and bronchospasm.
- *Nausea and vomiting* – the chemoreceptor trigger zone is stimulated via 5-HT$_3$ and dopamine receptors. The cells within the vomiting centre are depressed by morphine and do not stimulate vomiting.
- *Central nervous system* – sedation, euphoria and dysphoria occur with increasing doses.
- *Circulatory* – morphine may induce a mild bradycardia and hypotension secondary to histamine release and a reduction in sympathetic tone. It has no direct myocardial depressant effects.
- *Gut* – morphine constricts the sphincters of the gut. Constipation results from a state of spastic immobility of the bowel. Whilst the sphincter of Oddi is contracted by morphine thereby raising the pressure within the biliary tree, the clinical significance of this is unknown.

  Histamine release – reducing the rate of administration will help to limit histamine-induced bronchospasm and hypotension. Histamine release may result in a rash and pruritus but this may be reversed by naloxone.

  Pruritus – most marked following intrathecal or epidural use. However, this does not appear to be due to histamine release and is generally not associated with a rash. Paradoxically, antihistamines may be effective treatment for pruritus, possibly as a result of their sedative effects.

- *Muscle rigidity* – occasionally, morphine (and other opioids) can precipitate chest wall rigidity, which is thought to be due to opioid receptor interaction with dopaminergic and GABA pathways in the substantia nigra and striatum.
- *Miosis* – due to stimulation of the Edinger–Westphal nucleus, which can be reversed by atropine.
- *Endocrine* – morphine inhibits the release of adrenocorticotrophic hormone (ACTH), prolactin and gonadotrophic hormones. Antidiuretic hormone (ADH) secretion is increased and may cause impaired water excretion and hyponatraemia.
- *Urinary* – the tone of the bladder detrusor and vesical sphincter is increased and may precipitate urinary retention. Ureteric tone is also increased.

Kinetics

When given orally morphine is ionised in the acidic gastric environment (because it is a weak base, $pK_a = 8.0$) (see Table 10.3) so that absorption is delayed until it reaches the relatively alkaline environment of the small bowel where it becomes unionised. Its oral bioavailability of 30% is due to hepatic first-pass metabolism. Its peak effects following intravenous or intramuscular injection are reached after 10 and 30 minutes, respectively, and it has a duration of action of 3–4 hours. It has been given by the epidural (2–4 mg) and intrathecal (0.2–1.0 mg) routes but this has been associated with delayed respiratory depression.

Morphine concentration in the brain falls slowly due to its low lipid solubility, and consequently plasma concentrations do not correlate with its effects.

Morphine metabolism occurs mainly in the liver but also in the kidneys. Up to 70% is metabolised to morphine 3-glucuronide which appears to have effects on arousal and is possibly a μ-receptor antagonist. The other major metabolite is morphine 6-glucuronide, which is 13 times more potent than morphine and has a similar duration of action. They are both excreted in urine and accumulate in renal failure. Morphine is also N-demethylated. Neonates are more sensitive than adults to morphine due to reduced hepatic conjugating capacity, and in the elderly peak plasma levels are higher due to a reduced volume of distribution.

Diamorphine

Diamorphine is a diacetylated morphine derivative with no affinity for opioid receptors. It is a prodrug whose active metabolites are responsible for its effects. It is said to be approximately twice as potent as morphine (see Table 10.4).

Presentation and Uses

Diamorphine is available as 10 mg tablets and as a white powder for injection containing 5, 10, 30, 100 or 500 mg diamorphine hydrochloride, which is readily dissolved before administration. It is used parenterally for the relief of severe pain and dyspnoea associated with pulmonary oedema at 2.5–10 mg. It is used intrathecally (0.1–0.4 mg) and via the epidural route (1–3 mg) for analgesia where, due to a higher lipid solubility, it is theoretically less likely to cause delayed respiratory depression when compared with morphine.

Table 10.3 Various pharmacological properties of some opioids

	Elimination half-life (min)	Clearance (ml. $min^{-1}.kg^{-1}$)	Volume of distribution ($l.kg^{-1}$)	Plasma protein-bound (%)	pK_a	Percentage unionised (at pH 7.4)	Relative lipid solubility (from octanol:water coefficient)
Morphine	170	16	3.5	35	8.0	23	1
Pethidine	210	12	4.0	60	8.7	5	30
Fentanyl	190	13	4.0	83	8.4	9	600
Alfentanil	100	6	0.6	90	6.5	89	90
Remifentanil	10	40	0.3	70	7.1	68	20

Table 10.4 Equivalent doses of some opioids

	Route	Potency ratio with oral morphine	Equivalent dose to 10mg oral morphine
Codeine phosphate	po	0.1	100mg
Dihydrocodeine	po	0.1	100mg
Tramadol	po	0.15	67mg
Tapentadol	po	0.4	25mg
Oxycodone	po	1.5	6.6mg
Morphine	po	1	10mg
Morphine	im / iv / sc	2	5mg
Diamorphine	im / iv / sc	3.3	3mg

Kinetics

Owing to its high lipid solubility diamorphine is well absorbed from the gut but has a low oral bioavailability due to an extensive first-pass metabolism. Its high lipid solubility enables it to be administered effectively by the subcutaneous route. Once in the plasma it is 40% protein-bound. It has a $pK_a = 7.6$ so that 37% is in the unionised form at pH 7.4. Metabolism occurs rapidly in the liver, plasma and CNS by ester hydrolysis to 6-monoacetylmorphine and morphine, which confer its analgesic and other effects. The plasma half-life of diamorphine itself is approximately 5 minutes.

It produces the greatest degree of euphoria of the opioids and subsequently has become a drug of abuse.

Codeine

Codeine (3-methylmorphine) is 10 times less potent than morphine and not suitable for severe pain. The oral and intramuscular adult dose is 30–60 mg. Its use in children younger than 12 years has been restricted because of reports of morphine toxicity. The intravenous route tends to cause hypotension, probably via histamine release, and is therefore avoided. It has been suggested codeine acts as no more than a prodrug for morphine.

Uses

In addition to its analgesic uses it is used as an antitussive, antidiarrhoeal, hypnotic and anxiolytic.

Kinetics

Due to the presence of a methyl group that reduces hepatic first-pass metabolism the oral bioavailability of codeine (50%) is slightly higher than that of morphine.

A small proportion (5–15%) of codeine is eliminated unchanged in the urine while the remainder is eliminated via one of three metabolic pathways in the liver. The predominant metabolic pathway is 6-hydroxyglucuronidation to codeine-6-glucuronide, although 10–20%

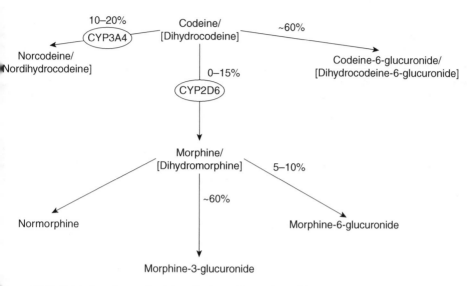

Figure 10.3 Metabolic pathway of codeine, dihydrocodeine and morphine.

undergoes N-demethylation to norcodeine, and up to 15% undergoes O-demethylation to morphine. A number of other metabolites, such as normorphine and hydrocodone, have also been identified. Of these metabolites only morphine has significant activity at μ-receptors. O-demethylation is dependent on the non-inducible CYP2D6, which exhibits genetic polymorphism so that poor metabolisers experience little pain relief. The frequency of poor metabolisers varies and is estimated at 9% of the UK population but 30% in the Hong Kong Chinese population. Fast metabolisers will generate increased amounts of morphine with its attendant side effects. This has lead to its restriction for children below 12 years.

Dihydrocodeine

Dihydrocodeine is a synthetic opioid, which is structurally similar to codeine but is very approximately twice as potent. It has an oral bioavailability of about 20%. While very little research has been completed on dihydrocodeine it does appear to have a greater efficacy than codeine for the μ receptor and as such is less dependent on CYP2D6 for its effects, making it more predictable than codeine. Its metabolic pathways are analogous to those of codeine (see Figure 10.3).

Fentanyl

Fentanyl is a synthetic phenylpiperidine derivative with a rapid onset of action. It is a μ-receptor agonist and as such shares morphine's effects. However, it is less likely to precipitate histamine release. High doses (50–150 μg.kg^{-1}) significantly reduce or even eliminate the metabolic stress response to surgery but are associated with bradycardia and chest wall rigidity.

Presentation

Fentanyl is prepared as a colourless solution for injection containing 50 μg.ml^{-1}, as transdermal patches that release between 25 and 100 μg per hour for 72 hours and as lozenges releasing 200 μg–1.6 mg over 15 minutes.

Uses

Doses vary enormously depending on the duration of analgesia and sedation required. For pain associated with minor surgery, 1–2 μg.kg^{-1} is used intravenously and has a duration of about 30 minutes. Higher doses are generally required to obtund the stimulation of laryngoscopy. High doses (50–100 μg.kg^{-1}) are used for an opioid-based anaesthetic (although a hypnotic is also required), and here its duration of action is extended to about 6 hours. Following prolonged administration by continuous infusion only its elimination half-life is apparent, leading to a significantly prolonged duration of action.

Fentanyl has also been used to augment the effects of local anaesthetics in spinal and epidural anaesthesia at 10–25 μg and 25–100 μg, respectively. Its high lipid solubility ensures that a typical intrathecal dose does not cause delayed respiratory depression as it diffuses rapidly from cerebrospinal fluid (CSF) into the spinal cord. This contrasts with morphine, which enters the spinal cord slowly, leaving some to be transported in the CSF by bulk flow up to the midbrain. However, respiratory depression is observed when epidural fentanyl is administered by continuous infusion or as repeated boluses.

Kinetics

Fentanyl's onset of action is rapid following intravenous administration due to its high lipid solubility (nearly 600 times more lipid-soluble than morphine). However, following the application of a transdermal patch, plasma levels take 12 hours to reach equilibrium. At low doses (< 3 μg.kg^{-1} intravenous) its short duration of action is due solely to distribution. However, following prolonged administration or with high doses, its duration of action is significantly prolonged as tissues become saturated. Its clearance is similar to and its elimination half-life is longer than that of morphine, reflecting its higher lipid solubility and volume of distribution. Fentanyl may become trapped in the acidic environment of the stomach where more than 99.9% is ionised. As it passes into the alkaline environment of the small bowel it becomes unionised and, therefore, available for systemic absorption. However, this is unlikely to raise systemic levels significantly due to a rapid hepatic first-pass metabolism, where it is N-demethylated to norfentanyl, which along with fentanyl is further hydroxylated. These inactive metabolites are excreted in the urine.

Alfentanil

Alfentanil is a synthetic phenylpiperidine derivative. It is a μ-receptor agonist but with some significant differences from fentanyl.

Presentation and Uses

Alfentanil is presented as a colourless solution containing 500 μg or 5 mg.ml^{-1}. For short-term analgesia it is used in boluses of 5–25 μg.kg^{-1}. It is also used by infusion for sedation where its duration of action is significantly prolonged.

Kinetics

Alfentanil has a pK$_a$ of 6.5; at a pH of 7.4, 89% is present in the unionised form and is, therefore, available to cross lipid membranes. Fentanyl has a pK$_a$ of 8.4, so only 9% is unionised at a pH of 7.4. So despite a significantly lower lipid solubility than fentanyl, it has a faster onset of action (when given in equipotent doses). Alfentanil has a much smaller initial volume of distribution so that despite a smaller clearance its elimination half-life is also shorter.

Metabolism occurs in the liver by N-demethylation to noralfentanil. This and other metabolites are conjugated and excreted in the urine. Midazolam is metabolised by the same hepatic enzymes (CYP3A3/4) so when administered concurrently both elimination half-lives are significantly increased. Erythromycin may prolong alfentanil's activity by inhibiting hepatic CYP450.

Remifentanil

The pure μ-receptor agonist remifentanil is a synthetic phenylpiperidine derivative of fentanyl with a similar potency. While it shares many of the effects associated with opioids its metabolism makes it unique in this class of drug.

Presentation

Remifentanil is presented as a crystalline white powder in glass vials containing 1, 2 or 5 mg remifentanil hydrochloride. The preparation also contains glycine and is not licensed for spinal or epidural administration.

Uses

Remifentanil is administered intravenously by infusion. Most crystalloid fluids or sterile water are suitable as a diluent, in which it is stable for 24 hours.

It is most commonly used as a co-induction agent alongside propofol and best administered using a target-controlled infusion (TCI) pump at 3–6 ng.ml^{-1} for patients 12 years or above. Where manual dosing is preferred (or in those < 12 years) a bolus dose of 0.5–1 μg.kg^{-1} given over at least 45 seconds, followed by an infusion of up to 0.25 μg.kg^{-1}.min^{-1} may be used. When plasma targets of > 5 ng.ml^{-1} or rates > 0.2 μg.kg^{-1}.min^{-1} are used this may cause opioid induced hyperalgesia, where larger than expected doses of opioid are required to control post-operative pain. Regardless of this, it should be remembered that due to its short duration of action it will not contribute to the patient's post-operative analgesia.

Effects

Remifentanil shares many of morphine's effects including respiratory depression and chest wall rigidity. However, due to its ultra-short duration of action, nausea and vomiting seem to be less common. It characteristically causes a fall in heart rate and blood pressure, which may be reversed by glycopyrrolate. Its analgesic effects are reversed by naloxone.

Kinetics

Remifentanil is rapidly broken down by non-specific plasma and tissue esterases resulting in an elimination half-life of 3–10 minutes. Its duration of action is, therefore, determined by metabolism and not distribution (cf. alfentanil and fentanyl). Owing to the abundance of these esterases the duration of administration does not significantly affect the duration of action, that is, the context-sensitive half-time (see p. 78) does not change significantly. This is in contrast to other opioids whose half-time is context-sensitive, being dependent on the duration of infusion. It is a poor substrate for plasma cholinesterases and as such is unaffected by cholinesterase deficiency. Anticholinesterase drugs do not alter its metabolism. An essentially inactive carboxylic acid metabolite (1/4600th as potent) is excreted in the urine. The half-life of this metabolite in the healthy adult is 2 hours. Impaired hepatic and renal function do not prolong its effects.

Oxycodone

Oxycodone may be thought of as an alternative to morphine. Both drugs have a similar profile but individual patients may tolerate one better than the other.

Combination Preparations

Oxycodone in combination with naloxone is sold under the trade name of *Targinact*. The dose combinations are fixed – oxycodone/naloxone, 5 mg/2.5 mg, 10 mg/5 mg, 20 mg/ 10 mg, 40 mg/20 mg – and are presented as prolonged release tablets.

Mechanism of Action

While the notion of mixing agonists and antagonists to the same receptor in one preparation seems strange, the concept becomes clearer when the pharmacokinetics are considered. Both are absorbed in the gut, but naloxone undergoes significant first-pass metabolism so that it has no systemic effects. In contrast, oxycodone has an oral bioavailability of 85% and exerts analgesic effects systemically. However, naloxone appears to have some local (pre-hepatic) effect on the gut and reduces constipation.

Uses

Targinact is used to treat severe pain with resistant constipation. Despite its prolonged-release formulation it may also have a role post-operatively in patients for whom constipation would be especially troublesome, including haemorrhoidectomy and pelvic floor repair.

Pethidine

Pethidine is a synthetic phenylpiperidine derivative originally designed as an anticholinergic agent but was subsequently shown to have analgesic properties.

Presentation

Pethidine is available as tablets and as a solution for injection containing 10–50 mg.ml^{-1}. The intravenous and intramuscular dose is 0.5–1.0 mg.kg^{-1} and may be repeated 2–3 hourly. In common with all opioids the dose should be titrated to effect.

Uses

Pethidine is often used during labour. Its high lipid solubility enables significant amounts to cross the placenta and reach the fetus. Following its metabolism, the less lipid-soluble norpethidine accumulates in the fetus, levels peaking about 4 hours after the initial maternal intramuscular dose. Owing to reduced fetal clearance, the half-lives of both pethidine and norpethidine are prolonged by a factor of three.

Effects

Pethidine shares the common opioid effects with morphine. However, differences are seen:
- *Anticholinergic effects* – it produces less marked miosis and possibly a degree of mydriasis, a dry mouth and sometimes tachycardia.

- *Gut* – it is said to produce less biliary tract spasm than morphine but the clinical significance of this is unclear.
- *Interactions* – pethidine may produce a serious interaction if administered with monoamine oxidase inhibitors (MAOI). This is probably due to central serotoninergic hyperactivity caused by pethidine's inhibition of serotonin re-uptake in combination with an MAOI-induced reduction in amine breakdown. Effects include coma, labile circulation, convulsions and hyperpyrexia. Other opioids are safe.

Kinetics

Pethidine is more lipid-soluble than morphine, resulting in a faster onset of action. It has an oral bioavailability of 50%. It is metabolised in the liver by ester hydrolysis to the inactive pethidinic acid and by N-demethylation to norpethidine, which has half the analgesic activity of pethidine. Norpethidine has a longer elimination half-life (14–21 hours) than pethidine and accumulates in renal failure. It has been associated with hallucinations and grand mal seizures following its accumulation. Its effects are not reversed by naloxone. Norpethidine and pethidinic acid are excreted in the urine along with small amounts of unchanged pethidine. The duration of action of pethidine is 120–150 minutes.

Methadone

The notable features of methadone are its relatively low first-pass metabolism resulting in a relatively high oral bioavailability of 75% and a long plasma half-life. It is used to treat opioid addicts on slow weaning programmes. It is less sedative than morphine.

Methadone may also act as an antagonist at the NMDA receptor and this is thought to be especially beneficial in the treatment of certain neuropathic pain that would be otherwise resistant to typical opioids.

Kinetics

Methadone is 90% plasma protein-bound and metabolism occurs in the liver to a number of inactive metabolites. Its plasma half-life is 18–36 hours. Up to 40% is excreted as unchanged drug in the urine, which is enhanced in acidic conditions.

Tramadol

Tramadol is a cyclohexanol derivative. It is a racemic mixture, each enantiomer producing specific actions.

Presentation

Tramadol is available as tablets, capsules or sachets in a variety of strengths (50–400 mg modified release) and as a solution for intravenous or intramuscular injection containing 100 mg in 2 ml. Its analgesic potency is one-fifth to one-tenth that of morphine.

Mechanism of Action

Tramadol has agonist properties at all opioid receptors but particularly at μ-receptors. It also inhibits the re-uptake of noradrenaline and 5-HT, and stimulates presynaptic 5-HT release, which provides an alternative pathway for analgesia involving the descending inhibitory pathways within the spinal cord.

Effects

In equi-analgesic doses to morphine, tramadol produces less respiratory depression and constipation. In other respects it has similar actions to morphine. Respiratory depression and analgesia are reversed by naloxone.

Interactions

Tramadol has the potential to interact with drugs that inhibit central 5-HT or noradrenaline re-uptake, that is, the tricyclic antidepressants and selective serotonin re-uptake inhibitors, resulting in seizures. It should not be used in patients with epilepsy.

Kinetics

Tramadol is well absorbed from the gut with an oral bioavailability of 70% which increases to more than 90% after repeated doses. It is metabolised by hepatic CPY2D6, CYP3A4 and CYP2B6 and subsequent glucuronidation to a number of metabolites, only one of which (O-desmethyltramadol) has been shown to have analgesic activity. These products are excreted in the urine. Its volume of distribution is 4 l.kg^{-1} and its elimination half-life is 5–6 hours.

Tapentadol

Tapentadol has an alkylbenzene structure. Of the four potential stereoisomers, only the R,R form is presented for medical use. It is used to treat moderate to severe pain in both the acute and chronic setting. The initial dose is 50 mg 4–6 hourly.

Presentation

Tapentadol is presented as 50–75 mg tablets and 20 mg.ml^{-1} oral solution for immediate release and also as a sustained release preparation containing 50–250 mg.

Mechanism of Action

It has a dual mode of action as a μ-receptor agonist and a noradrenaline re-uptake inhibitor (NARI). It has weak serotonin re-uptake inhibitor properties.

Interactions

Tapentadol can induce seizures and should be prescribed with caution in patients with a history of seizure disorders or epilepsy. Seizure risk may be increased in patients taking other medicines that lower seizure threshold, for example, antidepressants such as selective serotonin reuptake inhibitors (SSRIs), tricyclic antidepressants, and antipsychotics. Serotonin syndrome has been reported when tapentadol is used in combination with serotonergic antidepressants. Due to its NARI actions the manufacturers advise against the use of MAOIs within 14 days.

Kinetics

Tapentadol has a bioavailability of 30% due to extensive hepatic first-pass metabolism. Glucuronidation is the main metabolic pathway but oxidation by hepatic cytochromes (CYP2C9, CYP2C19 and CYP2D6) also play a limited role prior to further glucuronidation. None of the metabolites are active. Only 20% is protein bound in the plasma and the kidneys are the main route of excretion. It has a volume of distribution (Vd) of approximately 550 litres, and an elimination half-life of 4 hours.

Naloxone

Naloxone is a pure opioid antagonist and will reverse opioid effects at μ-, κ- and δ-receptors, although its affinity is highest for μ-receptors. Other occasional effects include hypertension, pulmonary oedema and cardiac arrhythmias and antanalgesia in opioid-naive subjects.

At 1–4 $μg.kg^{-1}$ intravenously it is the drug of choice in opioid overdose. However, its duration of action at 30–40 minutes is shorter than morphine and high-dose fentanyl so that supplementary doses or an infusion of naloxone may be required.

Opioid Partial Agonists

This group of drugs has been used to control pain and to reverse opioid-induced respiratory depression with variable success. They are not widely used.

Pentazocine produces analgesia with little respiratory depression. However, side effects including nausea, vomiting, hallucinations and dysphoria have meant that it is rarely used.

Buprenorphine is structurally similar to and more potent than morphine with a duration of up to 10 hours due to receptor binding. It is available as sublingual tablets and transdermal patches.

Due to its receptor-binding profile it produces analgesia at low concentrations (μ-receptor) but with increasing doses the NOP effects take over to produce anti-analgesic effects (see Table 10.5). It is metabolised by CYP3A4 and subsequently conjugated so that 70% is excreted in the bile, the rest in the urine. Nausea and vomiting are severe and prolonged.

Nalbuphine is equipotent to morphine but appears to have a ceiling effect with respect to its respiratory depression. Unfortunately it also appears to have a ceiling effect with respect to its analgesic actions, which may be reversed with naloxone.

Table 10.5 Summary of actions of some partial agonists at various opioid receptors

	Agonist action at:	Antagonist action at:
Nalorphine	κ	μ
Pentazocine	κ (partial), δ (partial)	μ
Buprenorphine	μ (partial), NOP (partial, very weak)	κ, δ
Nalbuphine	κ (partial)	μ (partial)

Non-Steroidal Anti-Inflammatory Drugs

Non-steroidal anti-inflammatory drugs (NSAIDs; see Table 10.6) are used widely to treat mild to moderate pain and also to reduce opioid consumption in the peri-operative period.

The route of administration is usually oral or rectal although some agents may be administered intravenously (diclofenac, ketorolac, parecoxib). Absorption is rapid through the small bowel. NSAIDs are highly protein-bound in the plasma and have low volumes of distribution. The effects of other highly protein-bound drugs (e.g. warfarin) may be

Table 10.6 Classification of NSAIDs

Group	Class	Drug
Non-specific COX inhibitors	salicylates	aspirin
	acetic acid derivatives	diclofenac, ketorolac, indomethacin
	anthralinic acids	mefanamic acid
	pyrazolones	phenylbutazone
	proprionic acids	ibuprofen, naproxen
	para-aminophenols	paracetamol
	oxicams	tenoxicam, piroxicam
Preferential COX-2 inhibitors	oxicams	meloxicam
Specific COX-2 inhibitors	pyrazole	parecoxib, celecoxib, (rofecoxib)
	methylsulfone	etoricoxib
	phenylacetic acid derivative	lumiracoxib

potentiated as they become displaced. Characteristically these drugs are metabolised in the liver and excreted in an inactive form in the urine and bile.

Mechanism of Action

Non-steroidal anti-inflammatory drugs inhibit the enzyme cyclo-oxygenase thereby preventing the production of both prostaglandins (including prostacyclin) and thromboxanes from membrane phospholipids (see Figure 10.4). Thromboxane is produced by platelets when activated by exposure to adenosine, collagen or adrenaline, and promotes haemostasis by vasoconstriction and platelet aggregation. Conversely, endothelial prostacyclin promotes vasodilatation and inhibits platelet aggregation.

Low-dose aspirin prevents arterial thromboembolism by selectively inhibiting platelet thromboxane production. Platelets have no nuclei and are therefore not able to regenerate new cyclo-oxygenase so that aspirin's effects last for the lifespan of the platelet. The production of prostacyclin in vascular endothelium is not affected in this way, so the overall effect is selective inhibition of thromboxane.

The other NSAIDs produce reversible enzyme inhibition, the activity of cyclo-oxygenase resuming when plasma levels fall. Decreased PGE_2 and $PGF_{2\alpha}$ synthesis account for their anti-inflammatory effect, while reduced thromboxane synthesis leads to reduced platelet aggregation and adhesiveness. Their antipyretic actions are due to inhibition of centrally produced prostaglandins that stimulate pyrexia. Reduced prostaglandin synthesis in gastric mucosal cells may lead to mucosal ulceration. Lipoxygenase is not inhibited by NSAIDs and the production of leukotrienes is unaltered.

Table 10.7 Clinical and kinetic data for selected NSAIDs

Drug	Maximum daily dose	Elimination half-life (h)	Plasma protein-binding (%)	Upper GI erosions	Coronary events	Stroke
Aspirin	4 g	variable*	85	+++	−	−
Paracetamol	4 g	2	10	0	0	0
Ibuprofen	1.2 g/2.4 g	2–3	99	++/++++	+/+++	+
Naproxen	1 g	12–17	99	++++	0	0
Ketorolac	40 mg	5	99	++++	?	+
Diclofenac	150 mg	1–2	99	++	+++	+
Tenoxicam	20 mg	72	99	+	?	0
Meloxicam	15 mg	20	99	+	?	0
Celecoxib	400 mg	11	97	+	+++	0
Etoricoxib	120 mg	22	92	+	+++	0
Parecoxib	80 mg	22 min	98	+	+++	0

* When obeying first-order kinetics the $t_{1/2}$ elimination as aspirin is short (15–30 minutes). However, this is significantly prolonged when enzyme systems become saturated and its kinetics become zero-order.

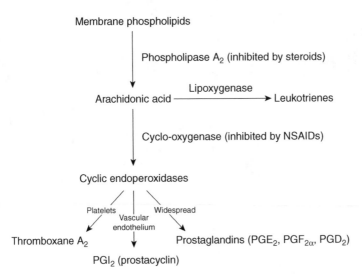

Figure 10.4 Prostaglandin synthesis.

Cyclo-oxygenase (COX) exists as two isoenzymes, COX-1 and COX-2. The main molecular difference between COX-1 and COX-2 lies in the substitution of isoleucine for valine, which allows access to a hydrophobic side pocket that acts as an alternative specific binding site for drugs.

COX-1 (the constitutive form) is responsible for the production of prostaglandins that control renal blood flow and form the protective gastric mucosal barrier. In addition COX-1 mediates synthesis of thromboxane. (A variant of COX-1, which has been called COX-3 and exists centrally, is possibly the mechanism by which paracetamol reduces pain and pyrexia.)

COX-2 (the inducible form) is produced in response to tissue damage and facilitates the inflammatory response. COX-2 also mediates production of prostacyclin (PGI_2) in vascular endothelium. As a result, COX-2 inhibitors may alter the delicate thromboxane/prostacyclin balance in favour of platelet aggregation, vasoconstriction and thromboembolism. However, it should be remembered that COX selectivity is relative not absolute.

Side Effects

- *Gastric irritation* – intestinal erosions not limited to the stomach are commonly encountered during prolonged administration of NSAIDs. These lesions result in a spectrum of adverse effects from mild pain to iron deficiency anaemia and fatal haemorrhage. Many elements (mucous layer, bicarbonate secretion, rapid cell turnover and an abundant blood supply) are involved in the protection of the intestinal mucosa against acid and enzyme attack. Prostaglandins are involved in many of these elements so that when their synthesis is inhibited, protection is reduced. During aspirin therapy acetylsalicylate and salicylate ions are trapped in the alkaline environment of the mucosal cells thereby increasing their potential for side effects. The potential for haemorrhage is increased due to its effect on platelet function. NSAIDs with the highest risk of serious gastrointestinal (GI) side effects are ketorolac and piroxicam, the intermediate risk drugs are diclofenac and naproxen, with ibuprofen (< 1.2 g.day^{-1}) having the lowest risk. COX-2 inhibitors have a lower risk than non-selective NSAIDs.

- *Major vascular events* – there has been much interest in this group of side effects, which comprise myocardial infarction, stroke, atrial fibrillation and heart failure. Initially, COX-2 inhibitors were shown to elevate the relative risk of major coronary events; however, diclofenac (150 mg.day^{-1}) and ibuprofen (2.4 g.day^{-1}) have similar risk profiles. For 1,000 patients receiving these drugs for 1 year there will be three extra coronary events, one of which will be fatal. More recent warnings state that there is no duration of NSAID use that is without increased risk. The risk of stroke appears higher in younger men and those with a prior history of stroke or TIA.

- *NSAID-sensitive asthma* – acute severe asthma may be precipitated in up to 20% of asthmatics when given NSAIDs and is associated with chronic rhinitis or nasal polyps. Those affected are usually middle-aged – children are relatively spared. By inhibiting cyclo-oxygenase, more arachidonic acid is converted to leukotrienes which are known to cause bronchospasm. Aspirin also causes an abnormal reaction to the platelets of susceptible patients, causing the release of cytotoxic mediators.

- *Renal function* – renally produced prostaglandins (PGE$_2$ and PGI$_2$) are essential in maintaining adequate renal perfusion when the level of circulating vasoconstrictors (renin, angiotensin, noradrenaline) is high. Aspirin and other NSAIDs may alter this delicate balance by inhibiting their production, reducing renal perfusion and potentially leading to acute renal failure. At low doses of aspirin (< 2 g.day^{-1}), urate is retained as its tubular secretion is inhibited. At higher doses (> 5 g.day^{-1}), aspirin becomes uricosuric as reabsorption of urates is inhibited to a greater degree. It is rarely used for this purpose as the side effects at higher doses are unacceptable. Analgesic nephropathy may develop after prolonged use of aspirin. The features are papillary necrosis and interstitial fibrosis. NSAIDs precipitate fluid retention and heart failure.

- *Platelet function* – while altered platelet function may be advantageous in certain circumstances (acute myocardial infarction and prevention of stroke), during the peri-operative period it may cause increased blood loss. The reduced production of cyclic endoperoxidases and thromboxane A$_2$ prevents platelet aggregation and vasoconstriction and, therefore, inhibits the haemostatic process. The effects of aspirin on platelets last for the lifespan of the platelet for two reasons: platelets are unable to generate new cyclo-oxygenase and the enzyme inhibition is irreversible. Up to 14 days are required to generate new platelets. COX-2 inhibition has no effect on platelet function even at high doses.

- *Drug interactions* – caution should be exercised when NSAIDs are administered with anticoagulants such as heparin or warfarin, especially as the latter may be displaced from its plasma protein-binding sites, increasing its effects. Serum lithium may be increased when administered with NSAIDs and its levels should, therefore, be monitored.

- *Hepatotoxicity* – this is normally observed following prolonged or excessive use of NSAIDs. Up to 15% of patients may experience a rise in serum transaminase levels, even following short courses.

Non-Specific COX Inhibitors

Aspirin

Uses

Aspirin (acetylsalicylic acid; see Figure 10.5) is widely used for its analgesic and anti-inflammatory effects. It is also used for its effects on platelet function in acute myocardial infarction and the prevention of stroke.

Mechanism of Action

At low dose, aspirin selectively inhibits platelet cyclo-oxygenase while preserving vessel wall cyclo-oxygenase. This has the effect of reducing TXA_2-induced vasoconstriction and platelet aggregation while leaving vessel wall synthesis of prostaglandins unaltered and, therefore, dilated.

Other Effects

• *Metabolic* – aspirin also has effects on the metabolic state, which are usually of little significance, but in overdose these become significant. It uncouples oxidative phosphorylation, thereby increasing oxygen consumption and carbon dioxide production. Initially minute ventilation is increased to keep $PaCO_2$ static. However, when aspirin levels are increased significantly the respiratory centre is stimulated directly causing a respiratory alkalosis. The picture is complicated in the premorbid state by a metabolic acidosis. However, in children the respiratory centre is depressed by rising aspirin levels, and a metabolic acidosis occurs earlier so that a mixed respiratory and metabolic acidosis is more common.

Features of Aspirin Overdose

Common

- Usually conscious – only unconscious in massive overdose
- Sweaty
- Tinnitus
- Blurred vision
- Tachycardia
- Pyrexia

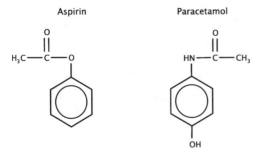

Aspirin Paracetamol

Figure 10.5 Structures of aspirin and paracetamol.

- Hyperventilation
- Respiratory alkalosis (subsequently complicated by metabolic acidosis).

Rare

- Nausea and vomiting, epigastric pain
- Oliguria
- GI bleed
- Pulmonary oedema (due to increased capillary permeability)
- Coagulopathy
- Hypokalaemia
- Hypo- or hyperglycaemia
- Encephalopathic, unconscious.

Treatment

- Activated charcoal
- Forced alkaline diuresis
- Haemofiltration/haemodialysis.

Reye's syndrome is uncommon and mainly affects children. Its aetiology has been linked to aspirin. It causes widespread mitochondrial damage, fatty changes in the liver progressing to hepatic failure, encephalopathy with cerebral oedema and has a mortality rate of up to 40%. Therefore, aspirin is only recommended for children below 12 years of age when specifically indicated, for example, for juvenile arthritis (Still's disease).

Kinetics

Aspirin is a weak acid with a pK_a of 3 and is present essentially in the unionised form in the stomach allowing gastric absorption, but due to the relatively alkaline nature of the mucosal cells salicylate ions may become trapped and unable to reach the systemic circulation. However, due to total surface area the small bowel absorbs more drug. Once in the systemic circulation, 85% is protein-bound, mainly by albumin. It is rapidly hydrolysed by intestinal and hepatic esterases to salicylate, which undergoes further hepatic metabolism to salicyluric acid and glucuronide derivatives. Salicylate and its metabolites are excreted in the urine (enhanced under alkaline conditions). The elimination half-life varies because glycine conjugation (converting salicylate to salicyluric acid) may become saturated in overdose resulting in zero-order kinetics.

Paracetamol

While paracetamol (see Figure 10.5) has essentially no effect on cyclo-oxygenase in vitro it has been classified as a NSAID because of its moderate analgesic and antipyretic properties. It has been proposed that its antipyretic actions are due to inhibition of prostaglandin synthesis within the CNS, by inhibition of COX-3, a COX-1 variant.

Presentation and Uses

Paracetamol is presented as 500 mg tablets alone and in combination with weak opioids. Suppositories contain 125 mg and 1 g and the paediatric elixir contains 120 mg in 5 ml.

A preparation containing 100 mg methionine and 500 mg paracetamol is available but at increased cost. A solution of 1 g or 500 mg in 100 ml is available for intravenous use.

Dose schedules have become more complicated with the advent of intravenous paracetamol. Patients weighing less than 50 kg should receive 15 mg.kg^{-1} and a maximum dose of 60 mg.kg^{-1}.day^{-1}. The initial paediatric dose is 15–30 mg.kg^{-1} which is then reduced to 10–15 mg.kg^{-1} every 4 hours with a maximum dose of 60 mg.kg^{-1}.day^{-1}.

Kinetics

Paracetamol is absorbed well from the small bowel and has an oral bioavailability of 80%. Unlike the other NSAIDs it does not cause gastric irritation, is less protein-bound (10%) and has a larger volume of distribution. Paracetamol is metabolised by the liver mainly to glucuronide conjugates but also to sulfate and cysteine conjugates. These are actively excreted in the urine, only a small fraction being excreted unchanged. N-acetyl-p-amino-benzoquinone imine is a highly toxic metabolite of paracetamol that is produced in small amounts following therapeutic doses. It is rapidly conjugated with hepatic glutathione to render it harmless.

Toxicity

Following a toxic dose, the normal hepatic conjugation pathways become saturated so that more N-acetyl-p-amino-benzoquinone imine is produced which rapidly exhausts hepatic glutathione. It is then free to form covalent bonds with sulfhydryl groups on hepatocytes resulting in cell death and centrilobular hepatic necrosis. Treatment with oral methionine and oral or intravenous acetylcysteine is directed at replenishing hepatic glutathione. Methionine enhances glutathione synthesis while acetylcysteine is hydrolysed to cysteine, which is a glutathione precursor. Intravenous acetylcysteine is preferred as vomiting is common in paracetamol overdose.

Features of Paracetamol Overdose

- Normally remain conscious
- Nausea and vomiting
- Epigastric pain
- Sweating
- Erythema, urticaria, mucosal lesions
- Acute haemolytic anaemia
- Peripheral vasodilatation and shock following massive overdose
- Delayed hyperglycaemia
- Hepatic failure after 48 hours
- Liver function and clotting worst at 3–5 days
- Cholestasis
- Fulminant hepatic failure at 3–7 days.

Treatment

- Activated charcoal within 1 hour of ingestion
- Early intravenous acetylcysteine
- Fluids and antiemetics
- Early referral to specialist centre.

Diclofenac

Diclofenac is a phenylacetic acid derivative.

Presentation

Diclofenac is available as an oral, rectal and parenteral formulation. The maximum adult dose is 150 mg.day^{-1} in divided doses. The paediatric dose is 1 mg.kg^{-1} tds for pain associated with minor surgery (tonsillectomy, inguinal herniotomy).

Uses

Diclofenac may be used alone to treat mild to moderate post-operative pain or to reduce opioid consumption when treating severe pain. It is particularly useful in treating renal colic. Side effects limit its use in major surgery.

Other Effects

- *Cardiovascular* – diclofenac is associated with an increased risk of coronary events at a rate similar to the COX-2 inhibitors during chronic use. It should not be considered a first-line agent.
  Renal – like all NSAIDs it may precipitate renal impairment, especially in major surgery.
  Gut – diclofenac produces less gastric irritation than both indomethacin and aspirin.
  Pain – the parenteral formulation is highly irritant and intramuscular injection may be very painful and is associated with muscle damage. Intravenous injection causes local thrombosis.
  Interactions – plasma concentrations of lithium and digoxin may be increased. In general it does not affect either oral anticoagulants or oral hypoglycaemic agents, but isolated reports would suggest that close monitoring is used.

Kinetics

In keeping with other drugs in its class, diclofenac is well absorbed from the gut, highly plasma protein-bound (99%) and has a small volume of distribution (0.15 l.kg^{-1}). It undergoes hepatic hydroxylation and conjugation to inactive metabolites that are excreted in the urine (60%) and bile (40%).

Ketorolac

Ketorolac is an acetic acid derivative with potent analgesic activity but limited anti-inflammatory activity. It is also a potent antipyretic. It may be given orally or parenterally and has a duration of action of up to 6 hours. It shares the side-effect profile common to all NSAIDs.

Phenylbutazone

Phenylbutazone is a potent anti-inflammatory agent. Its use has been limited to hospital patients with ankylosing spondylitis due to serious haematological side effects including granulocytosis and aplastic anaemia. It is significantly bound by plasma proteins and will interact with other highly bound drugs. It may also impair hepatic function, produce a rash, and cause sodium and water retention.

Ibuprofen

Ibuprofen use has increased as the adverse effects of other NSAIDs have been exposed. Like other proprionates, it has a chiral centre and forms a racemic mixture of 2 enantiomers. Much of the inactive (R) enantiomer is converted by an isomerase to the active (S) enantiomer, dexibuprofen, in the gut and liver.

Presentation

Ibuprofen is available as tablets, an oral suspension and in topical preparations. There is no parenteral or rectal preparation.

Dose

The normal adult dose is 400 mg tds, although this can be increased to 800 mg tds. The lower dose is not associated with an increase in prothrombotic events, the side effect which has changed the complexion of NSAID prescribing. The paediatric dose is 10 mg.kg^{-1} tds.

Side-Effect Profile

It has fewer side effects than many other NSAIDs but has weaker anti-inflammatory effects and at doses below 1.2 g.day^{-1} may not be effective in chronic inflammatory conditions.

Kinetics

Ibuprofen is rapidly absorbed from the gut and is highly plasma protein-bound. It is metabolised by hepatic cytochrome P450 to inactive hydroxy and carboxy metabolites. Glucuronidation forms a minor part of its metabolism. All metabolic products are eliminated renally.

Tenoxicam

Tenoxicam exhibits many of the features common with other NSAIDs. Two specific features make it particularly useful in the peri-operative period:

- It may be given intravenously resulting in a rapid onset of action.
- It has a long elimination half-life (72 hours) resulting in a long duration of action and allowing once-daily dosage.

However, these advantages may become disadvantages if side effects become significant.

Kinetics

Tenoxicam is well absorbed from the gut and has a high oral bioavailability. It is highly plasma protein-bound (99%). Clearance from the body is due to metabolism to an inactive metabolite that is excreted in the urine (66%) and in bile (33%). The dose is 20 mg.day^{-1}.

Preferential COX-2 Inhibitors

Meloxicam

Meloxicam is available as tablets and suppositories and the initial dose is 7.5 mg.day^{-1}, which may be doubled.

Meloxicam has limited preferential selectivity for COX-2 and is quoted as being between three and 50 times as potent against COX-2. At a dose of 7.5 mg.day^{-1} it has a reduced GI side-effect profile when compared with diclofenac, although its renal side-effect profile appears to be equivalent to other NSAIDs.

Kinetics

Meloxicam is slowly but almost completely absorbed from the gut with an oral bioavailability of 90%. It is 99% protein-bound, essentially to albumin. Metabolism occurs in the liver to inactive metabolites that are excreted in the urine (50%) and bile (50%). The elimination half-life is 20 hours.

Specific COX-2 Inhibitors

(See Figure 10.6.) The COX-2 enzyme was first discovered in 1988 and since then has generated legal fees in proportion to its potential to revolutionise the use of NSAIDs. The prospect of a new class of NSAID without GI side effects was a game changer. Unfortunately, not only was the improved GI side-effect profile not as good as hoped for, but another set of side effects – major vascular events – became evident. To make matters worse rofecoxib, the first licensed COX-2 inhibitor, had been prescribed to 80 million patients over 5 years (generating an annual revenue of USD 2.5 billion) prior to its withdrawal in 2004. Since that time the manufacturer has paid out hundreds of millions of dollars by way of compensation, legal settlement and fines.

The Committee on Safety of Medicines have advised that COX-2 use is contraindicated in patients with ischaemic heart disease, cerebrovascular disease, mild heart failure and peripheral vascular disease. Careful consideration should be given before their use in patients with risk factors for cardiovascular events (hypertension, hyperlipidaemia, diabetes, smoking).

Celecoxib

Celecoxib is presented as 100 mg tablets and used to a maximum dose of 200 mg bd for chronic pain associated with osteoarthritis and rheumatoid arthritis. It has also demonstrated efficacy in the post-operative setting. It has a COX-1:COX-2 inhibitory ratio of 1:30.

The CLASS trial demonstrated the incidence of ulcer complications in patients treated with celecoxib was similar to those treated with non-specific NSAIDs, although this may have been confused by concurrent aspirin therapy. Also the incidence of stroke and myocardial infarction was not increased by celecoxib. The picture is confused however by meta-analyses that have demonstrated that COX-2 inhibitors do increase coronary events. Like all COX-2 inhibitors it is recommended that it should be avoided in those with, or at risk of, ischaemic heart disease or cerebrovascular disease.

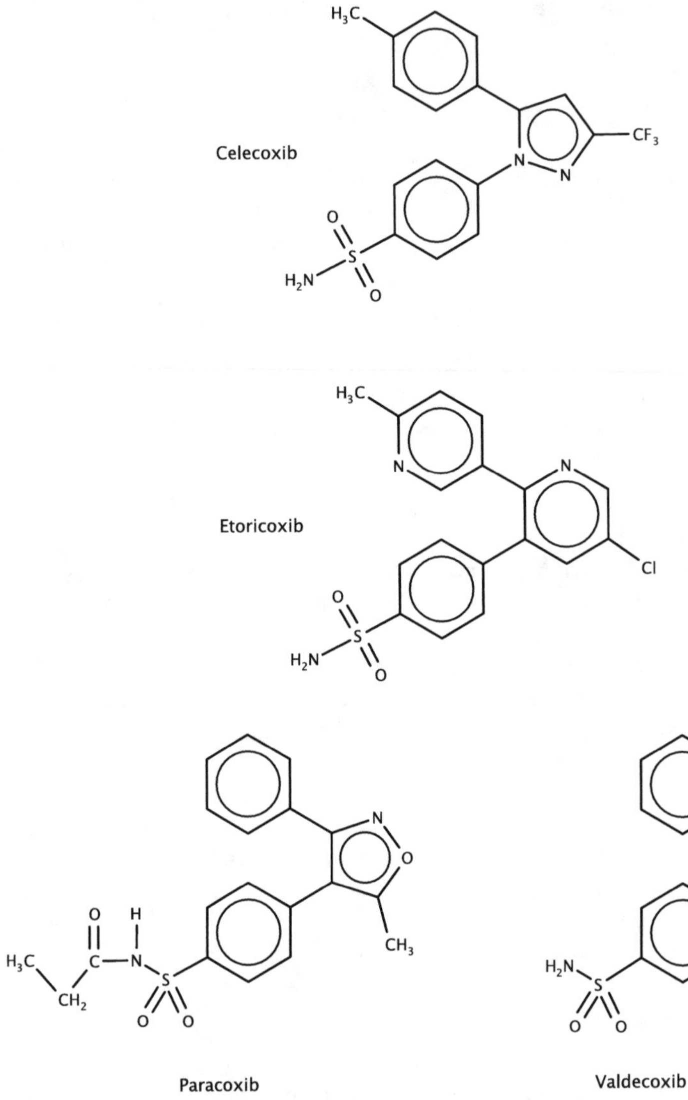

Figure 10.6 Structures of some COX-2 inhibitors.

Kinetics

Celecoxib reaches peak plasma concentration after 2–3 hours and has an elimination half-life of 8–12 hours. It is 97% protein-bound and has a volume of distribution of 5.7 l.kg^{-1}. It is metabolised by hepatic CYP2C9 to inactive metabolites so that only a small amount appears unchanged in the urine. Drugs that inhibit (omeprazole) or induce (carbamazepine) CYP2C9 will increase or decrease plasma concentrations.

Celecoxib has a sulfonamide group and therefore should not be used in patients with a sulfonamide allergy.

Valdecoxib and Parecoxib

Parecoxib is a prodrug that is converted to the active moiety valdecoxib. Its plasma half-life is 20 minutes and it has no actions of its own. Valdecoxib has been withdrawn (April 2005) due to serious dermatological side effects (see 'Kinetics' below). Parecoxib remains in use and has not been associated with similar dermatological side effects, probably due to its short-term use. It has a COX-1:COX-2 inhibitory ratio of 1:61.

Parecoxib is a parenteral COX-2 antagonist and should be reconstituted with 0.9% saline prior to administration. The initial dose is 40 mg followed by 20–40 mg 6–12 hourly up to a maximum dose of 80 mg.day^{-1}.

Kinetics

Parecoxib is converted to valdecoxib by enzymatic hydrolysis in the liver. Valdecoxib undergoes hepatic metabolism by CYP2C9, CYP3A4 and glucuronidation to many metabolites, one of which antagonises COX-2. Due to its hepatic elimination, renal impairment does not influence its kinetics, but it is not recommended in severe hepatic impairment.

The dose should be reduced when co-administered with fluconazole due to inhibition of CYP2C9, although no adjustment is necessary when co-administered with ketoconazole or midazolam which is metabolised by CYP3A4. Valdecoxib appears to inhibit other cytochrome P450 enzymes and may increase the plasma concentration of flecainide and metoprolol (CYP2D6 inhibition), and omeprazole, phenytoin and diazepam (CYP2C19 inhibition).

Parecoxib has a plasma half-life of 20 minutes while valdecoxib has an elimination half-life of 8 hours.

Hypersensitivity reactions including exfoliative dermatitis, Stevens–Johnson syndrome, toxic dermal necrolysis and angioedema have been reported following valdecoxib in those who also have sulfonamide sensitivity. The overall reporting rate is in the order of eight per million patients. It is, therefore, contraindicated in this group. However, parecoxib has a non-aromatic sulfonamide group similar to frusemide and tolbutamide, neither of which is contraindicated in sulfonamide sensitivity.

Etoricoxib

Etoricoxib is a highly selective COX-2 inhibitor that has a UK licence but is not currently approved for use in USA. It is a methylsulfone.

It has been shown to be efficacious in providing effective pain control when compared to COX-1 inhibitors. It has a COX-1:COX-2 inhibitory ratio of 1:344.

Kinetics

Etoricoxib is absorbed efficiently producing an oral bioavailability of > 95%. It has a volume of distribution of 1.5 l.kg^{-1} and is 90% plasma protein-bound. Its elimination half-life is 22 hours. It is metabolised in the liver through cytochrome P450 oxidation, CYP3A4 being the predominant isoenzyme. However, other isoenzymes are involved and may become more involved with specific CYP3A4 inhibition. It is a weak inhibitor of CYP-2D6, -3A, and -2C9. Its elimination half-life increases in hepatic failure, but in isolated renal failure no change is seen.

Its side effects (or lack of them) are predictable. Its rate of gastric irritation is similar to placebo and significantly lower than COX-1 inhibitors, although this effect decreases beyond 9–12 months of therapy. The little information that exists suggests that etoricoxib carries a similar major vascular event risk profile to diclofenac.

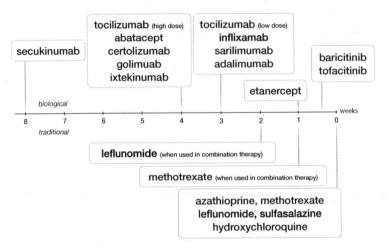

Figure 10.7 Summary of the number of weeks that certain agents should be withheld preoperatively. These values should be increased by a factor of 2.5 for high risk (abdominal & revision arthroplasty) surgery.

Disease Modifying Anti-Rheumatic Drugs

Disease modifying anti-rheumatic drugs (DMARDs) are not primarily analgesics, rather they modify the course of diseases that are often painful and thereby reduce pain. They are indicated in the treatment of rheumatoid arthritis as well as other types of autoimmune disease including vasculitis and inflammatory bowel disease. They have immunosuppressant properties and require careful peri-operative management (see Figure 10.7).

Traditional Disease Modifying Anti-Rheumatic Drugs

Traditional DMARDs include drugs that have been available for many years such as methotrexate, leflunomide, hydroxychloroquine, and sulfasalazine. Others include cyclophosphamide, cyclosporine, and tacrolimus.

Methotrexate can be given via the oral or parenteral route. Dosing is weekly, which has caused significant drug errors due to poor prescribing practice in the past. Its immunosuppressive properties come from its structural similarity to folate. It competitively inhibits the binding of dihydrofolate to the enzyme dihydrofolate reductase. This reduces the amount of active component available for metabolic pathways involving purine and pyrimidine metabolism, amino acid synthesis and polyamine synthesis. In addition, methotrexate works via extracellular dephosphorylation of adenine nucleosides to increase extracellular concentrations of adenosine, a potent anti-inflammatory. Methotrexate also has widespread effects on T cells and mononuclear cells. Methotrexate should be avoided in women who are pregnant or whom intend to become pregnant due to its teratogenic effects. It is directly embryotoxic and has been used in the management of ectopic pregnancy. It is contraindicated in those with renal disease and other side effects include pulmonary and hepatotoxicity. Bone marrow suppression can develop abruptly so regular blood tests are required and patients are advised to report the features of infection, bruising, mouth ulcers or shortness of breath which could indicate complications such as bone marrow suppression, infection or GI mucosal problems. Administration of folate may reduce these symptoms with no reduction in dose efficacy.

Sulfasalazine is a prodrug formed of 5-aminosalicylic acid (5-ASA) linked to sulfapyridine and is used in inflammatory bowel disease and rheumatoid arthritis. Metabolism in the large bowel results in its constituent parts. The mechanism of action is not entirely clear but it is known that the active ingredient in rheumatoid arthritis is sulfapyridine and in inflammatory bowel disease it is 5-ASA. Common side effects are insomnia, taste disturbance and tinnitus. Agranulocytosis is a rare but serious side effect and the blood count should be monitored regularly and patients encouraged to report any unexplained bruising, bleeding or signs of infection.

Hydroxychloroquine is an antimalarial drug also useful in the management of rheumatoid arthritis and systemic lupus. Common side effects include abdominal pain, diarrhoea and emotional lability. Retinal screening is recommended after long-term use. Hydroxychloroquine is extremely toxic in overdose. It causes sodium channel blockade resulting in neurological features including coma, and cardiac features that occur early and include prolonged QTc, Torsades des Pointes and cardiac arrest. The degree of toxicity is closely related to the ingested dose and to the degree of hypokalaemia on presentation to hospital.

Biological Disease Modifying Anti-Rheumatic Drugs

The biological agents are a more recent class of drugs developed to target various specific aspects of the immune system. Their mechanisms of action are varied and include interfering with cytokine function, signal transduction or production, inhibition of T-cell activation and depletion of B cells. A detailed discussion of these drugs is beyond the scope of this book, however, all have the potential to cause life-threatening myelosuppression and subsequent symptoms as well as reactivation of latent infections including TB and susceptibility to new infections. Wound healing may also be impaired.

Restarting Disease Modifying Anti-Rheumatic Drugs Post-Operatively

Disease modifying anti-rheumatic drugs can be recommended 2 weeks post-operatively as long as wound healing is satisfactory and there are no signs of infection. If in doubt these drugs should be withheld. Tocilizumab inhibits IL6 production which is the key cytokine involved with C reactive peptide (CRP) production, therefore a CRP rise may be delayed in patients presenting with post-operative infection.

Local Anaesthetics

Physiology

Individual nerve fibres are made up of a central core (axoplasm) and a phospholipid membrane containing integral proteins, some of which function as ion channels.

The Resting Membrane Potential

The neuronal membrane contains the enzyme Na^+/K^+ ATPase that actively maintains a thirty-fold K^+ concentration gradient (greater concentration inside) and a ten-fold Na^+ concentration gradient (greater concentration outside). K^+ tends to flow down its concentration gradient out of the cell due to the selective permeability of the membrane. However, intracellular anionic proteins tend to oppose this ionic flux, and the balance of these processes results in the resting membrane potential of -80 mV (negative inside). It can, therefore, be seen that the ratio of intracellular to extracellular K^+ alters the resting membrane potential. Hypokalaemia increases (makes more negative) the resting membrane potential while the Na^+ concentration has little effect, as the membrane is essentially impermeable to Na^+ when in the resting state.

The Action Potential

The action potential is generated by altered Na^+ permeability across the phospholipid membrane and lasts only 1–2 milliseconds. Electrical or chemical triggers initially cause a slow rise in membrane potential until the threshold potential (about -50 mV) is reached. Voltage-sensitive Na^+ channels then open, increasing Na^+ permeability dramatically and the membrane potential briefly reaches +30 mV (approaching the Na^+ equilibrium potential of +67 mV), at which point the Na^+ channels close. The membrane potential returns to its resting value with an increased efflux of K^+. The Na^+/K^+ ATPase restores the concentration gradients although the total number of ions moving across the membrane is small. Conduction along unmyelinated fibres is relatively slow compared with myelinated fibres where current jumps from one node of Ranvier to another (saltatory conduction) and reaches 120 m.s^{-1}. Retrograde conduction is not possible under normal circumstances due to inactive Na^+ channels following the action potential (see Figure 11.1).

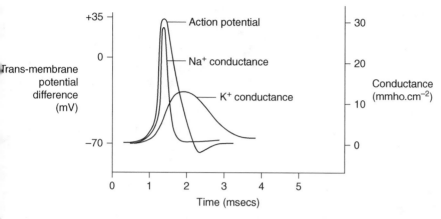

Figure 11.1 Changes in Na^+ and K^+ conductance during the action potential.

Local Anaesthetics

Preparations

Local anaesthetics are formulated as the hydrochloride salt to render them water-soluble. They often contain the preservative sodium metabisulfite and a fungicide. Multi-dose bottles contain 1 mg.ml^{-1} of the preservative methyl parahydroxybenzoate. Only the single-dose ampoules without additives (apart from glucose at 80 mg.ml^{-1} used in 'heavy' bupivacaine) are suitable for subarachnoid administration as the preservatives carry the risk of producing arachnoiditis. Adrenaline or felypressin (a synthetic derivative of vasopressin with no antidiuretic effect) are added to some local anaesthetic solutions in an attempt to slow down absorption from the site of injection and to prolong the duration of action. Lidocaine is available in a large range of concentrations varying from 0.5% to 10%. The high concentrations are used as a spray to anaesthetise mucous membranes (note $1\% = 10$ mg.ml^{-1}).

Mechanism of Action

Local anaesthetic action is dependent on blockade of the Na^+ channel. Unionised lipid-soluble drug passes through the phospholipid membrane where in the axoplasm it is protonated. In this ionised form it binds to the internal surface of a Na^+ channel, preventing it from leaving the inactive state. The degree of blockade in vitro is proportional to the rate of stimulation due to the attraction of local anaesthetic to 'open' Na^+ channels (see Figure 11.2).

Alternatively, 'membrane expansion' may offer an additional mechanism of action. Unionised drug dissolves into the phospholipid membrane and may cause swelling of the Na^+ channel/lipoprotein matrix resulting in its inactivation.

Physiochemical Characteristics

Local anaesthetics are weak bases and exist predominantly in the ionised form at neutral pH as their pK$_a$ exceeds 7.4. They fall into one of two chemical groupings, ester or amide, which

Local anaesthetic

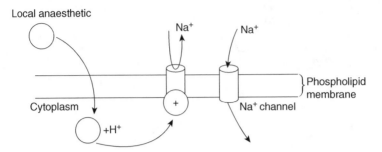

Figure 11.2 Mechanism of action of local anaesthetics.

Table 11.1 Classification of local anaesthetics

Esters –CO.O–	Amides –NH.CO–
Procaine	Lidocaine
Amethocaine	Prilocaine
Cocaine	Bupivacaine
	Ropivacaine
	Dibucaine

describes the linkage between the aromatic lipophilic group and the hydrophilic group that each group possesses. Esters are comparatively unstable in solution, unlike amides that have a shelf-life of up to 2 years (see Table 11.1; Figure 11.3).

The individual structures confer different physiochemical and clinical characteristics.

- **Potency** is closely correlated to **lipid solubility** in vitro, but less so in vivo. Other factors such as vasodilator properties and tissue distribution determine the amount of local anaesthetic that is available at the nerve.
- **The duration of action** is closely associated with the extent of **protein binding**. Local anaesthetics with limited protein binding have a short duration of action, and conversely those with more extensive protein binding have a longer duration of action.
- **The onset of action** is closely related to pK_a. Local anaesthetics are weak bases and exist mainly in the ionised form at normal pH. Those with a high pK_a have a greater fraction present in the ionised form, which is unable to penetrate the phospholipid membrane, resulting in a slow onset of action. Conversely, a low pK_a reflects a higher fraction present in the unionised form and, therefore, a faster onset of action as more is available to cross the phospholipid membrane.
- The intrinsic **vasodilator activity** varies between drugs and influences **potency** and **duration of action**. In general, local anaesthetics cause vasodilatation in low concentrations (prilocaine > lidocaine > bupivacaine > ropivacaine) and vasoconstriction at higher concentrations. However, cocaine has solely vasoconstrictor actions by inhibiting neuronal uptake of catecholamines (uptake 1) and inhibiting monoamine oxidase MAOs.

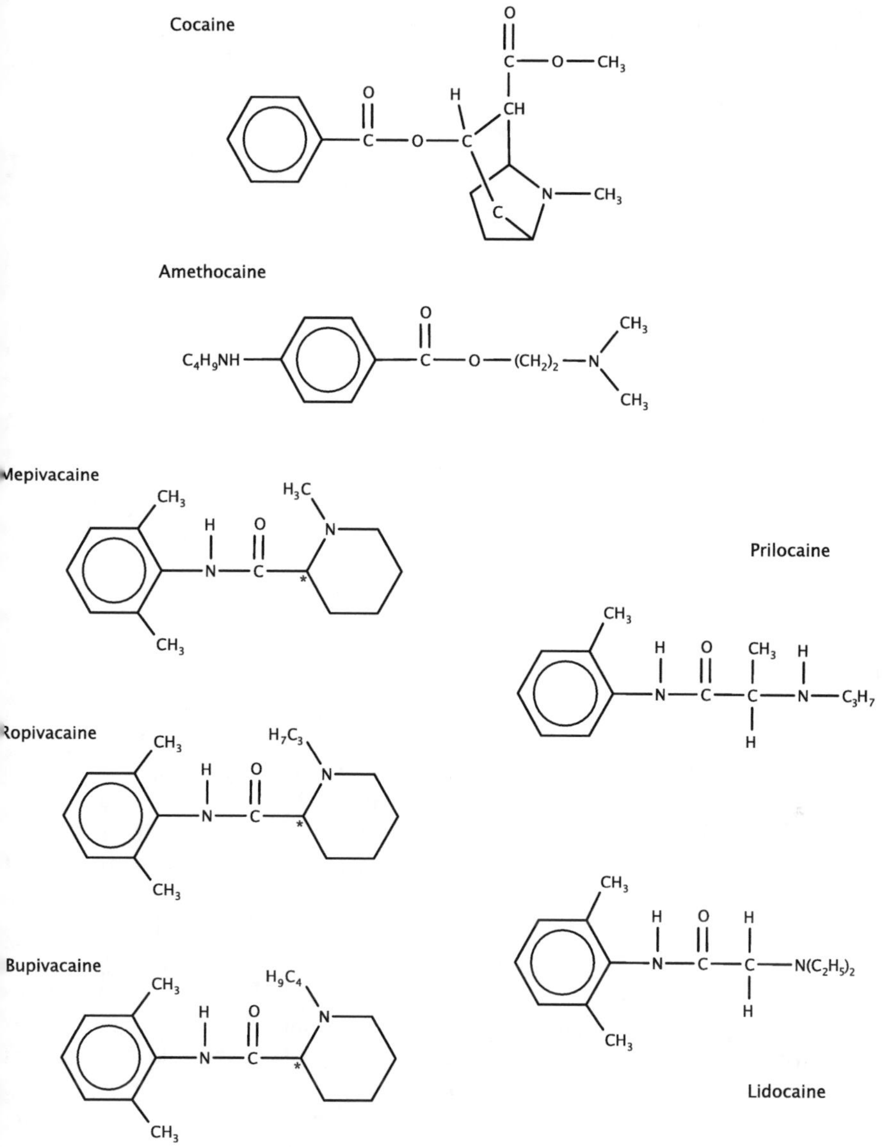

Figure 11.3 Structure of some local anaesthetics. Asterisk marks chiral centre.

However, total dose and concentration of administered local anaesthetic will also have a significant effect on a given clinical situation.

Local anaesthetics are generally ineffective when used to anaesthetise infected tissue. The acidic environment further reduces the unionised fraction of drug available to diffuse into and block the nerve. There may also be increased local vascularity, which increases removal of drug from the site.

Lidocaine: $pK_a = 7.9$

At pH 7.4

$$pH = pKa + \log\left\{\frac{[B]}{[BH^+]}\right\}$$

$$7.4 = 7.9 + \log\left\{\frac{[B]}{[BH^+]}\right\}$$

$$-0.5 = \log\left\{\frac{[B]}{[BH^+]}\right\}$$

$$0.3 = \left\{\frac{[B]}{[BH^+]}\right\}$$

so 75% ionised and 25% unionised.
   At pH of 7.1

$$7.1 = 7.9 + \log\left\{\frac{[B]}{[BH^+]}\right\}$$

$$0.16 = \left\{\frac{[B]}{[BH^+]}\right\}$$

so 86% ionised and 14% unionised (i.e. less available to penetrate nerves).

Other Effects

- *Cardiac* – lidocaine may be used to treat ventricular arrhythmias, while bupivacaine is not. Both drugs block cardiac Na^+ channels and decrease the maximum rate of increase of phase 0 of the cardiac action potential (see Chapter 15). They also have direct myocardial depressant properties (bupivacaine > lidocaine). The PR and QRS intervals are also increased and the refractory period prolonged. However, bupivacaine is 10 times slower at dissociating from the Na^+ channels, resulting in persistent depression. This may lead to re-entrant arrhythmias and ventricular fibrillation. In addition, tachycardia may enhance frequency-dependent blockade by bupivacaine, which adds to its cardiac toxicity. Life-threatening arrhythmias may also reflect disruption of Ca^{2+} and K^+ channels. Ropivacaine differs from bupivacaine both in the substitution of a propyl for a butyl group and in its preparation as a single, S, enantiomer. It dissociates more rapidly from cardiac Na^+ channels and produces less direct myocardial depression than bupivacaine, and is, therefore, less toxic. However, it has a slightly shorter duration of action and is slightly less potent than bupivacaine, resulting in a slightly larger dose requirement for an equivalent block.
- *Central nervous system* – local anaesthetics penetrate the brain rapidly and have a bi-phasic effect. Initially inhibitory interneurones are blocked, resulting in excitatory phenomena – circumoral tingling, visual disturbance, tremors and dizziness. This is followed by convulsions. Finally, all central neurones are depressed leading to coma and apnoea.

Kinetics

Absorption

The absorption of local anaesthetics into the systemic circulation varies depending on the characteristics of the agent used, the presence of added vasoconstrictor and the site of injection.

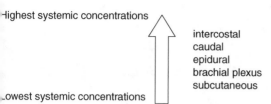

Highest systemic concentrations

intercostal
caudal
epidural
brachial plexus
subcutaneous

Lowest systemic concentrations

Clearly, if local anaesthetic is inadvertently injected into a vein or artery, very high systemic levels will result and possibly cause CNS or cardiovascular toxicity. Less than 10 mg lidocaine inadvertently injected into the carotid or vertebral artery will result in a rapid rise in CNS concentrations and will cause coma and possibly apnoea and cardiac arrest.

Distribution

Ester local anaesthetics are minimally bound while amides are more extensively bound (bupivacaine > ropivacaine > lidocaine > prilocaine) in the plasma. α_1-Acid glycoprotein binds local anaesthetic with high affinity although albumin binds a greater quantity due to its relative abundance. When protein binding is increased (pregnancy, myocardial infarction, renal failure, post-operatively and in infancy) the free fraction of drug is reduced.

The degree of protein binding will affect the degree of placental transfer. Bupivacaine is more highly bound than lidocaine, so less crosses the placenta. If the fetus becomes acidotic there will be an increase in the ionised fraction and local anaesthetic will accumulate in the fetus (ion trapping). Ester local anaesthetics do not cross the placenta in significant amounts due to their rapid metabolism.

Metabolism and Elimination

Esters are hydrolysed rapidly by plasma cholinesterases and other esterases to inactive compounds. Para-aminobenzoate is one of the main metabolites and has been associated with hypersensitivity reactions especially in the atopic patient. This rapid hydrolysis results in a short elimination half-life. Cocaine is the exception, undergoing hepatic hydrolysis to water-soluble metabolites that are excreted in the urine.

Amides undergo hepatic metabolism by amidases. Amidase metabolism is much slower than plasma hydrolysis and so amides are more prone to accumulation when administered by continuous infusion. Reduced hepatic blood flow or hepatic dysfunction can decrease amide metabolism.

Toxicity

Raised systemic blood levels of local anaesthetic lead initially to the CNS and then to cardiovascular toxicity. However, the absorption of local anaesthetic varies widely depending on the site of administration and presence of vasoconstrictors. Therefore, the concept of a toxic dose without regard to the site of administration is meaningless. The toxic plasma levels are given in Table 11.2.

Table 11.2 Some pharmacological properties of various local anaesthetics

	Relative potency	Onset	Duration of action	Toxic plasma concentration ($\mu g.ml^{-1}$)	pK_a	Percentage unionised (at pH 7.4)	Plasma protein-bound (%)	Relative lipid solubility	Elimination half-life (mins)
Amethocaine	8	slow	long		8.5	7	75	200	80
Cocaine		moderate	short	0.5	8.6	5	95		100
Lidocaine	2	fast	moderate	> 5	7.9	25	70	150	100
Prilocaine	2	fast	moderate	> 5	7.7	33	55	50	100
Bupivacaine	8	moderate	long	> 1.5	8.1	15	95	1000	160
Ropivacaine	8	moderate	long	> 4	8.1	15	94	300	120

Intralipid

In cases of toxicity supportive treatment has been superseded by treatment with intravenous lipid emulsion (e.g. intralipid, a component of parenteral nutrition). Its mechanism of action centres around its ability to function as a 'lipid sink'. As such it binds the local anaesthetic (and many other drugs with high lipid solubility), effectively removing it from its target organ. In addition lipids may provide an alternative energy substrate, offsetting LA inhibition of fatty acid metabolism and may prevent Na^+ channel inhibition.

Dose

Initial bolus of 20% intralipid of 1.5 $mg.kg^{-1}$ over 1 minute, followed by an infusion of 0.25 $ml.kg^{-1}.min^{-1}$. The bolus may be repeated and the infusion rate doubled in resistant cases. The maximum dose over the first 30 minutes is 10 $ml.kg^{-1}$.

Adverse Effects

The adverse effects associated with acute infusion of intralipid includes acute kidney injury, cardiac arrest, ventilation perfusion mismatch, acute lung injury, venous thromboembolism, hypersensitivity, fat embolism, fat overload syndrome, pancreatitis, allergic reaction, and increased susceptibility to infection. These appear to be related to both the rate of infusion as well as the total dose administered.

Intravenous Regional Anaesthesia

Bupivacaine has been used for intravenous regional techniques, but following a number of deaths attributed to cardiac toxicity it is no longer used in this way. Prilocaine (0.5%) is commonly used in this setting although lidocaine may also be used.

Lidocaine

Lidocaine is an amide local anaesthetic that is also used to control ventricular tachyarrhythmias. It has class Ib anti-arrhythmic actions (see Chapter 15).

Preparations

Lidocaine is formulated as the hydrochloride and is presented as a colourless solution 0.5–2%) with or without adrenaline (1 in 80–200,000); a 2% gel; a 5% ointment; a spray delivering 10 mg per dose and a 4% solution for topical use on mucous membranes.

Kinetics

Lidocaine is 70% protein-bound to α_1-acid glycoprotein. It is extensively metabolised in the liver by dealkylation to monoethylglycine-xylidide and acetaldehyde. The former is further hydrolysed while the latter is hydroxylated to 4-hydroxy-2,6-xylidine forming the main metabolite, which is excreted in the urine. Some of the metabolic products of lidocaine have anti-arrhythmic properties while others may potentiate lidocaine-induced seizures.

Clearance is reduced in the presence of hepatic or cardiac failure.

Eutectic Mixture of Local Anaesthetic

When two compounds are mixed to produce a substance that behaves with a single set of physical characteristics, it is said to be eutectic. Eutectic mixture of local anaesthetic (EMLA) (5%) contains a mixture of crystalline bases of 2.5% lidocaine and 2.5% prilocaine in a white oil:water emulsion. The mixture has a lower melting point, being an oil at room temperature, while the individual components would be crystalline solids.

Presentation and Uses

Eutectic mixture of local anaesthetic is presented as an emulsion in tubes containing 5 g or 30 g. It is used to anaesthetise skin before vascular cannulation or harvesting for skin grafts. It should be applied to intact skin under an occlusive dressing for at least 60 minutes to ensure adequate anaesthesia.

Cautions

Eutectic mixture of local anaesthetic cream should be avoided in patients with congenital or idiopathic methaemoglobinaemia, or in infants less than 12 months of age who are receiving treatment with methaemoglobin-inducing drugs. Patients taking drugs associated with methaemoglobinaemia (e.g. sulfonamides or phenytoin) are at greater risk of developing methaemoglobinaemia if concurrently treated with EMLA cream. Methaemoglobinaemia is caused by o-toluidine, a metabolite of prilocaine.

EMLA should not be used on mucous membranes due to rapid systemic absorption. EMLA should be used with caution in patients receiving class I anti-arrhythmic drugs (e.g. tocainide, mexiletine) because the toxic effects are additive and potentially synergistic.

Bupivacaine

Presentation and Uses

Bupivacaine is prepared as a 0.25% and 0.5% (with or without 1:200,000 adrenaline) solution. A 0.5% preparation containing 80 $mg.ml^{-1}$ glucose (specific gravity 1.026) is available for subarachnoid block.

Bupivacaine remains the mainstay of epidural infusions in labour and postoperatively despite concerns regarding its potential cardiac toxicity and the availability of newer drugs (ropivacaine and levobupivacaine). The maximum dose is said to be 2 $mg.kg^{-1}$.

Kinetics

The onset of action is intermediate or slow and significantly slower than that of lidocaine. It is the most highly protein-bound amide local anaesthetic and is metabolised in the liver by dealkylation to pipecolic acid and pipecolylxylidine.

Levobupivacaine

Levobupivacaine is the S-enantiomer of bupivacaine, which is the racemic mixture of the S- and R-enantiomer.

Presentation and Uses

Levobupivacaine is prepared as a 2.5, 5 and 7.5 $mg.ml^{-1}$ solution. It is used in a manner similar to that of bupivacaine. A maximum single dose of 150 mg is recommended with a maximum dose over 24 hours of 400 mg.

Toxicity Profile

The single advantage of levobupivacaine over bupivacaine and other local anaes-thetics is its potential for reduced toxicity. While extrapolation of research from animal models to humans may be confusing, combined with limited human volun-teer work it appears that levobupivacaine has two potentially useful properties. First, the dose required to produce myocardial depression (by blocking cardiac K^+ chan-nels) is higher for levobupivacaine compared with bupivacaine, and second, excita-tory CNS effects or convulsions occur at lower doses with bupivacaine than levobupivacaine.

Ropivacaine

Presentation and Uses

The amide local anaesthetic ropivacaine is prepared in three concentrations (2, 7.5 and 10 mg.ml^{-1}), in two volumes (10 and 100 ml) and as the pure S-enantiomer. It is not prepared in combination with a vasoconstrictor as this does not alter its duration of action or uptake from tissues. The R-enantiomer is less potent and more toxic. It has a propyl group on its piperidine nitrogen in contrast to the butyl group present in bupivacaine and the methyl group present in mepivacaine (see Figure 11.3).

The main differences from bupivacaine lie in its pure enantiomeric formulation, improved toxic profile and lower lipid solubility. Its lower lipid solubility may result in reduced penetration of the large myelinated Aβ motor fibres, so that initially these fibres are relatively spared from local anaesthetic. However, during continuous infusion they too will become blocked by local anaesthetic resulting in similar degrees of block between Aβ fibres and the smaller unmyelinated C fibres. Therefore, the motor block produced by ropivacaine is slower in onset, less dense and of shorter duration when compared with an equivalent dose of bupivacaine. Theoretically it would appear more appropriate than bupivacaine for epidural infu-sion due to its sensory/motor discrimination and greater clearance.

Kinetics

Ropivacaine is metabolised in the liver by aromatic hydroxylation, mainly to 3-hydroxy-ropivacaine, but also to 4-hydroxy-ropivacaine, both of which have some local anaesthetic activity.

Prilocaine

Presentation and Uses

Prilocaine is presented as a 0.5–2.0% solution, and a hyperbaric 2% solution for spinal anaesthesia. It is also available as a 3% solution with felypressin (0.03 unit.ml^{-1}) for dental use. It has similar indications to lidocaine but is most frequently used in situations where large volumes of local anaesthetic are required. The maximum dose is 6 mg.kg^{-1} or 8 mg.kg^{-1} when administered with felypressin. The 2% hyperbaric spinal preparation is most commonly used at doses of 40–60 mg (2–3 ml) where return of motor function is faster than seen with spinal bupivacaine.

Kinetics

Prilocaine is the most rapidly metabolised amide local anaesthetic, metabolism occurring not only in the liver, but also in the kidney and lung. When given in large doses one of its metabolites, o-toluidine, may precipitate methaemoglobinaemia. This may require treatment with ascorbic acid or methylene blue, which act as reducing agents. The neonate is at special risk as its red blood cells are deficient in methaemoglobin reductase. EMLA cream may precipitate the same reaction.

Cocaine

Presentation and Uses

Cocaine is an ester local anaesthetic derived from the leaves of *Erythroxylon coca*, a plant indigenous to Bolivia and Peru. It is used for topical anaesthesia and local vasoconstriction. Moffatt's solution (2 ml 8% cocaine, 2 ml 1% sodium bicarbonate, 1 ml 1:1,000 adrenaline) has been used in the nasal cavities, although its potential for side effects has rendered it less popular. Cocaine is also formulated as a paste ranging from 1% to 4%. A maximum dose of 1.5 mg.kg^{-1} or 100 mg is currently recommended.

Mechanism of Action

Cocaine blocks uptake 1 and MAO while also stimulating the CNS. These combined effects increase the likelihood of precipitating hypertension and arrhythmias. Its use also provokes hyperthermia.

Side Effects

When taken or administered in high doses it can cause confusion, hallucinations, seizures, arrhythmias and cardiac rupture.

Kinetics

Cocaine is absorbed well from mucous membranes and is highly protein-bound (about 95%). Unlike other esters it undergoes significant hepatic hydrolysis to inactive products, which are excreted in the urine.

Amethocaine

Amethocaine is an ester local anaesthetic used for topical anaesthesia. It is presented as 0.5% and 1% drops for topical use before local anaesthetic block or as a sole agent for lens surgery. It may produce a burning sensation on initial instillation. It is also available as a 4% cream for topical anaesthesia to the skin and is used in a similar fashion to EMLA cream. However, it has a faster onset of action, producing good topical anaesthesia by 30 minutes, following which it may be removed. Its effects last for 4–6 hours. It produces some local vasodilatation and erythema, which may assist venous cannulation.

Chloroprocaine

Chloroprocaine is an ultra-short acting ester local anaesthetic. It was first introduced in 1952 and used successfully as a neuraxial anaesthetic. However, following the addition of preservatives (sodium bisulphite) its use was abandoned following reports of neurological injuries in women receiving large epidural doses. The current preparations are preservative free. 30–60 mg of the 1% or 2% solutions appear useful for surgical procedures with a duration of less than 60 minutes. The recovery times are shorter than compared with bupivacaine and consequently they may be useful in the ambulatory setting.

Muscle Relaxants and Reversal Agents

Physiology

The neuromuscular junction (NMJ) forms a chemical bridge between the motor neurone and skeletal muscle. The final short section of the motor nerve is unmyelinated and comes to lie in a gutter on the surface of the muscle fibre at its mid-point – each being innervated by a single axonal terminal from a fast Aα neurone (*en plaque* appearance). However, for the intra-ocular, intrinsic laryngeal and some facial muscles the pattern of innervation is different with multiple terminals from slower Aγ neurones scattered over the muscle surface (*en grappe* appearance). Here, muscle contraction depends on a wave of impulses throughout the terminals.

The postsynaptic membrane has many folds; the shoulders contain acetylcholine (ACh) receptors while the clefts contain the enzyme acetylcholinesterase (AChE), which is responsible for the hydrolysis of ACh (see Figure 12.1).

Acetylcholine

Synthesis

The synthesis of ACh (see Figure 12.2) is dependent on acetyl-coenzyme A and choline, which is derived from the diet and recycled from the breakdown of ACh. Once synthesised in the axoplasm it is transferred into small synaptic vesicles where it is stored prior to release.

Release

When an action potential arrives at a nerve terminal it triggers Ca^{2+} influx, which then combines with various proteins to trigger the release of vesicular ACh. About 200 such vesicles (each containing about 10,000 ACh molecules) are released in response to each action potential.

Acetylcholine Receptor

Nicotinic ACh receptors are in groups on the edges of the junctional folds on the postsynaptic membrane. They are integral membrane proteins with a molecular weight of 250,000 Da and consist of five subunits (two α, and a single β, ε and δ in adults). They are configured with a central ion channel that opens when the α subunits (each of 40,000 Da) bind ACh. Binding the initial molecule of ACh increases the affinity of the second α subunit for ACh. It is the quaternary nitrogen group, $-N^+(CH_3)_3$, of ACh (and all neuromuscular

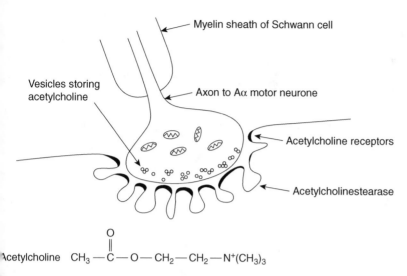

Acetylcholine $CH_3 - \overset{\overset{\displaystyle O}{\displaystyle \|}}{C} - O - CH_2 - CH_2 - N^+(CH_3)_3$

Figure 12.1 Neuromuscular junction (NMJ) and structure of acetylcholine (ACh).

blocking drugs) which is attracted to the α subunit. The ACh receptors are also present on the prejunctional membrane and provide positive feedback to maintain transmitter release during periods of high activity. When blocked by non-depolarising muscle relaxants they may be responsible for 'fade' (see Figure 12.3).

The ACh receptor ion channel is non-specific, allowing Na^+, K^+ and Ca^{2+} across the membrane, generating a miniature end-plate potential. These summate until the threshold potential is reached at which point voltage-gated Na^+ channels are opened, causing a rapid depolarisation, leading to the propagation of an action potential across the muscle surface. On reaching the T tubular system, Ca^{2+} is released from the sarcoplasmic reticulum which initiates muscle contraction.

Metabolism

ACh is metabolised by AChE, which is located on the junctional clefts of the postsynaptic membrane. AChE has an anionic and an esteratic binding site. The anionic site binds with the positively charged quaternary ammonium moiety while the esteratic site binds the ester

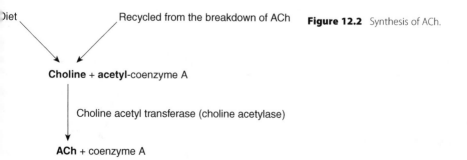

Diet   Recycled from the breakdown of ACh   **Figure 12.2** Synthesis of ACh.

Choline + **acetyl**-coenzyme A

Choline acetyl transferase (choline acetylase)

ACh + coenzyme A

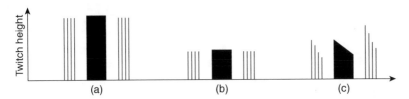

Figure 12.3 Types of neuromuscular block in response to a train-of-four (TOF), tetanic stimulus, repeat TOF. (a) Control, no muscle relaxant present; (b) partial depolarising block, reduced but equal twitch height, no post-tetanic facilitation; (c) partial non-depolarising block, reducing twitch height, fade on tetanic stimulation, post-tetanic facilitation.

group of ACh. At the point of ACh breakdown choline is released and AChE becomes acetylated. The acetylated enzyme is rapidly hydrolysed and acetic acid is produced.

Monitoring Neuromuscular Block

Muscle relaxants are monitored by examining the effect they have on muscle contraction following stimulation of the relevant nerve. Nerve stimulators must generate a supramaximal stimulus (60–80 mA) to ensure that all the composite nerve fibres are depolarised. The duration of the stimulus is 0.1 milliseconds. The negative electrode should be directly over the nerve while the positive electrode should be placed where it cannot affect the muscle in question.

There are five main patterns of stimulation that are used and the characteristic responses observed in the relevant muscle reveal information about the block.

Single Twitch Stimulation

This is the simplest form of neurostimulation and requires a baseline twitch height for it to reveal useful information. It should be remembered that no reduction in twitch height will be observed until 75% of NMJ receptors have been occupied by muscle relaxant (see Figure 12.4). This margin of safety exists because only a small number of receptors are required to generate a summated mini end-plate potential, which triggers an action potential within the muscle. Partial NMJ block with depolarising muscle relaxants (DMRs) and non-depolarising muscle relaxants (NDMRs) reduce the height of single twitch stimulation.

Tetanic Stimulation

When individual stimuli are applied at a frequency > 30 Hz the twitches observed in the muscle become fused into a sustained muscle contraction – tetany. The response may be larger in magnitude than a single stimulus as the elastic forces of the muscle do not need to be overcome for each twitch. Most stimulators deliver stimuli of 0.1 milliseconds duration at a frequency of 50 Hz, which provides maximum sensitivity. In the presence of a partial NDMR the tetanic stimulation fades with time. This is due to blockade by the NDMR of presynaptic ACh receptors, thereby preventing the positive feedback (see above) used to mobilise ACh at times of peak activity. Partial DMR block reduces but does not exhibit fade in response to tetanic stimulation.

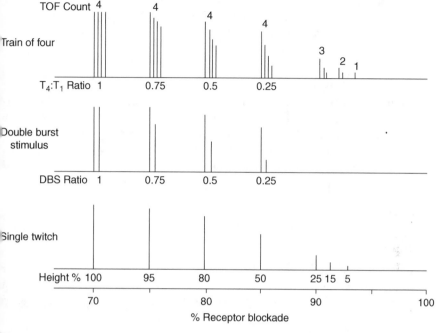

Figure 12.4 Patterns of non-depolarising muscle-relaxant (NDMR) block against increasing NMJ, receptor blockade.

Post-Tetanic Potentiation and Count

Following tetanic stimulation, subsequent twitches are seen to be larger. This may be due to increased synthesis and mobilisation of ACh and/or increased Ca^{2+} in the synaptic terminal. Post-tetanic potentiation forms the basis of the post-tetanic count where stimuli at 1 Hz are started 3 seconds after a tetanic stimulation. The number of twitches is inversely related to the depth of block. It is best used when the degree of receptor blockade is > 95%, that is, when single twitch or train-of-four (TOF) are unable to evoke muscle twitches. It should be remembered that the effects of tetanic stimulation may last for up to 6 minutes and may therefore give a false impression of inadequate block to single twitch or TOF analysis. Partial NMR block does not exhibit post-tetanic potentiation.

Train-of-Four

The TOF is four 0.1 millisecond stimuli delivered at 2 Hz. The ratio of the fourth twitch height to the first twitch height ($T_4:T_1$), or the number of twitches may be recorded, leading to the TOF ratio or the TOF count, respectively (see Figure 12.4). It does not require a baseline twitch height.

In a manner similar to that seen with tetanic stimulation, the rapid stimuli lead to a reducing twitch height in the presence of partial NDMR blockade, that is, $T_4 < T_1$. As receptor occupancy rises above 70%, T_4 will start to decrease in size. When T_4 has decreased by 25%, T_1 starts to decrease, corresponding to 75–80% receptor occupancy. T_4 disappears when T_1 is approximately 25% of its original height. TOF ratio is difficult to assess in practice.

The TOF count records the number of twitches in response to a TOF. As receptor occupancy exceeds 90%, T_4 disappears and only T_1 is present at 95% receptor occupancy. So the TOF count assesses the degree of deep NDMR block.

TOF ratio in the presence of partial DMR block is 1.

Double Burst Stimulation

Double burst stimulation (DBS) describes the delivery of two bursts of stimulation separated by 0.75 seconds. Each burst consists of three 0.2 millisecond stimuli separated by 20 milliseconds (i.e. at a 50 Hz). DBS was developed to allow easy manual detection of small amounts of residual NMJ blockade so that, when the magnitude of the two stimuli are equal, clinically significant residual NMJ blockade does not exist. However, when assessed mechanically, DBS is no more sensitive than TOF (see Figure 12.4).

Depolarising Muscle Relaxants

Suxamethonium

Suxamethonium was first introduced in 1952 and provided a significant advantage over tubocurarine as profound muscle relaxation of short duration was achieved rapidly. It can be thought of as two molecules of ACh joined back-to-back through their acetyl groups.

$$H_2C-\overset{\overset{\text{O}}{\|}}{C}-O-CH_2-CH_2-N^+(CH_3)_3$$
$$H_2C-\underset{\underset{\text{O}}{\|}}{C}-O-CH_2-CH_2-N^+(CH_3)_3$$

Presentation and Uses

Suxamethonium is formulated as a colourless solution containing $50\ mg.ml^{-1}$ and should be stored at 4°C. It is used to achieve rapid muscle relaxation required during rapid sequence induction and has also been used by infusion to facilitate short surgical procedures.

Mechanism of Action

Suxamethonium mimics the action of ACh by attaching to the nicotinic ACh receptor and causing membrane depolarisation. However, because its hydrolysing enzyme (plasma or pseudo-cholinesterase) is not present at the NMJ its duration of action is longer than that of ACh. The persistent depolarisation produced initiates local current circuits that render the voltage-sensitive Na^+ channels within 1–2 millimetres inactive. This area of electrical inexcitability prevents the transmission of further action potentials resulting in muscle relaxation. The concentration gradient from plasma to NMJ, down which ACh initially moved, is reversed by the actions of plasma cholinesterase, so that ACh moves in the opposite direction, away from the NMJ allowing recovery of NMJ signal transmission.

Initially this depolarising block is described as a Phase I block; however, if further doses of suxamethonium are given it may become a Phase II block. The characteristics of a Phase II block are similar to those of a non-depolarising block, but the mechanism is thought to be different (probably a presynaptic effect) (see Table 12.1; Figure 12.3).

Table 12.1 Characteristics of partial neuromuscular blockade

	Partial depolarising or Phase I block	Partial non-depolarising or Phase II block
Single twitch	reduced	reduced
Train-of-four ratio $(T_4:T_1)$	> 0.7	< 0.7
1 Hz stimulus	Sustained	fade
Post-tetanic potentiation	no	yes
Effect of anticholinesterases	block augmented	block antagonised

Kinetics

Suxamethonium is rapidly hydrolysed by plasma or pseudo-cholinesterase (an enzyme of the liver and plasma – none being present at the NMJ), to such an extent that only 20% of the initial intravenous dose reaches the NMJ, so that the rate of hydrolysis becomes a critical factor in determining the duration of the neuromuscular block. Suxamethonium is hydrolysed to choline and succinylmonocholine, which is weakly active. Succinylmonocholine is metabolised further by plasma cholinesterase to succinic acid and choline. Because metabolism is rapid, less than 10% is excreted in the urine (see Figure 12.5).

Other Effects

Apart from its useful effects at the NMJ, suxamethonium has many other effects, all of which are detrimental:

Arrhythmias – sinus or nodal bradycardia, and ventricular arrhythmias can occur following suxamethonium, via stimulation of the muscarinic receptors in the sinus node. The bradycardia is often more severe after a second dose but may be prevented by atropine. This phenomenon is often more pronounced in children.

Hyperkalaemia – a small rise in serum K^+ is expected following suxamethonium in the normal subject as depolarisation involves K^+ efflux into extracellular fluid. Patients with burns (of > 10%) or neuromuscular disorders are susceptible to a sudden release of K^+, which may be large enough to provoke cardiac arrest. Burn patients are at risk from about 24 hours after injury and for up to 18 months. Extra-junctional ACh receptors (which contain a fetal γ subunit in place of an adult ε subunit) proliferate over the surface of the muscle, and when activated release K^+ into the circulation. Patients with paraplegia, progressive muscle disease or trauma-induced immobility are at risk via a similar mechanism. The period of particular risk in those with paraplegia is during the first 6 months but it continues in those with progressive muscle disease, becoming more severe as more muscle is involved.

Those with renal failure are not at increased risk of a sudden hyperkalaemic response to suxamethonium per se. However, serum K^+ may be grossly deranged in acute renal failure leading to an increased risk of arrhythmias.

Myalgia – muscle pains are commonest in young females mobilising rapidly in the post-operative period. Pre-treatment with a small dose of NDMR (e.g. vecuronium), diazepam or dantrolene have all been used with limited success in an attempt to reduce this unpleasant side effect.

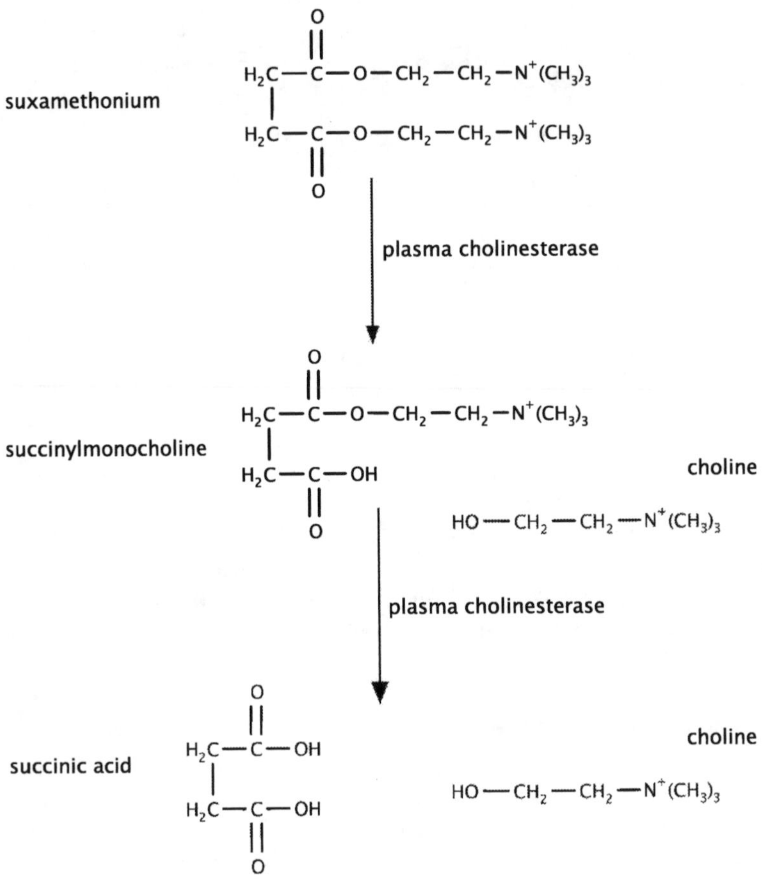

Figure 12.5
Metabolism of suxamethonium.

suxamethonium

$$H_2C-C(=O)-O-CH_2-CH_2-N^+(CH_3)_3$$
$$H_2C-C(=O)-O-CH_2-CH_2-N^+(CH_3)_3$$

plasma cholinesterase

succinylmonocholine

$$H_2C-C(=O)-O-CH_2-CH_2-N^+(CH_3)_3$$
$$H_2C-C(=O)-OH$$

choline

$$HO-CH_2-CH_2-N^+(CH_3)_3$$

plasma cholinesterase

choline

$$HO-CH_2-CH_2-N^+(CH_3)_3$$

succinic acid

$$H_2C-C(=O)-OH$$
$$H_2C-C(=O)-OH$$

- *Intra-ocular pressure (IOP)* – is raised by about 10 mmHg for a matter of minutes following suxamethonium (normal range 10–15 mmHg) and is significant in the presence of a globe perforation. However, concurrently administered thiopental will offset this rise so that IOP remains static or may even fall. The mechanism by which suxamethonium increases IOP has not been clearly defined, but it is known to involve contraction of tonic myofibrils and transient dilation of choroidal blood vessels.
- *Intragastric pressure* – rises by about 10 cmH$_2$O, but as the lower oesophageal sphincter tone increases simultaneously there is no increased risk of reflux.
- *Anaphylaxis* – suxamethonium is twice as likely to cause anaphylaxis compared to NDMRs, with a rate of approximately 1 per 10,000 administrations.
- *Malignant hyperthermia* (see 'Malignant Hyperthermia' below).
- Prolonged neuromuscular block (see 'Prolonged Block (Suxamethonium Apnoea)' below).

Malignant Hyperthermia

Malignant hyperthermia (MH) is a rare (incidence of 1 in 50,000–70,000 in the UK) autosomal dominant condition, affecting males (62%) more than females (38%) and may occur after many previous anaesthetics.

Mechanism

The exact mechanism has not been fully elucidated but the ryanodine receptor located on the membrane of the sarcoplasmic reticulum and encoded on chromosome 19 is intimately involved. There are three isoforms of the ryanodine receptor encoded by three distinct genes. Isoform 1 (RYR1) is located primarily in skeletal muscle, isoform 2 (RYR2) is located primarily in heart muscle and isoform 3 (RYR3) is located primarily in the brain. The RYR1 receptor functions as the main Ca^{2+} channel allowing stored Ca^{2+} from the sarcoplasmic reticulum into the cytoplasm, which in turn activates the contractile mechanisms within muscle. Abnormal RYR1 receptors allow excessive amounts of Ca^{2+} to pass, resulting in generalised muscle rigidity. ATP consumption is high as it is used in the process to return Ca^{2+} to the sarcoplasmic reticulum and as a result there is increased CO_2, heat and lactate production. Cells eventually break down resulting in myoglobinaemia and hyperkalaemia.

Treatment

This requires intravenous dantrolene (increments of 1 mg.kg^{-1} up to 10 mg.kg^{-1}), aggressive cooling (using ice-cold saline to lavage bladder and peritoneum – if open) and correction of abnormal biochemical and haematological parameters. Treatment should continue on the ICU and should only stop when symptoms have completely resolved, otherwise it may recur. Before the introduction of dantrolene in 1979 the mortality rate was as high as 70% but is now less than 5%.

Diagnosis

The diagnosis of MH is based on the response of biopsied muscle to 2% halothane and caffeine (2 mmol.l^{-1}). Patients are labelled either 'susceptible' (MHS) – when positive to both halothane and caffeine, 'equivocal' (MHE) – when positive to either halothane or caffeine, or 'non-susceptible' (MHN) – when negative to halothane and caffeine.

Safe Drugs

These include opioids, thiopental, propofol, etomidate, ketamine, benzodiazepines, atropine, local anaesthetics and N_2O. Patients suspected of having MH should be referred to the UK malignant hyperthermia investigation unit in Leeds.

Dantrolene

Dantrolene is used in the treatment (and prophylaxis) of MH, neuroleptic malignant syndrome, chronic spasticity of voluntary muscle and ecstasy intoxication. It is available as capsules and in vials as an orange powder containing dantrolene 20 mg, mannitol 3 g and sodium hydroxide. Each vial should be reconstituted with 60 ml water producing a solution of pH 9.5. It is highly irritant when extravasated and a diuresis follows intravenous administration reflecting its formulation with mannitol. Treatment of suspected MH starts with a dose of 2.5 mg.kg^{-1}, followed by 1 mg.kg^{-1} every 5 minutes until the metabolic signs start to resolve. Although there is no upper dose limit, little benefit is seen with doses above 10 mg.kg^{-1}. Chronic use is associated with hepatitis and pleural effusion.

Mechanism of Action   Dantrolene uncouples the excitation contraction process by binding to the ryanodine receptor, thereby preventing the release of Ca^{2+} from the sarcoplasmic reticulum in striated muscle. As vascular smooth muscle and cardiac muscle are not primarily dependent on Ca^{2+} release for contraction, they are not usually affected. It has no effect on the muscle action potential and usually has little effect on the clinical duration of the NDMRs. It may, however, produce respiratory failure secondary to skeletal muscle weakness.

Kinetics Oral bioavailability is variable and it is approximately 85% bound in the plasma to albumin. It is metabolised in the liver and excreted in the urine.

Prolonged Block (Suxamethonium Apnoea)

Plasma cholinesterase activity may be reduced due to genetic variability or acquired conditions, leading to prolonged neuromuscular block. Single amino acid substitutions are responsible for genetically altered enzymatic activity. Four alleles – usual (normal), atypical (dibucaine-resistant), silent (absent) and fluoride-resistant – have been identified at a single locus on chromosome 3 and make up the 10 genotypes.

Ninety-six percent of the population is homozygous for the normal Eu gene and metabolise suxamethonium rapidly. Up to 4% may be heterozygotes resulting in a mildly prolonged block of up to 10 minutes, while a very small fraction may have a genotype that confers a block of a few hours. This prolonged block may be reversed by administration of fresh frozen plasma, which provides a source of plasma cholinesterase. Alternatively the patient may be sedated and ventilated while the block wears off naturally.

Dibucaine (cinchocaine) is an amide local anaesthetic that inhibits normal plasma cholinesterase. However, it inhibits the variant forms of plasma cholinesterase less effectively. At a concentration of 10^{-5} mol.l^{-1}, using benzylcholine as a substrate, dibucaine inhibits the Eu:Eu form by 80% but the Ea:Ea form by only 20%. Other combinations are inhibited by 20–80% depending on the type involved. The percentage inhibition is known as the 'Dibucaine number' and indicates the genetic makeup for an individual but makes no assessment of the quantity of enzyme in the plasma (see Table 12.2).

Acquired factors associated with reduced plasma cholinesterase activity include:

• Pregnancy
• Liver disease

Table 12.2 Some genetic variants of plasma cholinesterase

Genotype	Incidence	Duration of block	Dibucaine number
Eu:Eu	96%	normal	80
Eu:Ea	1:25	+	60
Eu:Es	1:90	+	80
Eu:Ef	1:200	+	75
Ea:Ea	1:2,800	++++	20
Ea:Ef	1:20,000	++	50
Es:Ea	1:29,000	++++	20
Es:Es	1:100,000	++++	–
Ef:Es	1:150,000	++	60
Ef:Ef	1:154,000	++	70

- Renal failure
- Cardiac failure
- Thyrotoxicosis
- Cancer
- Drugs – either directly or by acting as substrate or inhibitor to AChE. Metoclopramide, ketamine, the oral contraceptive pill, lithium, lidocaine, ester local anaesthetics, cytotoxic agents, edrophonium, neostigmine and trimetaphan.

Non-Depolarising Muscle Relaxants

Non-depolarising muscle relaxants inhibit the actions of ACh at the NMJ by binding competitively to the α subunit of the nicotinic ACh receptor on the post-junctional membrane, through its quaternary ammonium group. Drugs with two quaternary ammonium groups (bisquaternary ammonium) are more potent than those with one (monoquaternary ammonium).

There is a wide safety margin at the NMJ to ensure muscle contraction, so that more than 70% of receptors need to be occupied by muscle relaxant before neuromuscular blockade can be detected by a peripheral nerve stimulator. The non-depolarising block has essentially the same characteristics as the Phase II block (see Table 12.1).

NDMRs (see Figure 12.6) fall into one of two chemical groupings:

- Aminosteroidal compounds – vecuronium, rocuronium, pancuronium
- Benzylisoquinolinium compounds – atracurium, mivacurium, tubocurarine

Across the two chemical groups the drugs can be divided according to their duration of action:

- Short – mivacurium
- Intermediate – atracurium
- Long – pancuronium.

Owing to their relatively polar nature, non-depolarising drugs are unable to cross lipid membranes, resulting in a small volume of distribution. Some are hydrolysed in the plasma (atracurium, mivacurium) while others undergo a degree of hepatic metabolism (pancuronium, vecuronium). The unmetabolised fraction is excreted in the urine or bile.

Muscle relaxants are never given in isolation and so their potential for drug interaction should be considered (see Table 12.3).

Vecuronium

Vecuronium is a 'clean' drug, so called because it does not affect the cardiovascular system or precipitate the release of histamine. Its chemical structure differs from pancuronium by a single methyl group, making it the monoquaternary analogue.

Presentation and Uses

Vecuronium is potentially unstable in solution and so is presented as 10 mg freeze-dried powder containing mannitol and sodium hydroxide and is dissolved in 5 ml water before administration. At 0.1 mg.kg^{-1} satisfactory intubating conditions are reached in about 90–120 seconds. It has a medium duration of action (see Table 12.4).

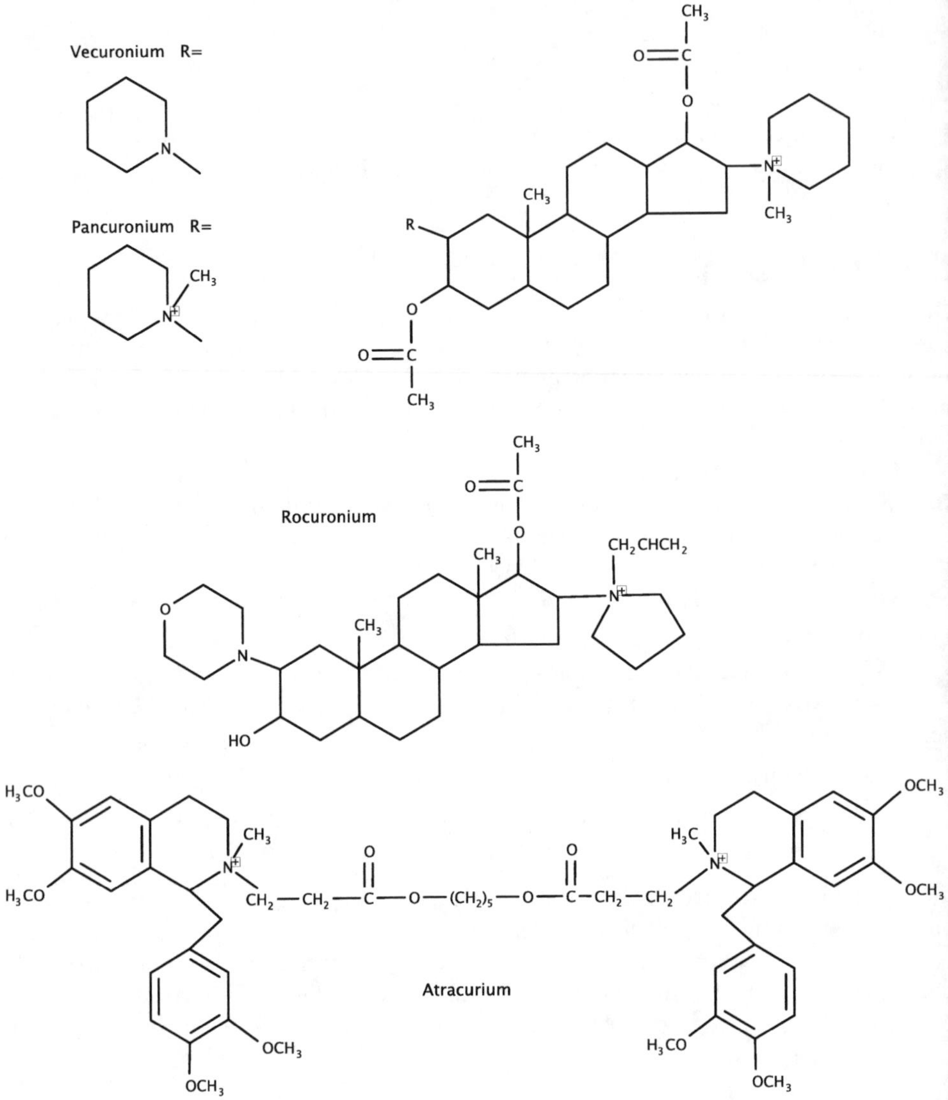

Figure 12.6 Structure of some NDMRs.

Other Effects

- *Cardiovascular* – vecuronium has no cardiac effects but, unlike pancuronium or tubocurarine, it may leave unchecked the bradycardia associated with fentanyl and propofol.
- *Critical illness myopathy* – this is seen most frequently in critically ill patients in association with corticosteroids and/or muscle relaxants and may involve a prolonged recovery.

Table 12.3 Pharmacological and physiological interactions of muscle relaxants

	Effect on blockade	Mechanism
Pharmacological		
Volatile anaesthetics	prolonged	Depression of somatic reflexes in CNS (reducing transmitter release at the NMJ)
Aminoglycosides (large intraperitoneal doses), polymyxins and tetracycline	prolonged	Decreased ACh release possibly by competition with Ca^{2+} (which unpredictably reverses the block)
Local anaesthetics	variable	Low doses of local anaesthetic may enhance blockade by causing a degree of Na^+ channel blockade
Lithium	prolonged	Na^+ channel blockade
Diuretics	variable	Variable effect on cAMP. May have effects via serum K^+
Ca^{2+} channel antagonists	prolonged	Reduced Ca^{2+} influx leading to reduced ACh release
Physiological		
Hypothermia	prolonged	Reduced metabolism of muscle relaxant
Acidosis	variable	Prolonged in most, but reduced for gallamine. The tertiary amine group of dTC becomes protonated, increasing its affinity for the ACh receptor
Hypokalaemia	variable	Acute hypokalaemia increases (i.e. makes more negative) the resting membrane potential. Non-depolarising relaxants are potentiated while depolarising relaxants are antagonised. The reverse is true in hyperkalaemia
Hypermagnesaemia	prolonged	Decreased ACh release by competition with Ca^{2+}, and stabilisation of the post-junctional membrane. When used at supranormal levels (e.g. pre-eclampsia) Mg^{2+} can cause apnoea via a similar mechanism

Kinetics

Like pancuronium, vecuronium is metabolised in the liver by de-acetylation to 3- and 17-hydroxy and 3,17-dihydroxy-vecuronium. Again the 3-hydroxy metabolite carries significant muscle-relaxant properties, but unlike 3-hydroxypancuronium it has a very short half-life and is of little clinical significance with normal renal function. With only a single charged quaternary ammonium group, it is more lipid-soluble than pancuronium and,

Table 12.4 Properties of some non-depolarising muscle relaxants

	Intubating dose (mg.kg^{-1})	Speed of onset	Duration	Cardiovascular effects	Histamine release
Vecuronium	0.1	medium	medium	none/ bradycardia	rare
Rocuronium	0.6	rapid	medium	none	rare
Pancuronium	0.1	medium	long	tachycardia	rare
Atracurium	0.5	medium	medium	none	slight
Cis-atracurium	0.2	medium	medium	none	rare
Mivacurium	0.2	medium	short	none	slight

despite the metabolism of a similar proportion in the liver, a far greater proportion is excreted in the bile. It may accumulate during administration by infusion.

Rocuronium

This aminosteroidal drug was developed from vecuronium and is structurally different at only four positions. Its main advantage is its rapid onset (hence its name, 'RO – curonium') with intubating conditions at 60–90 seconds, which in turn is due to its low potency. Its effects are reversed not only by anticholinesterases but also by sugammadex (see below).

A muscle relaxant with a low potency must be given at a higher dose to achieve a clinically significant effect. A higher number of molecules result in a greater concentration gradient from the plasma to the NMJ so that diffusion is faster and onset time is reduced.

Presentation and Uses

Rocuronium is prepared as a colourless solution containing 50 mg in 5 ml. At 0.6 mg.kg^{-1} intubating conditions are reached within 100–120 seconds, although this may be reduced to 60 seconds with higher doses (0.9–1.2 mg.kg^{-1}). Its duration of action is similar to that of vecuronium although higher doses increase this significantly.

Other Effects

- *Cardiovascular* – like vecuronium it has minimal cardiovascular effects, although at high doses when used to facilitate a more rapid tracheal intubation, it may cause an increase in heart rate.

Kinetics

Rocuronium is mainly excreted unchanged in the bile and to a lesser extent in the urine, although some de-acetylated metabolites may be produced. Its duration of action may be prolonged in hepatic and renal failure.

Pancuronium

Pancuronium is a bisquaternary aminosteroidal compound.

Presentation and Uses

Pancuronium is presented as a colourless solution containing 4 mg in 2 ml and should be stored at 4°C. At 0.1 mg.kg^{-1} intubating conditions are reached within 90–150 seconds. Its duration of action is about 45 minutes.

Other Effects

- *Cardiovascular* – pancuronium causes a tachycardia by blocking cardiac muscarinic receptors. It may also have indirect sympathomimetic actions by preventing the uptake of noradrenaline at post-ganglionic nerve endings.

Kinetics

Between 10% and 40% is plasma protein-bound, and in keeping with other drugs in its class, pancuronium has a low volume of distribution. About 35% is metabolised in the liver by de-acetylation to 3- and 17-hydroxy and 3,17-dihydroxy-pancuronium, the former of which is half as potent as pancuronium. Unchanged drug is eliminated mainly in the urine while its metabolites are excreted in bile.

Atracurium

Atracurium is a benzylisoquinolinium compound that is formulated as a mixture of 10 stereoisomers, resulting from the presence of four chiral centres.

Presentation and Uses

Atracurium is presented as a colourless solution containing 10 mg.ml^{-1} in 2.5, 5 and 25 ml vials and should be stored at 4°C. At 0.5 mg.kg^{-1} intubating conditions are reached within 90–120 seconds.

Other Effects

- *Cardiorespiratory* – following rapid administration it may precipitate the release of histamine, which may be localised to the site of injection but may be generalised resulting in bronchospasm and hypotension. Slow intravenous injection minimises these effects.
- *Myopathy* – in a manner similar to that of vecuronium, atracurium is associated with critical illness myopathy.

Kinetics

Atracurium has a unique metabolic pathway, undergoing ester hydrolysis and Hofmann elimination.

- *Ester hydrolysis* – non-specific esterases unrelated to plasma cholinesterase are responsible for hydrolysis and account for 60% of atracurium's metabolism. The breakdown products are a quaternary alcohol, a quaternary acid and laudanosine. Unlike Hofmann elimination, acidic conditions accelerate this metabolic pathway. However, pH changes in the clinical range probably do not alter the rate of ester hydrolysis of atracurium.
- *Hofmann elimination* – while atracurium is stable at pH 4 and at 4°C, Hofmann elimination describes its spontaneous breakdown to laudanosine and a

quaternary monoacrylate when placed at normal body temperature and pH. Acidosis and hypothermia will slow the process. Both breakdown products have been shown to have potentially serious side effects (i.e. seizures), but at concentrations in excess of those encountered clinically. Laudanosine, while being a glycine antagonist, has no neuromuscular-blocking properties and is cleared by the kidneys.

These metabolic pathways result in a drug whose elimination is independent of hepatic or renal function, which in certain clinical situations is advantageous.

Cisatracurium

Cisatracurium is one of the 10 stereoisomers present in atracurium.

Presentation and Uses

Cisatracurium is presented as a colourless solution containing 2 or 5 mg.ml^{-1} and should be stored at 4°C. It is about three to four times more potent than atracurium and, therefore, has a slower onset time. However, the onset time can be improved by increasing the dose as its potential for histamine release is extremely low.

Kinetics

Cisatracurium has a similar kinetic profile to atracurium. However, it does not undergo direct hydrolysis by plasma esterases and the predominant pathway for its elimination is Hofmann elimination to laudanosine and a monoquaternary acrylate. This is then hydrolysed by non-specific plasma esterases to a monoquaternary alcohol and acrylic acid. All of its metabolites are void of neuromuscular-blocking properties.

It has been used safely in children from 2 years of age and in elderly patients with minimal alteration of its kinetics. There is no change in its kinetic profile in patients with end-stage renal or hepatic impairment (see Table 12.5).

Table 12.5 Kinetics of some non-depolarising muscle relaxants

	Protein bound (%)	Volume of distribution (l.kg^{-1})	Metabolised (%)	Elimination (%)	
				Bile	Urine
Pancuronium	20–60	0.27	30	20	80
Vecuronium	10	0.23	20	70	30
Rocuronium	10	0.20	< 5	60	40
Atracurium	15	0.15	90	0	10
Cis-atracurium	15	0.15	95	0	5
Mivacurium	10	*0.21–0.32	90	0	5

* Isomer specific

Mivacurium

Mivacurium (a benzylisoquinolinium ester – similar to atracurium) is a chiral mixture of three stereospecific isomers in the following proportions:

- 36% cis-trans
- 58% trans-trans
- 6% cis-cis.

The cis-cis isomer has about 10% of the potency of the other two isomers and is not metabolised enzymatically. Its half-life is 10 times that of the other two isomers.

The main advantage of mivacurium is its short duration of action. Routine reversal of mivacurium with neostigmine may not be required due to its rapid enzymatic metabolism. In addition, neostigmine inhibits plasma cholinesterase and may prevent its metabolism. Edrophonium may be a more suitable agent for the reversal of neuromuscular block secondary to mivacurium.

Presentation and Uses

Mivacurium is presented as an acidic (pH 3.5–5.0) aqueous solution containing 2 mg.ml^{-1} in 5 and 10 ml ampoules. It has a shelf-life of 18 months when stored below 25°C.

Effects

- *Cardiorespiratory* – high doses may release histamine, resulting in a fall in blood pressure and bronchospasm.

Kinetics

Plasma cholinesterase is responsible for the metabolism of the cis-trans and trans-trans isomers, so those patients with genetically low plasma cholinesterase levels (see 'Suxamethonium Apnoea', p. 176) are subject to prolonged neuromuscular blockade. Its duration of action is significantly prolonged in patients with end-stage liver disease, mainly due to reduced plasma cholinesterase activity.

Reversal Agents

Until recently anticholinesterases have been the only means of reversing non-depolarising neuromuscular blockade. However, the cyclodextrin sugammadex offers a completely different mechanism of action.

Anticholinesterases

The enzyme AChE is responsible for the hydrolysis of ACh. Anticholinesterases (Figure 12.8) antagonise AChE, slowing down this reaction, so that more ACh is available at the NMJ. As AChE is present at sites other than the NMJ, it is no surprise that anticholinesterases have effects other than reversal of NDMRs. For this reason an anticholinergic agent (glycopyrrolate or atropine) is often given with an anticholinesterase to prevent bradycardia or excessive salivation.

The differing mechanism of action of anticholinesterases allows three groups to emerge.

Easily reversible inhibition

Formation of a carbamylated enzyme complex

Irreversible inactivation.

Easily Reversible Inhibition

Edrophonium

Edrophonium is the only drug in this group. It is a phenolic quaternary amine.

Uses

At an intravenous dose of 2–10 mg it rapidly distinguishes between a myasthenic crisis (where muscle power is improved) and a cholinergic crisis (where the clinical picture is worsened).

Mechanism of Action

The quaternary amine group of edrophonium is attracted to the anionic site of AChE while its hydroxyl group forms a hydrogen bond at the esteratic site and stabilises the complex (see Figure 12.7). ACh is now unable to reach the active site of AChE. However, ACh competes with edrophonium for AChE because a true covalent bond is not formed between edrophonium and AChE. Edrophonium also causes increased ACh release.

Kinetics

Owing to its quaternary amine structure edrophonium has a low lipid solubility and is not absorbed following oral administration. For similar reasons, it does not cross the blood–brain barrier or the placenta. It has a faster onset of action than neostigmine. Up to 65% is excreted unchanged in the urine; the rest undergoes glucuronidation in the liver and subsequent excretion in the bile. It has only slight muscarinic side effects but may still cause a bradycardia and salivation.

Formation of a Carbamylated Enzyme Complex

Neostigmine, pyridostigmine, physostigmine

Mechanism of Action

Both ACh and the carbamate esters are hydrolysed when they react with AChE. However, ACh acetylates AChE while the carbamate esters produce a carbamylated enzyme (see Figure 12.9). The later has a much slower rate of hydrolysis and so is unable to work for longer, hence, it stops AChE hydrolysing ACh. The carbamate esters are also known as acid-transferring or time-dependent AChE inhibitors. Neostigmine also inhibits plasma cholinesterase and as such may prolong the actions of suxamethonium.

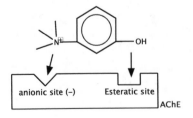

Figure 12.7 Edrophonium forms an easily reversible enzyme complex.

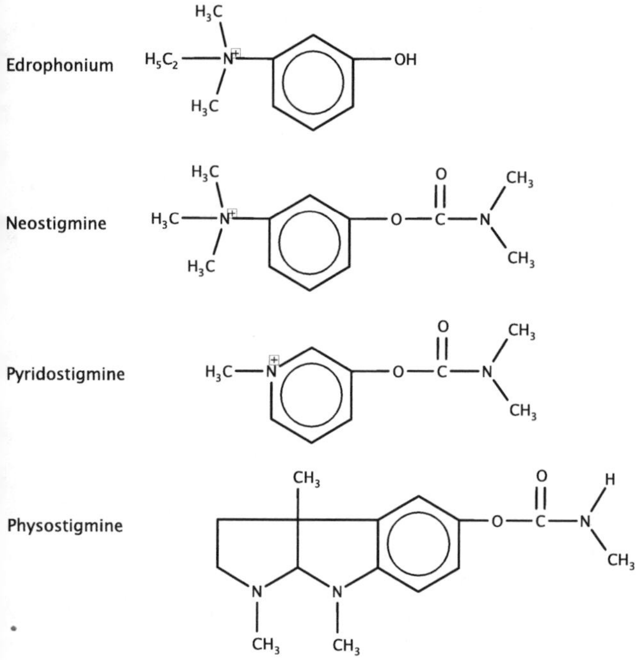

Edrophonium

Neostigmine

Pyridostigmine

Physostigmine

Figure 12.8 Chemical structure of some anticholinesterases.

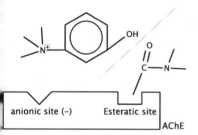

Figure 12.9 Neostigmine forms a carbamylated enzyme complex.

anionic site (−)   Esteratic site

AChE

Neostigmine

Neostigmine is a quaternary amine.

Presentation and Uses

Neostigmine is available as tablets and in solution for intravenous injection (and in combination with glycopyrrolate). It is used to reverse the effects of non-depolarising muscle relaxants (0.05 mg.kg^{-1} intravenously), in the treatment of myasthenia gravis (15–30 mg orally where effects last up to 4 hours) and in urinary retention.

Effects

- *Cardiovascular* – if administered alone it will precipitate a bradycardia. It has a limited role in the treatment of supraventricular tachycardia.

- *Respiratory* – it may precipitate bronchospasm in asthmatics.
- *Gut* – it increases salivation and intestinal motility, which may result in abdominal cramps.

Kinetics

Neostigmine is poorly absorbed from the gut and has a low oral bioavailability. It is minimally protein-bound, has a low volume of distribution and is partially metabolised in the liver. Approximately 55% is excreted unchanged in the urine.

Pyridostigmine

Pyridostigmine is also a quaternary amine used mainly in the treatment of myasthenia gravis, where it is preferred to neostigmine because it has a longer duration of action and fewer autonomic effects.

Kinetics

Pyridostigmine has a slower onset of action than neostigmine and its duration of action is longer. It relies on renal elimination more than neostigmine (75% excreted unchanged).

Like neostigmine it does not cross the blood–brain barrier.

Physostigmine has a tertiary amine structure and it, therefore, has different properties. It is well absorbed from the gut and crosses the blood–brain barrier. In the past it has been used in the treatment of anticholinergic poisoning.

Organophosphorous Compounds

Organophosphorous compounds are highly toxic and are mainly used as insecticides (e.g. tetraethylpyrophosphate; TEPP), or nerve gases (sarin; GB). However, ecothiopate iodide has been used to treat glaucoma by relaxing the ciliary muscle and thereby improving drainage channels of the trabecular meshwork.

These agents are highly lipid-soluble and are, therefore, rapidly absorbed across skin.

Mechanism of Action

The esteratic site of AChE is phosphorylated by organophosphorous compounds resulting in inhibition of the enzyme (see Figure 12.10). The complex that is formed is very stable and, unlike the carbamate esters, is resistant to hydrolysis or reactivation. In practice recovery depends on synthesis of new enzyme. These drugs also inhibit plasma cholinesterase.

Toxic manifestations include nicotinic and muscarinic effects, autonomic instability and initially central excitation progressing to depression, coma and apnoea.

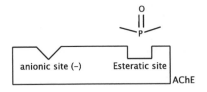

Figure 12.10 Organophosphorous compounds phosphorylate AChE, forming a very stable complex.

Pralidoxime and **obidoxine** are reactivators of phosphorylated AChE by promoting hydrolysis. Atropine, anticonvulsants and ventilation may also be necessary in organophosphorous poisoning.

Cyclodextrins

Cyclodextrins are a family of compounds that have a wide range of uses. Chemically, they comprise a ring structure made up of 6 (α), 7 (β) or 8 (γ) sugars. The inside of the ring is relatively hydrophobic while the outside is hydrophilic. As a result hydrophobic drugs form complexes with cyclodextrins, increasing their solubility and bioavailability. Other uses include the preparation of cholesterol-free products (where cholesterol is attracted to the inside of the cyclodextrin and then the whole complex is removed) and complexing of fragrances and toxins, both their release and consumption.

Sugammadex

Sugammadex is a γ cyclodextrin and is sometimes referred to as a selective relaxant binding agent (SRBA). It was approved for use in Europe in 2008, and the USA in 2015, the difference being due to concerns over hypersensitivity reactions.

Uses and Mechanism of Action

Its licensed indication is the reversal of neuromuscular blockade induced by rocuronium or vecuronium. It selectively encapsulates these aminosteroidal NDMRs and effectively removes them from the plasma and the NMJ. As such their mechanism of action is specific and generally without the predictable side effects of anticholinesterases (see above). It has been used to treat suspected rocuronium-induced anaphylaxis but does not currently form part of any approved anaphylaxis guideline.

Presentation and Dose

It is presented as a 100 mg.ml^{-1} solution in 2 or 5 ml vials. The dose required depends on the depth of neuromuscular blockade. It has a shelf-life of 3 years.

Routine Reversal

Dose is 4 mg.kg^{-1} if there is some post-tetanic twitch activity; 2 mg.kg^{-1} when during a TOF, T2 is visible. Both rocuronium- and vecuronium-induced neuromuscular blockade may be reversed.

Emergency Reversal

Dose (immediately following 1.2 mg.kg^{-1} rocuronium) is 16 mg.kg^{-1}. As a result, numerous vials will be required.

Interactions

The main interactions relate to displacement or capture. Displacement of rocuronium or vecuronium are possible with the following drugs; flucloxacillin, diclofenac, fusidic acid and toremifene (a selective estrogen receptor modulator), leading to the potential for recurisation. Capture of other medicines into the γ cyclodextrin may reduce their efficacy. The most significant is the potential reduction in efficacy of oral contraceptives. This should be discussed with those concerned and they should be advised to use additional contraception for seven days following administration of sugammadex.

Kinetics

It has a volume of distribution of 11–14 litres and demonstrates linear kinetics at therapeutic doses. It is not metabolised and is excreted solely via the kidneys with an effective half-life of 2.5 hours.

Side Effects

Hypersensitivity reactions remain a cause of concern and a single case of sugammadex - induced anaphylaxis was identified in NAP6. Severe bradycardia is seen very rarely following its use.

Chapter

13

Sympathomimetics

Physiology

Autonomic Nervous System

The autonomic nervous system (ANS) is a complex system of neurones that controls the body's internal milieu. It is not under voluntary control and is anatomically distinct from the somatic nervous system. Its efferent limb controls individual organs and smooth muscle, while its afferent limb relays information (occasionally in somatic nerves) concerning visceral sensation and may result in reflex arcs.

The hypothalamus is the central point of integration of the ANS, but is itself under the control of the neocortex. However, not all autonomic activity involves the hypothalamus: locally, the gut coordinates its secretions; some reflex activity is processed within the spinal cord; and the control of vital functions by baroreceptors is processed within the medulla. The ANS is divided into the parasympathetic and sympathetic nervous systems.

Parasympathetic Nervous System

The parasympathetic nervous system (PNS) is made up of pre- and post-ganglionic fibres. The pre-ganglionic fibres arise from two locations (see Figure 13.1):

- Cranial nerves (III, VII, IX, X) – which supply the eye, salivary glands, heart, bronchi, upper gastrointestinal (GI) tract (to the splenic flexure) and ureters
- Sacral fibres (S2, 3, 4) – which supply distal bowel, bladder and genitals.

All these fibres synapse within ganglia that are close to, or within, the effector organ. The post-ganglionic neurone releases acetylcholine (ACh), which acts via nicotinic receptors.

The PNS may be modulated by anticholinergics (see Chapter 19) and anticholinesterases (see Chapter 12).

Sympathetic Nervous System

The sympathetic nervous system (SNS) is also made up of pre- and post-ganglionic fibres. The pre-ganglionic fibres arise within the lateral horns of the spinal cord at the thoracic and upper lumbar levels (T1–L2) and pass into the anterior primary rami, and via the white rami communicans into the sympathetic chain or ganglia where they may either synapse at that or an adjacent level, or pass anteriorly through a splanchnic nerve to synapse in a prevertebral ganglion (see Figure 13.2). The unmyelinated post-ganglionic fibres then

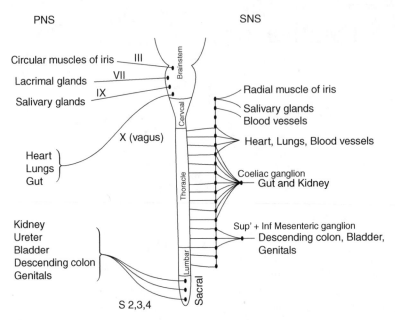

PNS   SNS

Circular muscles of iris — III
Lacrimal glands — VII
                IX
Salivary glands

X (vagus)

Heart
Lungs
Gut

Kidney
Ureter
Bladder
Descending colon
Genitals

S 2,3,4

Brainstem
Cervical
Thoracic
Lumbar
Sacral

Radial muscle of iris
Salivary glands
Blood vessels

Heart, Lungs, Blood vessels

Coeliac ganglion
Gut and Kidney

Sup' + Inf Mesenteric ganglion
Descending colon, Bladder,
Genitals

Figure 13.1
Simplified diagram
of the autonomic
nervous
system (ANS).

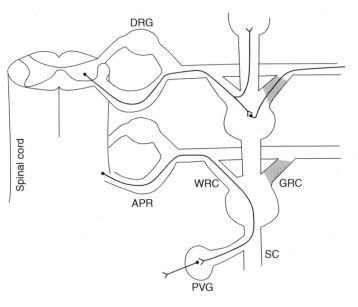

DRG

Spinal cord

WRC   GRC

APR

SC

PVG

Figure 13.2 Various
connections of the
sympathetic nervous system
(SNS). DRG, dorsal root
ganglion; APR, anterior
primary rami; WRC, white
rami communicans; GRC,
grey rami communicans;
PVG, prevertebral ganglion;
SC, sympathetic chain.

pass into the adjacent spinal nerve via the grey rami communicans. They release noradrenaline, which acts via adrenoceptors.

The adrenal medulla receives presynaptic fibres that synapse directly with its chromaffin cells using ACh as the transmitter. It releases adrenaline into the circulation, which, therefore, acts as a hormone, not a transmitter.

Post-ganglionic sympathetic fibres release ACh to innervate sweat glands.

All pre-ganglionic ANS fibres are myelinated and release ACh, which acts via nicotinic receptors (see Table 13.1).

Sympathomimetics

Sympathomimetics exert their effects via adrenoceptors or dopamine receptors either directly or indirectly. **Direct-acting** sympathomimetics attach to and act directly via these receptors, while **indirect-acting** sympathomimetics cause the release of noradrenaline to produce their effects via these receptors.

The structure of sympathomimetics is based on a benzene ring with various amine side chains attached at the C1 position. Where a hydroxyl group is present at the C3 and C4 positions the agent is known as a **catechol**amine (because 3,4-dihydroxybenzene is otherwise known as 'catechol').

Sympathomimetic and other inotropic agents will be discussed under the following headings:

- **Naturally occurring catecholamines**
- **Synthetic agents**
- **Other inotropic agents.**

Naturally Occurring Catecholamines

Adrenaline, noradrenaline and dopamine are the naturally occurring catecholamines and their synthesis is interrelated (see Figure 13.3). They act via adrenergic and dopaminergic receptors, which are summarised in Table 13.2.

Adrenaline

Presentation and Uses

Adrenaline is presented as a clear solution containing $0.1-1$ mg.ml^{-1} for administration as a bolus in asystole or anaphylaxis or by infusion (dose range $0.01-0.5$ μg.kg^{-1}.min^{-1}) in the critically ill with circulatory failure. It may also be nebulised into the upper airway where its vasoconstrictor properties will temporarily reduce the swelling associated with acute upper airway obstruction. A 1% ophthalmic solution is used in open-angle glaucoma, and a metered dose inhaler delivering 280 μg for treatment of anaphylaxis associated with insect stings or drugs. In addition, it is presented in combination with local anaesthetic solutions at a strength of 1 in 80,000–200,000.

Table 13.1 Summary of transmitters within the autonomic nervous system

	Pre-ganglionic	Post-ganglionic
PNS	ACh	ACh
SNS	ACh	noradrenaline
Adrenal medulla	ACh	–
Sweat glands	ACh	ACh

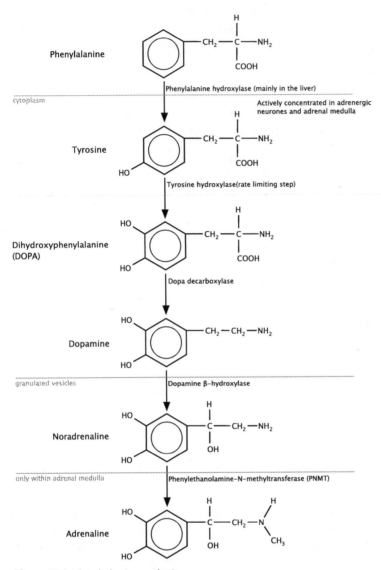

Figure 13.3 Catecholamine synthesis.

Mechanism of Action

Adrenaline exerts its effects via α- and β-adrenoceptors. $α_1$-Adrenoceptor activation stimulates phospholipase C (via G_q), which hydrolyses phosphatidylinositol bisphosphate (PIP_2). Inositol triphosphate (IP_3) is released, which leads to increased Ca^{2+} availability within the cell. $α_2$-Adrenoceptor activation is coupled to G_i-proteins that inhibit adenylate cyclase and reduce cAMP concentration. β-Adrenoceptors are coupled to G_s-proteins that activate adenylate cyclase, leading to an increase in cAMP and specific phosphorylation depending on the site of the adrenoceptor.

Table 13.2 Actions and mechanisms of adrenoceptors

Receptor	Subtype	Location	Actions when stimulated	Mechanism
α	1	vascular smooth muscle	vasoconstriction	G_q-coupled phospholipase C activated $\rightarrow\uparrow IP_3 \rightarrow\uparrow Ca^{2+}$
	2	widespread throughout the nervous system	sedation, analgesia, attenuation of sympathetically mediated responses	G_i-coupled adenylate cyclase inhibited $\rightarrow\downarrow$ cAMP
β	1	platelets	platelet aggregation	
		heart	+ ve inotropic and chronotropic effect	G_s-coupled adenylate cyclase activated $\rightarrow\uparrow$ cAMP
	2	bronchi, vascular smooth muscle, uterus (and heart)	relaxation of smooth muscle	G_s-coupled adenylate cyclase activated $\rightarrow\uparrow$ cAMP $\rightarrow\uparrow Na^+/K^+$ ATPase activity and hyperpolarisation
	3	adipose tissue	lipolysis	G_s-coupled adenylate cyclase activated $\rightarrow\uparrow$ cAMP
D	1	within the CNS	modulates extrapyramidal activity	G_s-coupled adenylate cyclase activated $\rightarrow\uparrow$ cAMP
		peripherally	vasodilatation of renal and mesenteric vasculature	
	2	within the CNS	reduced pituitary hormone output	G_i-coupled adenylate cyclase inhibited $\rightarrow\downarrow$ cAMP
		peripherally	inhibit further noradrenaline release	

Effects

- *Cardiovascular* – the effects of adrenaline vary according to dose. When administered as a low-dose infusion, β effects predominate. This produces an increase in cardiac output, myocardial oxygen consumption, coronary artery dilatation and reduces the threshold for arrhythmias. Peripheral β effects may result in a fall in diastolic blood pressure and peripheral vascular resistance. At high doses by infusion or when given as a 1 mg bolus during cardiac arrest, α_1 effects predominate causing a rise in systemic vascular resistance. It is often used in combination with local anaesthetics to produce vasoconstriction before dissection during surgery. When used with halothane, the dose should be restricted to 100 μg per 10 minutes to avoid arrhythmias. It should not be infiltrated into areas supplied by end arteries lest their vascular supply become compromised. Extravasation can cause tissue necrosis.
- *Respiratory* – adrenaline produces a small increase in minute volume. It has potent bronchodilator effects although secretions may become more tenacious. Pulmonary vascular resistance is increased.
- *Metabolic* – adrenaline increases the basal metabolic rate. It raises plasma glucose by stimulating glycogenolysis (in liver and skeletal muscle), lipolysis and gluconeogenesis. Initially insulin secretion is increased (a β_2 effect) but is often overridden by an α effect, which inhibits its release and compounds the increased glucose production. Glucagon secretion and plasma lactate are also raised. Lipase activity is augmented resulting in increased free fatty acids, which leads to increased fatty acid oxidation in the liver and ketogenesis. These metabolic effects limit its use, especially in those with diabetes. Na^+ reabsorption is increased by direct stimulation of tubular Na^+ transport and by stimulating renin and, therefore, aldosterone production. β_2-Receptors are responsible for the increased transport of K^+ into cells, which follows an initial temporary rise as K^+ is released from the liver.
- *Central nervous system* – it increases MAC and increases the peripheral pain threshold.
- *Renal* – renal blood flow is moderately decreased and the increase in bladder sphincter tone may result in difficulty in micturition.

Kinetics

Adrenaline is not given orally due to inactivation. Subcutaneous absorption is less rapid than intramuscular. Tracheal absorption is erratic but may be used in emergencies where intravenous access is not available.

Adrenaline is metabolised by mitochondrial MAO and catechol O-methyl transferase (COMT) within the liver, kidney and blood to the inactive 3-methoxy-4-hydroxymandelic acid (vanillylmandelic acid or VMA) and metadrenaline, which is conjugated with glucuronic acid or sulfates, both of which are excreted in the urine. It has a short half-life (about 2 minutes) due to rapid metabolism.

Noradrenaline

Presentation and Uses

Noradrenaline is presented as a clear solution containing 0.2–2 mg.ml^{-1} noradrenaline acid tartrate, which is equivalent to 0.1–1 mg.ml^{-1} of noradrenaline base, and contains the preservative sodium metabisulfite. It is used as an intravenous infusion (dose range $0.05–0.5$ μg.kg^{-1}.min^{-1}) to increase the systemic vascular resistance.

Mechanism of Action

Its actions are mediated mainly via stimulation of $α_1$-adrenoceptors but also β-adrenoceptors.

Effects

- *Cardiovascular* – the effects of systemically infused noradrenaline are slightly different from those of endogenous noradrenaline. Systemically infused noradrenaline causes peripheral vasoconstriction, increases systolic and diastolic blood pressure and may cause a reflex bradycardia. Cardiac output may fall and myocardial oxygen consumption is increased. A vasodilated coronary circulation carries an increased coronary blood flow. Pulmonary vascular resistance may be increased and venous return is increased by venoconstriction. In excess it produces hypertension, bradycardia, headache and excessive peripheral vasoconstriction, occasionally leading to ischaemia and gangrene of extremities. Extravasation can cause tissue necrosis. Endogenously released noradrenaline causes tachycardia and a rise in cardiac output.
- *Splanchnic* – renal and hepatic blood flow falls due to vasoconstriction.
- *Uterus* – blood flow to the pregnant uterus is reduced and may result in fetal bradycardia. It may also exert a contractile effect and cause fetal asphyxia.
- *Interactions* – despite being a direct-acting sympathomimetic amine, noradrenaline should be used with caution in patients taking monoamine oxidase inhibitors (MAOIs) as its effects may be exaggerated and prolonged.

Kinetics

For endogenously released noradrenaline, Uptake 1 describes its active uptake back into the nerve terminal where it is metabolised by MAO (COMT is not present in sympathetic nerves) or recycled. It forms the main mechanism by which noradrenaline is inactivated. Uptake 2 describes the diffusion away from the nerve and is less important. Noradrenaline reaches the circulation in this way and is metabolised by COMT to the inactive VMA and normetadrenaline, which is conjugated with glucuronic acid or sulfates, both of which are excreted in the urine. It has a short half-life (about 2 minutes) due to rapid metabolism. Unlike adrenaline and dopamine, up to 25% is taken up as it passes through the lungs.

Dopamine

In certain cells within the brain and interneurones of the autonomic ganglia, dopamine is not converted to noradrenaline and is released as a neurotransmitter.

Presentation and Uses

Dopamine is presented as a clear solution containing 200 or 800 mg in 5 ml water with sodium metabisulfite. It is used to improve haemodynamic parameters and urine output.

Mechanism of Action

In addition to its effects on α- and β-adrenoceptors, dopamine also acts via dopamine (D_1 and D_2) receptors via G_s and G_i coupled adenylate cyclase leading to increased or decreased levels of cAMP.

Effects

*   *Cardiovascular* – these depend on its rate of infusion and vary between patients. At lower rates (up to 10 $\mu g.kg^{-1}.min^{-1}$) β_1 effects predominate leading to increased contractility, heart rate, cardiac output and coronary blood flow. In addition to its direct effects, it also stimulates the release of endogenous noradrenaline. At higher rates (> 10 $\mu g.kg^{-1}.min^{-1}$) α effects tend to predominate leading to increased systemic vascular resistance and venous return. In keeping with other inotropes an adequate preload is essential to help control tachycardia. It is less arrhythmogenic than adrenaline. Extravasation can cause tissue necrosis.
*   *Respiratory* – infusions of dopamine attenuate the response of the carotid body to hypoxaemia. Pulmonary vascular resistance is increased.
*   *Splanchnic* – dopamine has been shown to vasodilate mesenteric vessels via D_1 receptors. However, the improvement in urine output may be entirely due to inhibition of proximal tubule Na^+ reabsorption and an improved cardiac output and blood pressure.
*   *Central nervous system* – dopamine modulates extrapyramidal movement and inhibits the secretion of prolactin from the pituitary gland. It cannot cross the blood–brain barrier, although its precursor, L-dopa, can.
*   *Miscellaneous* – owing to stimulation of the chemoreceptor trigger zone it causes nausea and vomiting. Gastric transit time is also increased.
*   *Interactions* – despite being a direct-acting sympathomimetic amine the effects of dopamine may be significantly exaggerated and prolonged during MAOI therapy.

Kinetics

Dopamine is only administered intravenously and preferably via a central vein. It acts within 5 minutes and has a duration of 10 minutes. Metabolism is via MAO and COMT in the liver, kidneys and plasma to inactive compounds (3,4-dihydroxyphenylacetic acid and homovanillic acid; HVA) which are excreted in the urine as sulfate and glucuronide conjugates. About 25% of an administered dose is converted to noradrenaline in sympathetic nerve terminals. Its half-life is about 3 minutes.

Synthetic Agents

Of the synthetic agents, only isoprenaline, dobutamine and dopexamine are classified as catecholamines as only they contain hydroxyl groups on the 3- and 4- positions of the benzene ring (see Figure 13.4).

α$_1$-Agonists

Phenylephrine

Phenylephrine is a direct-acting sympathomimetic amine with potent α$_1$-agonist actions. It causes a rapid rise in systemic vascular resistance and blood pressure. It has no effect on β-adrenoceptors.

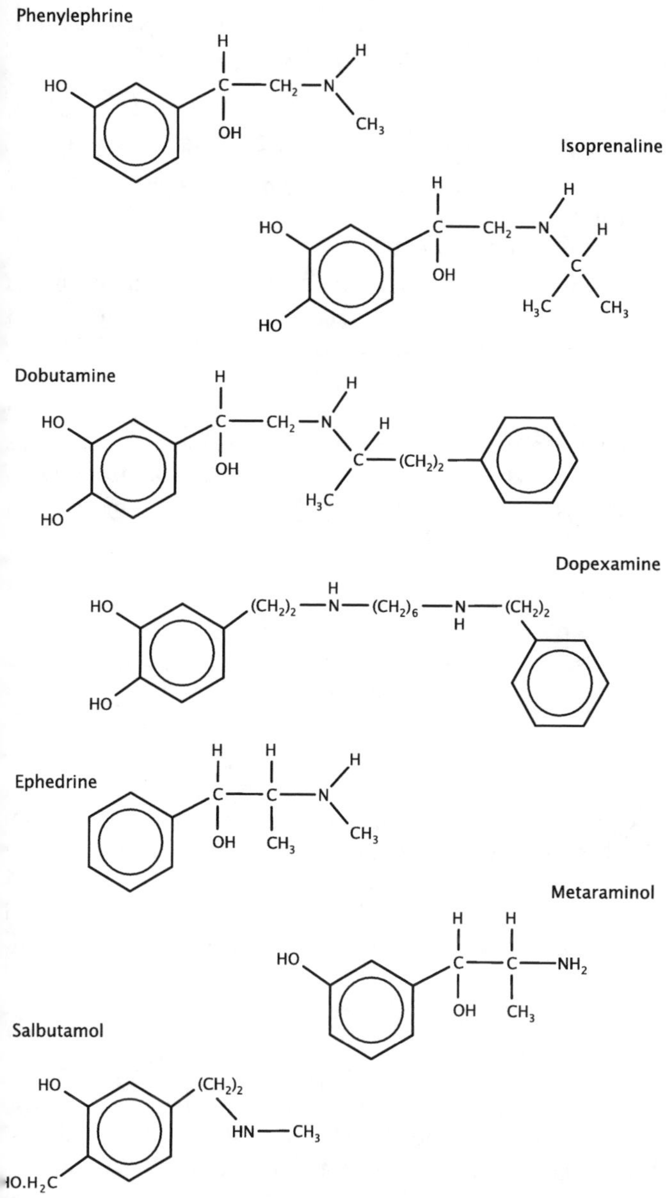

Phenylephrine

Isoprenaline

Dobutamine

Dopexamine

Ephedrine

Metaraminol

Salbutamol

Figure 13.4 Structure of some synthetic sympathomimetic amines.

Presentation and Uses

Phenylephrine is presented as a clear solution containing 10 mg in 1 ml. Bolus doses of 50–100 μg are used intravenously although 2–5 mg may be administered intramuscularly or subcutaneously for a more prolonged duration. It is used to increase a low systemic vascular resistance associated with spinal anaesthesia or systemically administered drugs. In certain patients, general anaesthesia may drop the systemic vascular resistance and reverse a left-to-right intracardiac shunt; this may be reversed by phenylephrine. It is also available for use as a nasal decongestant and mydriatic agent. It may have a limited use in the treatment of supraventricular tachycardia associated with hypotension.

Effects

- *Cardiovascular* – phenylephrine raises the systemic vascular resistance and blood pressure and may result in a reflex bradycardia, all of which results in a drop in cardiac output. It is not arrhythmogenic.
- *Central nervous system* – it has no stimulatory effects.
- *Renal* – blood flow falls in a manner similar to that demonstrated by noradrenaline.
- *Uterus* – its use in obstetrics to treat hypotension associated with spinal anaesthesia results in a more favourable cord gas profile compared to ephedrine.

Kinetics

Intravenous administration results in a rapid rise in blood pressure, which lasts 5–10 minutes, while intramuscular or subcutaneous injection takes 15 minutes to work but lasts up to 1 hour. It is metabolised in the liver by MAO. The products of metabolism and their route of elimination have not been identified.

β-Agonists
Isoprenaline

Isoprenaline is a highly potent synthetic catecholamine with actions at β_1- and β_2-adrenoceptors. It has no α effects.

Presentation and Uses

Isoprenaline is presented as a clear solution containing 1 mg.ml^{-1} for intravenous infusion and as a metered dose inhaler delivering 80 or 400 µg. It is no longer used to treat reversible airway obstruction as this was associated with an increased mortality. More specific β_2-agonists are now used (e.g. salbutamol). The 30 mg tablets are very rarely used. It is used intravenously to treat severe bradycardia associated with atrioventricular (AV) block or β-blockers (dose range 0.5–10 µg.min^{-1}).

Effects

- *Cardiovascular* – stimulation of β_1-adrenoceptors increases heart rate, myocardial contractility, automaticity and cardiac output. The effects on blood pressure are varied. The β_2 effects may drop the systemic vascular resistance so that the increase in cardiac output is insufficient to maintain blood pressure. Myocardial oxygen delivery may decrease significantly when tachycardia reduces diastolic coronary filling time and the reduced diastolic blood pressure reduces coronary perfusion. Some coronary vasodilatation occurs to attenuate this.
- *Respiratory* – isoprenaline is a potent bronchodilator and inhibits histamine release in the lungs, improving mucous flow. Anatomical dead space and ventilation perfusion mismatching increases which may lead to systemic hypoxaemia.
- *Central nervous system* – isoprenaline has stimulant effects on the CNS.
- *Splanchnic* – mesenteric and renal blood flow is increased.
- *Metabolic* – its β effects lead to a raised blood glucose and free fatty acids.

Kinetics

When administered orally it is well absorbed but extensive first-pass metabolism results in a low oral bioavailability, being rapidly metabolised by COMT within the liver. A significant fraction is excreted unchanged in the urine along with conjugated metabolites.

Dobutamine

Dobutamine is a direct-acting synthetic catecholamine derivative of isoprenaline. β_1 effects predominate but it retains a small effect at β_2-adrenoceptors.

Presentation and Uses

Dobutamine is presented in 20 ml water containing 250 mg dobutamine and sodium metabisulfite or in 5 ml water containing 250 mg dobutamine and ascorbic acid. It is used to augment low cardiac output states associated with myocardial infarction, cardiac surgery and cardiogenic shock (dose range 0.5–20 $\mu g.kg^{-1}.min^{-1}$). It is also used in cardiac stress testing as an alternative to exercise.

Effects

- *Cardiovascular* – its main actions are direct stimulation of β_1-receptors resulting in increased contractility, heart rate and myocardial oxygen requirement. The blood pressure is usually increased despite a limited fall in systemic vascular resistance via β_2 stimulation. It may precipitate arrhythmias including an increased ventricular response rate in patients with atrial fibrillation or flutter, due to increased AV conduction. It should be avoided in patients with cardiac outflow obstruction (e.g. aortic stenosis, cardiac tamponade).
- *Splanchnic* – it has no effect on the splanchnic circulation although urine output may increase following a rise in cardiac output.

Kinetics

Dobutamine is only administered intravenously. It is rapidly metabolised by COMT to inactive metabolites that are conjugated and excreted in the urine. It has a half-life of 2 minutes.

Dopexamine

Dopexamine is a synthetic analogue of dopamine.

Presentation and Uses

Dopexamine is presented as 50 mg in 5 ml (at pH 2.5) for intravenous use. It is used to improve cardiac output and improve mesenteric perfusion (dose range 0.5–6 $\mu g.kg^{-1}.min^{-1}$).

Mechanism of Action

Dopexamine stimulates β_2-adrenoceptors and dopamine (D_1) receptors and may also inhibit the re-uptake of noradrenaline. It has only minimal effect on D_2 and β_1-adrenoceptors, and no effect on α-adrenoceptors.

Effects

- *Cardiovascular* – while it has positive inotropic effects (due to cardiac β_2-receptors), improvements in cardiac output are aided by a reduced afterload due to peripheral β_2 stimulation, which may reduce the blood pressure. It produces a small increase in coronary blood flow and there is no change in myocardial oxygen extraction. The alterations in heart rate are varied and it only rarely precipitates arrhythmias.
- *Mesenteric and renal* – blood flow to the gut and kidneys increases due to an increased cardiac output and reduced regional vascular resistance. Urine output increases. It may cause nausea and vomiting.
- *Respiratory* – bronchodilation is mediated via β_2 stimulation.
- *Miscellaneous* – tremor and headache have been reported.

Kinetics

Dopexamine is cleared rapidly from the blood and has a half-life of 7 minutes.

Salbutamol

Salbutamol is a synthetic sympathomimetic amine with actions mainly at β_2-adrenoceptors.

Presentation and Uses

Salbutamol is presented as a clear solution containing 50–500 $\mu g.ml^{-1}$ for intravenous infusion after dilution, a metered dose inhaler (100 μg) and a dry powder (200–400 μg) for inhalation, a solution containing 2.5–5 $mg.ml^{-1}$ for nebulisation, and oral preparations (syrup 0.4 $mg.ml^{-1}$ and 2, 4 or 8 mg tablets). It is used in the treatment of reversible lower airway obstruction and occasionally in premature labour.

Effects

- *Respiratory* – its main effects are relaxation of bronchial smooth muscle. It reverses hypoxic pulmonary vasoconstriction, increasing shunt, and may lead to hypoxaemia. Adequate oxygen should, therefore, be administered with nebulised salbutamol.
- *Cardiovascular* – the administration of high doses, particularly intravenously, can cause stimulation of β_1-adrenoceptors resulting in tachycardia, which may limit the dose. Lower doses are sometimes associated with β_2-mediated vasodilatation, which may reduce the blood pressure. It may also precipitate arrhythmias, especially in the presence of hypokalaemia.
- *Metabolic* – Na^+/K^+ ATPase is stimulated and transports K^+ into cells resulting in hypokalaemia. Blood sugar rises especially in diabetic patients and is exacerbated by concurrently administered steroids.
- *Uterus* – it relaxes the gravid uterus. A small amount crosses the placenta to reach the fetus.
- *Miscellaneous* – a direct effect on skeletal muscle may produce tremor.

Kinetics

The absorption of salbutamol from the gut is incomplete and is subject to a significant hepatic first-pass metabolism. Following inhalation or intravenous administration, it has a rapid onset of action. It is 10% protein-bound and has a half-life of 4–6 hours. It is metabolised in the liver to the inactive 4-O-sulfate, which is excreted along with salbutamol in the urine.

Salmeterol

Salmeterol is a long-acting β_2-agonist used in the treatment of nocturnal and exercise-induced asthma. It should not be used during acute attacks due to a relatively slow onset.

It has a long non-polar side chain, which binds to the β_2-adrenoceptor giving it a long duration of action (about 12 hours). It is 15 times more potent than salbutamol at the β_2-adrenoceptor, but four times less potent at the β_1-adrenoceptor. It prevents the release of histamine, leukotrienes and prostaglandin D_2 from mast cells, and also has additional anti-inflammatory effects that differ from those induced by steroids.

Its effects are similar to those of salbutamol.

Ritodrine

Ritodrine is a β_2-agonist that is used to treat premature labour. Tachycardia (β_1 effect) is often seen during treatment. It crosses the placenta and may result in fetal tachycardia.

Ritodrine has been associated with fatal maternal pulmonary oedema. It also causes hypokalaemia, hyperglycaemia and, at higher levels, vomiting, restlessness and seizures.

Terbutaline

Terbutaline is a β_2-agonist with some activity at β_1-adrenoceptors. It is used in the treatment of asthma and uncomplicated pre-term labour. It has a similar side-effect profile to other drugs in its class.

Mixed (α and β)
Ephedrine

Ephedrine is found naturally in certain plants but is synthesised for medical use.

Presentation and Uses

Ephedrine is formulated as tablets, an elixir, nasal drops and as a solution for injection containing 30 mg.ml^{-1}. It can exist as four isomers but only the L-isomer is active. It is used intravenously to treat hypotension associated with regional anaesthesia. In the obstetric setting this is now known to result in a poorer cord gas pH when compared to purer α-agonists, but it is still preferred in the presence of relative maternal bradycardia. It is also used to treat bronchospasm, nocturnal enuresis and narcolepsy.

Mechanism of Action

Ephedrine has both direct and indirect sympathomimetic actions. It also inhibits the actions of MAO on noradrenaline. Owing to its indirect actions it is prone to tachyphylaxis as noradrenaline stores in sympathetic nerves become depleted.

Effects

- *Cardiovascular* – it increases the cardiac output, heart rate, blood pressure, coronary blood flow and myocardial oxygen consumption. Its use may precipitate arrhythmias.

- *Respiratory* – it is a respiratory stimulant and causes bronchodilation.
- *Renal* – renal blood flow is decreased and the glomerular filtration rate falls.
- *Interactions* – it should be used with extreme caution in those patients taking MAOI.

Kinetics

Ephedrine is well absorbed orally, intramuscularly and subcutaneously. Unlike adrenaline it is not metabolised by MAO or COMT and, therefore, has a longer duration of action and an elimination half-life of 4 hours. Some is metabolised in the liver but 65% is excreted unchanged in the urine.

Metaraminol

Metaraminol is a synthetic amine with both direct and indirect sympathomimetic actions. It acts mainly via α_1-adrenoceptors but also retains some β-adrenoceptor activity.

Presentation and Uses

Metaraminol is presented as a clear solution containing 10 mg.ml^{-1}. It is used to correct hypotension associated with spinal or epidural anaesthesia. An intravenous bolus of 0.5–2 mg is usually sufficient.

Effects

- *Cardiovascular* – its main actions are to increase systemic vascular resistance, which leads to an increased blood pressure. Despite its activity at β-adrenoceptors the cardiac output often drops in the face of the raised systemic vascular resistance. Coronary artery flow increases by an indirect mechanism. Pulmonary vascular resistance is also increased leading to raised pulmonary artery pressure.

Other Inotropic Agents

Non-Selective Phosphodiesterase Inhibitors
Aminophylline

Aminophylline is a methylxanthine derivative. It is a complex of 80% theophylline and 20% ethylenediamine (which has no therapeutic effect but improves solubility) (see Figure 13.5).

Presentation and Uses

Aminophylline is available as tablets and as a solution for injection containing 25 mg.ml^{-1}. Oral preparations are often formulated as slow release due to its half-life of about 6 hours. It is used in the treatment of asthma where the dose ranges from 450 to 1250 mg daily. When given intravenously during acute severe asthma a loading dose of 6 mg.kg^{-1} over 20 minutes is given, followed by an infusion of 0.5 mg.kg^{-1}.hour^{-1}. It may also be used to reduce the frequency of episodes of central apnoea in premature neonates. It is very occasionally used in the treatment of heart failure.

Mechanism of Action

Aminophylline is a non-selective inhibitor of all five phosphodiesterase isoenzymes, which hydrolyse cAMP and possibly cGMP, thereby increasing their intracellular levels. It may also directly release noradrenaline from sympathetic neurones and demonstrate synergy

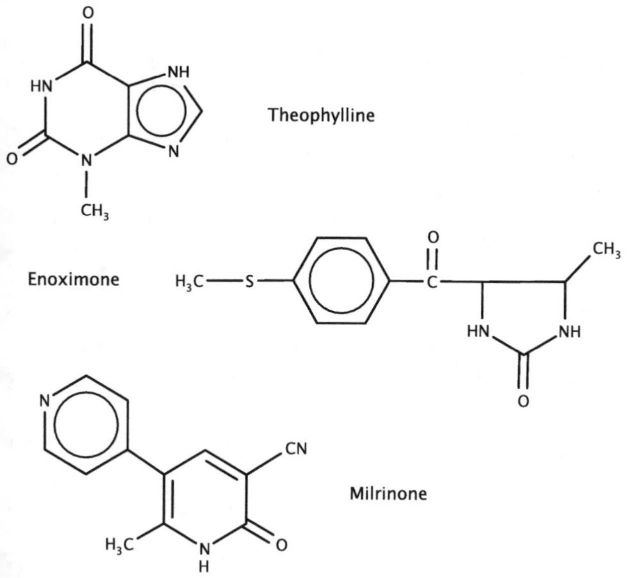

Figure 13.5 Structure of some phosphodiesterase inhibitors.

with catecholamines, which act via adrenoceptors to increase intracellular cAMP. In addition it interferes with the translocation of Ca^{2+} into smooth muscle, inhibits the degranulation of mast cells by blocking their adenosine receptors and potentiates prostaglandin synthetase activity.

Effects

- *Respiratory* – aminophylline causes bronchodilation, improves the contractility of the diaphragm and increases the sensitivity of the respiratory centre to carbon dioxide. It works well in combination with β_2-agonists due to the different pathway used to increase cAMP.
- *Cardiovascular* – it has mild positive inotropic and chronotropic effects and causes some coronary and peripheral vasodilatation. It lowers the threshold for arrhythmias (particularly ventricular) especially in the presence of halothane.
- *Central nervous system* – the alkyl group at the 1-position (also present in caffeine) is responsible for its CNS stimulation, resulting in a reduced seizure threshold.
- *Renal* – the alkyl group at the 1-position is also responsible for its weak diuretic effects. Inhibition of tubular Na^+ reabsorption leads to a natriuresis and may precipitate hypokalaemia.
- *Interactions* – co-administration of drugs that inhibit hepatic cytochrome P450 (cimetidine, erythromycin, ciprofloxacin and oral contraceptives) tend to delay the elimination of aminophylline and a reduction in dose is recommended. The use of certain selective serotonin re-uptake inhibitors (fluvoxamine) should be avoided with aminophylline as levels of the latter may rise sharply. Drugs that induce hepatic cytochrome P450 (phenytoin, carbamazepine, barbiturates and rifampicin) increase aminophylline clearance and the dose may need to be increased.

Kinetics

Aminophylline is well absorbed from the gut with a high oral bioavailability (> 90%). About 50% is plasma protein-bound. It is metabolised in the liver by cytochrome P450 to inactive metabolites and interacts with the metabolism of other drugs undergoing metabolism by a similar route. Owing to its low hepatic extraction ratio its metabolism is independent of liver blood flow. Approximately 10% is excreted unchanged in the urine. The effective therapeutic plasma concentration is 10–20 μg.ml^{-1}. Cigarette smoking increases the clearance of aminophylline.

Toxicity

Above 35 μg.ml^{-1}, hepatic enzymes become saturated and its kinetics change from first- to zero-order resulting in toxicity. Cardiac toxicity manifests itself as tachyarrhythmias including ventricular fibrillation. CNS toxicity includes tremor, insomnia and seizures (especially following rapid intravenous administration). Nausea and vomiting are also a feature, as is rhabdomyolysis.

Selective Phosphodiesterase Inhibitors
Enoximone

The imidazolone derivative enoximone is a selective phosphodiesterase III inhibitor.

Presentation and Uses

Enoximone is available as a yellow liquid (pH 12) for intravenous use containing 5 mg.ml^{-1}. It is supplied in propyl glycol and ethanol and should be stored between 5°C and 8°C. It is used to treat congestive heart failure and low cardiac output states associated with cardiac surgery. It should be diluted with an equal volume of water or 0.9% saline in plastic syringes (crystal formation is seen when mixed in glass syringes) and administered as an infusion of 5–20 μg. kg^{-1}.min^{-1}, which may be preceded by a loading dose of 0.5 mg.kg^{-1}, and can be repeated up to a maximum of 3 mg.kg^{-1}. Unlike catecholamines it may take up to 30 minutes to act.

Mechanism of Action

Enoximone works by preventing the degradation of cAMP and possibly cGMP in cardiac and vascular smooth muscle. By effectively increasing cAMP within the myocardium, it increases the slow Ca^{2+} inward current during the cardiac action potential. This produces an increase in Ca^{2+} release from intracellular stores and an increase in the Ca^{2+} concentration in the vicinity of the contractile proteins, and hence to a positive inotropic effect. By interfering with Ca^{2+} flux into vascular smooth muscle it causes vasodilatation.

Effects

- *Cardiovascular* – enoximone has been termed an 'inodilator' due to its positive inotropic and vasodilator effects on the heart and vascular system. In patients with heart failure the cardiac output increases by about 30% while end diastolic filling pressures decrease by about 35%. The myocardial oxygen extraction ratio remains unchanged by virtue of a reduced ventricular wall tension and improved coronary artery perfusion. The blood pressure may remain unchanged or fall, the heart rate remains unchanged or rises slightly and arrhythmias occur only rarely. It shortens atrial, AV node and ventricular refractoriness. When used in patients with ischaemic heart disease, a reduction in coronary perfusion pressure and a rise in heart rate may outweigh the benefits of improved myocardial blood flow so that further ischaemia ensues.

- *Miscellaneous* – agranulocytosis has been reported.

Kinetics

While enoximone is well absorbed from the gut an extensive first-pass metabolism renders it useless when given orally. About 70% is plasma protein-bound and metabolism occurs in the liver to a renally excreted active sulfoxide metabolite with 10% of the activity of enoximone and a terminal half-life of 7.5 hours. Only small amounts are excreted unchanged in the urine and by infusion enoximone has a terminal half-life of 4.5 hours. It has a wide therapeutic ratio and the risks of toxicity are low. The dose should be reduced in renal failure.

Milrinone

Milrinone is a bipyridine derivative and a selective phosphodiesterase III inhibitor with similar effects to enoximone. However, it has been associated with an increased mortality rate when administered orally to patients with severe heart failure.

Preparation and Uses

Milrinone is formulated as a yellow solution containing 1 mg.ml^{-1} and may be stored at room temperature. It should be diluted before administration and should only be used intravenously for the short-term management of cardiac failure.

Kinetics

Approximately 70% is plasma protein-bound. It has an elimination half-life of 1–2.5 hours and is 80% excreted in the urine unchanged. The dose should be reduced in renal failure.

Levosimendan

Levosimendan is a calcium sensitiser of troponin C. It has also been described as an inodilator due to its ability to relax smooth muscle by opening ATP-sensitive K$^+$ channels. It is improves both the symptoms and survival of patients with acute heart failure. It is given by intravenous infusion, which may follow an initial loading dose.

Effects

Cardiovascular – It increases cardiac contractility and output, stroke volume, heart rate and coronary blood flow but decreases systemic vascular resistance, natriuretic peptide blood pressure and myocardial oxygen consumption. It can produce atrial fibrillation.

Kinetics

It has an oral bioavailability of 85%, is highly protein-bound and extensively metabolised in the liver to active metabolites. It is excreted in both the bile and urine and the dose should be adjusted in renal impairment.

Glucagon

Within the pancreas, α-cells secrete the polypeptide glucagon. The activation of glucagon receptors, via G-protein-mediated mechanisms, stimulates adenylate cyclase and increases intracellular cAMP. It has only a limited role in cardiac failure, occasionally being used in the treatment of β-blocker overdose by an initial bolus of 10 mg followed by infusion of up to 5 mg.hr^{-1}. Hyperglycaemia and hyperkalaemia may complicate its use.

Ca^{2+}

While intravenously administered Ca^{2+} salts often improve blood pressure for a few minutes, their use should be restricted to circulatory collapse due to hyperkalaemia and Ca^{2+} channel antagonist overdose.

T3

Thyroxine (T_4) and triiodothyronine (T_3) have positive inotropic and chronotropic effects via intracellular mechanisms. They are only used to treat hypothyroidism and are discussed in more detail in Chapter 26.

Adrenoceptor Antagonists

α-Adrenoceptor Antagonists

α-Adrenoceptor antagonists (α-blockers) prevent the actions of sympathomimetic agents at α-adrenoceptors. Certain α-blockers (phentolamine, phenoxybenzamine) are non-specific and inhibit both α_1- and α_2-receptors, whereas others selectively inhibit α_1-receptors (prazosin) or α_2-receptors (yohimbine). The actions of specific α-adrenoceptor stimulation are shown in Table 14.1.

Non-Selective α-Blockade
Phentolamine

Phentolamine (an imidazolone) is a competitive non-selective α-blocker. Its affinity for α_1-adrenoceptors is three times that for α_2-adrenoceptors.

Presentation

It is presented as 10 mg phentolamine mesylate in 1 ml clear pale-yellow solution. The intravenous dose is 1–5 mg and should be titrated to effect. The onset of action is 1–2 minutes and its duration of action is 5–20 minutes.

Uses

Phentolamine is used in the treatment of hypertensive crises due to excessive sympathomimetics, monoamine oxidase inhibitor (MAOI) reactions with tyramine and phaeochromocytoma, especially during tumour manipulation. It has a role in the assessment of sympathetically mediated chronic pain and has previously been used to treat pulmonary hypertension. Injection into the corpus cavernosum has been used to treat impotence due to erectile failure.

Effects

- *Cardiovascular* – α_1-blockade results in vasodilatation and hypotension while α_2-blockade facilitates noradrenaline release leading to tachycardia and a raised cardiac output. Pulmonary artery pressure is also reduced. Vasodilatation of vessels in the nasal mucosa leads to marked nasal congestion.
- *Respiratory* – the presence of sulfites in phentolamine ampoules may lead to hypersensitivity reactions, which are manifest as acute bronchospasm in susceptible asthmatics.
- *Gut* – phentolamine increases secretions and motility of the gastrointestinal (GI) tract.
- *Metabolic* – it may precipitate hypoglycaemia secondary to increased insulin secretion.

Table 14.1 Actions of specific α-adrenoceptor stimulation

Receptor type	Action
Postsynaptic	
α_1-Receptors	vasoconstriction
	mydriasis
	contraction of bladder sphincter
α_2-Receptors	platelet aggregation
	hyperpolarisation of some CNS neurones
Presynaptic	
α_2-Receptors	inhibit noradrenaline release

Kinetics

The oral route is rarely used and has a bioavailability of 20%. It is 50% plasma protein-bound and extensively metabolised, leaving about 10% to be excreted unchanged in the urine. Its elimination half-life is 20 minutes.

Phenoxybenzamine

Phenoxybenzamine is a long-acting non-selective α-blocker. It has a high affinity for α_1-adrenoceptors.

Presentation

It is presented as capsules containing 10 mg and as a clear, faintly straw-coloured solution for injection containing 100 mg/2 ml phenoxybenzamine hydrochloride with ethyl alcohol, hydrochloric acid and propylene glycol.

Uses

Phenoxybenzamine is used in the pre-operative management of phaeochromocytoma (to allow expansion of the intravascular compartment), peri-operative management of some neonates undergoing cardiac surgery, hypertensive crises and occasionally as an adjunct to the treatment of severe shock. The oral dose starts at 10 mg and is increased daily until hypertension is controlled, the usual dose is $1-2$ mg.kg^{-1}.day^{-1}. Intravenous administration should be via a central cannula and the usual dose is 1 mg.kg^{-1}.day^{-1} given as a slow infusion in at least 200 ml 0.9% saline. β-blockade may be required to limit reflex tachycardia.

Mechanism of Action

Its effects are mediated by a reactive intermediate that forms a covalent bond to the α-adrenoceptor resulting in irreversible blockade. In addition to receptor blockade, phenoxybenzamine inhibits neuronal and extra-neuronal uptake of catecholamines.

Effects

• *Cardiovascular* – hypotension, which may be orthostatic, and reflex tachycardia are characteristic. Overdose should be treated with noradrenaline. Adrenaline will lead to unopposed β effects thereby compounding the hypotension and tachycardia. There is an increase in cardiac output and blood flow to skin, viscera and nasal mucosa leading to nasal congestion.

- *Central nervous system* – it usually causes marked sedation although convulsions have been reported after rapid intravenous infusion. Miosis is also seen.
- *Miscellaneous* – impotence, contact dermatitis.

Kinetics

Phenoxybenzamine is incompletely and variably absorbed from the gut (oral bioavailability about 25%). Its maximum effect is seen at 1 hour following an intravenous dose. The plasma half-life is about 24 hours and its effects may persist for 3 days while new α-adrenoceptors are synthesised. It is metabolised in the liver and excreted in urine and bile.

Selective α_1-Blockade
Prazosin

Prazosin (a quinazoline derivative) is a highly selective α_1-adrenoceptor antagonist.

Presentation and Uses

Prazosin is available as 0.5–2 mg tablets. It is used in the treatment of essential hypertension, congestive heart failure, Raynaud's syndrome and benign prostatic hypertrophy. The initial dose is 0.5 mg tds, which may be increased to 20 mg per day.

Effects

- *Cardiovascular* – prazosin produces vasodilatation of arteries and veins and a reduction of systemic vascular resistance with little or no reflex tachycardia. Diastolic pressures fall the most. Severe postural hypotension and syncope may follow the first dose. Cardiac output may increase in those with heart failure secondary to reduced filling pressures.
- *Urinary* – it relaxes the bladder trigone and sphincter muscle thereby improving urine flow in those with benign prostatic hypertrophy. Impotence and priapism have been reported.
- *Central nervous system* – fatigue, headache, vertigo and nausea all decrease with continued use.
- *Miscellaneous* – it may produce a false-positive when screening urine for metabolites of noradrenaline (VMA and MHPG seen in phaeochromocytoma).

Kinetics

Plasma levels peak about 90 minutes following an oral dose with a variable oral bioavailability of 50–80%. It is highly protein-bound, mainly to albumin, and is extensively metabolised in the liver by demethylation and conjugation. Some of the metabolites are active. It has a plasma half-life of 3 hours. It may be used safely in patients with renal impairment as it is largely excreted in the bile.

Selective α_2-Blockade
Yohimbine

The principal alkaloid of the bark of the yohimbe tree is formulated as the hydrochloride and has been used in the treatment of impotence. It has a variable effect on the cardiovascular system, resulting in a raised heart rate and blood pressure, but may precipitate orthostatic hypotension. In vitro it blocks the hypotensive responses of clonidine. It has an antidiuretic effect and can cause anxiety and manic reactions. It is contraindicated in renal or hepatic disease.

β-Adrenoceptor Antagonists

β-Adrenoceptor antagonists (β-blockers) are used widely in the treatment of hypertension, angina and peri-myocardial infarction.

They are also used in patients with phaeochromocytoma (preventing the reflex tachycardia associated with α-blockade), hyperthyroidism (propranolol), hypertrophic obstructive cardiomyopathy (to control infundibular spasm), anxiety associated with high levels of catecholamines, topically in glaucoma, in the prophylaxis of migraine and to suppress the response to laryngoscopy and at extubation (esmolol).

They are all competitive antagonists with varying degrees of receptor selectivity. In addition some have intrinsic sympathomimetic activity (i.e. are partial agonists), whereas others demonstrate membrane stabilising activity. These three features form the basis of their differing pharmacological profiles (see Table 14.2). Prolonged administration may result in an increase in the number of β-adrenoceptors.

Receptor Selectivity

In suitable patients, the useful effects of β-blockers are mediated via antagonism of $β_1$-adrenoceptors, while antagonism of $β_2$-adrenoceptors results in unwanted effects. Atenolol, esmolol and metoprolol demonstrate $β_1$-adrenoceptor selectivity (cardioselectivity) although when given in high dose $β_2$-antagonism may also be seen. All β-blockers should be used with extreme caution in patients with poor ventricular function as they may precipitate serious cardiac failure.

Table 14.2 Comparison between receptor selectivity, intrinsic sympathomimetic activity and membrane stabilising activity of various β-blockers

	$β_1$-receptor selectivity (cardioselectivity)	Intrinsic sympathomimetic activity	Membrane stabilising activity
Acebutolol	+	+	+
Atenolol	++	−	−
Esmolol	++	−	−
Metoprolol	++	−	+
Pindolol	−	++	+
Propranolol	−	−	++
Sotalol	−	−	−
Timolol	−	+	+
Labetalol	−	±	+

Intrinsic Sympathomimetic Activity – Partial Agonist Activity

Partial agonists are drugs that are unable to elicit the same maximum response as a full agonist despite adequate receptor affinity. In theory, β-blockers with partial agonist activity will produce sympathomimetic effects when circulating levels of catecholamines are low, while producing antagonist effects when sympathetic tone is high. In patients with mild cardiac failure they should be less likely to induce bradycardia and heart failure. However, they should not be used in those with more severe heart failure as β-blockade will further reduce cardiac output.

Membrane Stabilising Activity

These effects are probably of little clinical significance as the doses required to elicit them are higher than those seen in vivo.

Other Effects

- *Cardiac* – β-blockers have negative inotropic and chronotropic properties on cardiac muscle; sino-atrial (SA) node automaticity is decreased and atrioventricular (AV) node conduction time is prolonged leading to a bradycardia, while contractility is also reduced. The bradycardia lengthens the coronary artery perfusion time (during diastole) thereby increasing oxygen supply while reduced contractility diminishes oxygen demand. These effects are more important than those that tend to compromise the supply/demand equation, that is, prolonged systolic ejection time, dilation of the ventricles and increased coronary vascular resistance (due to antagonism of the vasodilatory β_2 coronary receptors). The improvement in the balance of oxygen supply/demand forms the basis for their use in angina and peri-myocardial infarction. However, in patients with poor left ventricular function β-blockade may lead to cardiac failure. β-blockers are class II anti-arrhythmic agents and are mainly used to treat arrhythmias associated with high levels of catecholamines (see Chapter 15).
- *Circulatory* – the mechanism by which β-blockers control blood pressure is not yet fully elucidated but probably includes a reduced heart rate and cardiac output, and inhibition of the renin–angiotensin system. Inhibition of β_1-receptors at the juxtaglomerular apparatus reduces renin release leading ultimately to a reduction in angiotensin II and its effects (vasoconstriction and augmenting aldosterone production). In addition, the baroreceptors may be set at a lower level, presynaptic β_2-receptors may inhibit noradrenaline release and some β-blockers may have central effects. However, due to antagonism of peripheral β_2-receptors there will be an element of vasoconstriction, which appears to have little hypertensive effect but may result in poor peripheral circulation and cold hands.
- *Respiratory* – all β-blockers given in sufficient dose will precipitate bronchospasm via β_2-antagonism. The relatively cardioselective drugs (atenolol, esmolol and metoprolol) are preferred but should still be used with extreme caution in patients with asthma.
- *Metabolic* – the control of blood sugar is complicated, involving different tissue types (liver, pancreas, adipose), receptors (α-, β-adrenoceptors) and hormones (insulin, glucagon, catecholamines). Non-selective β-blockade may obtund the normal blood sugar response to exercise and hypoglycaemia although it may also increase the resting blood sugar levels in diabetics with hypertension. Therefore, non-selective β-blockers

should not be used with hypoglycaemic agents. In addition, β-blockade may mask the normal symptoms of hypoglycaemia. Lipid metabolism may be altered resulting in increased triglycerides and reduced high density lipoproteins.

- *Central nervous system* – the more lipid-soluble β-blockers (metoprolol, propranolol) are more likely to produce CNS side effects. These include depression, hallucination, nightmares, paranoia and fatigue.
- *Ocular* – intra-ocular pressure is reduced, probably as a result of decreased production of aqueous humour.
- *Gut* – dry mouth and GI disturbances.

Kinetics

Varying lipid solubility confers the main differences seen in the kinetics of β-blockers (see Table 14.3). Those with low lipid solubility (atenolol) are poorly absorbed from the gut, undergo little hepatic metabolism and are excreted largely unchanged in the urine. However, those with high lipid solubility are well absorbed from the gut and are extensively metabolised in the liver. They have a shorter half-life and consequently need more frequent administration. In addition, they cross the blood–brain barrier, resulting in sedation and nightmares. Protein binding is variable.

Individual β-Blockers
Acebutolol

Acebutolol is a relatively cardioselective β-blocker that is only available orally. It has limited intrinsic sympathomimetic activity and some membrane stabilising properties. The adult dose is 400 mg bd but may be increased to 1.2 g.day^{-1} if required.

Kinetics

Acebutolol is well absorbed from the gut due to its moderately high lipid solubility, but due to a high first-pass metabolism its oral bioavailability is only 40%. Despite its lipid solubility it does not cross the blood–brain barrier to any great extent. Hepatic metabolism produces the active metabolite diacetol, which has a longer half-life, and is less cardioselective than acebutolol. Both are excreted in bile and may undergo enterohepatic recycling. They are also excreted in urine and the dose should be reduced in the presence of renal impairment.

Atenolol

Atenolol is a relatively cardioselective β-blocker that is available as 25–100 mg tablets, a syrup containing 5 mg.ml^{-1} and as a colourless solution for intravenous use containing 5 mg in 10 ml. The oral dose is 50–100 mg.day^{-1} while the intravenous dose is 2.5 mg slowly, repeated up to a maximum of 10 mg, which may then be followed by an infusion.

Kinetics

Atenolol is incompletely absorbed from the gut. It is not significantly metabolised and has an oral bioavailability of 45%. Only 5% is protein-bound. It is excreted unchanged in the urine and, therefore, the dose should be reduced in patients with renal impairment. It has an elimination half-life of 7 hours but its actions appear to persist for longer than this would suggest.

Table 14.3 Various pharmacological properties of some ß-blockers

Drug	Lipid solubility	Absorption (%)	Bioavailability (%)	Protein binding (%)	Elimination half-life (h)	Clearance	Active metabolites
Acebutolol	++	90	40	25	6	hepatic metabolism and renal excretion	yes
Atenolol	+	45	45	5	7	Renal	no
Esmolol	+++	n/a	n/a	60	0.15	plasma hydrolysis	no
Metoprolol	+++	95	50	20	3–7*	hepatic metabolism	no
Oxprenolol	+++	80	40	80	2	hepatic metabolism	no
Pindolol	++	90	90	50	4	hepatic metabolism	no
Propranolol	+++	90	30	90	4	hepatic metabolism	yes
Sotalol	+	85	85	0	15	Renal	no
Timolol	+++	90	50	10	4	hepatic metabolism and renal excretion	no
Labetalol	+++	70	25	50	5	hepatic metabolism	no

* Depends on genetic polymorphism – may be fast or slow hydroxylators.

Esmolol

Esmolol is a highly lipophilic, cardioselective β-blocker with a rapid onset and offset. It is presented as a clear liquid with either 2.5 g or 100 mg in 10 ml. The former should be diluted before administration as an infusion (dose range 50–200 $\mu g.kg^{-1}.min^{-1}$), while the latter is titrated in 10 mg boluses to effect. It is used in the short-term management of tachycardia and hypertension in the peri-operative period, and for acute supraventricular tachycardia. It has no intrinsic sympathomimetic activity or membrane stabilising properties.

Kinetics

Esmolol is only available intravenously and is 60% protein-bound. Its volume of distribution is 3.5 $l.kg^{-1}$. It is rapidly metabolised by red blood cell esterases to an essentially inactive acid metabolite (with a long half-life) and methyl alcohol. Its rapid metabolism ensures a short half-life of 10 minutes. The esterases responsible for its hydrolysis are distinct from plasma cholinesterase so that it does not prolong the actions of suxamethonium.

Like other β-blockers it may also precipitate heart failure and bronchospasm, although its short duration of action limits these side effects.

It is irritant to veins and extravasation may lead to tissue necrosis.

Metoprolol

Metoprolol is a relatively cardioselective β-blocker with no intrinsic sympathomimetic activity. Early use of metoprolol in myocardial infarction reduces infarct size and the incidence of ventricular fibrillation. It is also used in hypertension, as an adjunct in thyrotoxicosis and for migraine prophylaxis. The dose is 50–200 mg daily. Up to 5 mg may be given intravenously for arrhythmias and in myocardial infarction.

Kinetics

Absorption is rapid and complete but, due to hepatic first-pass metabolism, its oral bioavailability is only 50%. However, this increases to 70% during continuous administration and is also increased when given with food. Hepatic metabolism may exhibit genetic polymorphism resulting in two different half-life profiles of 3 and 7 hours. Its high lipid solubility enables it to cross the blood–brain barrier and also into breast milk. Only 20% is plasma protein-bound.

Propranolol

Propranolol is a non-selective β-blocker without intrinsic sympathomimetic activity. It exhibits the full range of effects described above at therapeutic concentrations. It is a racemic mixture, the S-isomer conferring most of its effects, although the R-isomer is responsible for preventing the peripheral conversion of T_4 to T_3.

Uses

Propranolol is used to treat hypertension, angina, essential tremor and in the prophylaxis of migraine. It is the β-blocker of choice in thyrotoxicosis as it not only inhibits the effects of the thyroid hormones, but also prevents the peripheral conversion of T_4 to T_3. Intravenous doses of 0.5 mg (up to 10 mg) are titrated to effect. The oral dose ranges from 160 mg to

320 mg daily, but due to increased clearance in thyrotoxicosis even higher doses may be required.

Kinetics

Owing to its high lipid solubility it is well absorbed from the gut but a high first-pass metabolism reduces its oral bioavailability to 30%. It is highly protein-bound although this may be reduced by heparin. Hepatic metabolism of the R-isomer is more rapid than the S-isomer and one of their metabolites, 4-hydroxypropranolol, retains some activity. Its elimination is dependent on hepatic metabolism but is impaired in renal failure by an unknown mechanism. The duration of action is longer than its half-life of 4 hours would suggest.

Sotalol

Sotalol is a non-selective β-blocker with no intrinsic sympathomimetic properties. It also has class III anti-arrhythmic properties (see Chapter 15). It is a racemic mixture, the D-isomer conferring the class III activity while the L-isomer has both class III and class II (β-blocking) actions.

Uses

Sotalol is used to treat ventricular tachyarrhythmias and for the prophylaxis of paroxysmal supraventricular tachycardias following direct current (DC) cardioversion. The ventricular rate is also well controlled if sinus rhythm degenerates back into atrial fibrillation. The Committee on Safety of Medicines states that sotalol should not be used for angina, hypertension, thyrotoxicosis or peri-myocardial infarction. The oral dose is 80–160 mg bd and the intravenous dose is 50–100 mg over 20 minutes.

Other Effects

The most serious side effect is precipitation of torsades de pointes, which is rare, occurring in less than 2% of those being treated for sustained ventricular tachycardia or fibrillation. It is more common with higher doses, a prolonged QT interval and electrolyte imbalance. It may precipitate heart failure.

Kinetics

Sotalol is completely absorbed from the gut and its oral bioavailability exceeds 90%. It is not protein-bound or metabolised. Approximately 90% is excreted unchanged in urine while the remainder is excreted in bile. Renal impairment significantly reduces clearance.

Combined α- and β-Adrenoceptor Antagonists

Labetalol

Labetalol, as its name indicates, is an α- and β-adrenoceptor antagonist; α-blockade is specific to α_1-receptors while β-blockade is non-specific. It contains two asymmetric centres and exists as a mixture of four stereoisomers present in equal proportions. The (SR)-stereoisomer is probably responsible for the α_1 effects while the (RR)-stereoisomer probably confers the β-blockade. The ratio of α_1:β-blocking effects is dependent on the route of administration: 1:3 for oral, 1:7 for intravenous.

Presentation and Uses

Labetalol is available as 50–400 mg tablets and as a colourless solution containing 5 mg.ml^{-1}. It is used to treat hypertensive crises and to facilitate hypotension during anaesthesia. The intravenous dose is 5–20 mg titrated up to a maximum of 200 mg. The oral form is used to treat hypertension associated with angina and during pregnancy where the dose is 100–800 mg bd but may be increased to a maximum of 2.4 g daily.

Mechanism of Action

Selective α_1-blockade produces peripheral vasodilatation while β-blockade prevents reflex tachycardia. Myocardial afterload and oxygen demand are decreased providing favourable conditions for those with angina.

Kinetics

Labetalol is well absorbed from the gut but due to an extensive hepatic first-pass metabolism its oral bioavailability is only 25%. However, this may increase markedly with increasing age and when administered with food. It is 50% protein-bound. Metabolism occurs in the liver and produces several inactive conjugates.

Chapter 15

Anti-Arrhythmics

Physiology

Cardiac Action Potential

The heart is composed of pacemaker, conducting and contractile tissue. Each has a different action potential morphology allowing the heart to function as a coordinated unit.

The sino-atrial (SA) node is in the right atrium, and of all cardiac tissue it has the fastest rate of spontaneous depolarisation so that it sets the heart rate. The slow spontaneous depolarisation (pre-potential or pacemaker potential) of the membrane potential is due to increased Ca^{2+} conductance (directed inward). At -40 mV, slow voltage-gated Ca^{2+} channels (L channels) open, resulting in membrane depolarisation. Na^+ conductance changes very little. Repolarisation is due to increased K^+ conductance while Ca^{2+} channels close (see Figure 15.1a).

Contractile cardiac tissue has a more stable resting potential at -80 mV. Its action potential has been divided into five phases (see Figure 15.1b):

- Phase 0 – describes the rapid depolarisation (duration < 1 millisecond) of the membrane, resulting from increased Na^+ (and possibly some Ca^{2+}) conductance through voltage-gated Na^+ channels.
- Phase 1 – represents closure of the Na^+ channels while Cl^- is expelled.
- Plateau phase 2 – due to Ca^{2+} influx via voltage-sensitive type-L Ca^{2+} channels and lasts up to 150 milliseconds. This period is also known as the absolute refractory period in which the myocyte cannot be further depolarised. This prevents myocardial tetany.
- Phase 3 – commences when the Ca^{2+} channels are inactivated and there is an increase in K^+ conductance that returns the membrane potential to its resting value. This period is also known as the relative refractory period in which the myocyte requires a greater than normal stimulus to provoke a contraction.
- Phase 4 – during this the Na^+/K^+ ATPase maintains the ionic concentration gradient at about -80 mV, although there will be variable spontaneous 'diastolic' depolarisation.

Arrhythmias

Tachyarrhythmias

- These may originate from **enhanced automaticity** where the resting potential of contractile tissue loses its stability and may reach its threshold for depolarisation before that of the SA node. This is seen during ischaemia and hypokalaemia.

- Ischaemic myocardium may result in oscillations of the membrane potential. These **after-potentials** may reach the threshold potential and precipitate tachyarrhythmias.
- **Re-entry** or **circus** mechanisms describe how an ectopic focus may originate, leading to tachyarrhythmias (see Figure 15.2).

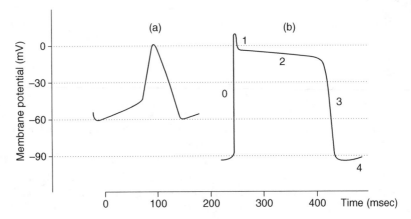

Figure 15.1 Action potentials of (a) pacemaker and (b) contractile tissue.

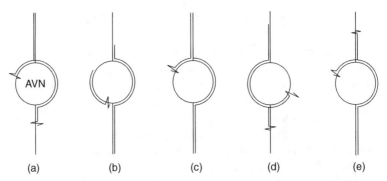

Figure 15.2 Atrioventricular nodal re-entrant tachycardia (action potential followed by refractory period). In this situation, there are two anatomically and physiologically distinct conduction pathways within the atrioventricular node (AVN). The fast pathway has a long refractory period, whereas the slow pathway has a short refractory period. (a) A normal atrial action potential (AP) travels at different velocities through the two pathways. The AP in the slow pathway arrives at the refractory final common pathway and is therefore terminated (b). (b) also demonstrates how the slow pathway recovers from its refractory state more quickly than the fast pathway. If a premature atrial impulse arrives at the origins of the two pathways and finds the fast pathway still refractory, it will only travel down the slow pathway (c). Because it travels slowly down the slow pathway it is not terminated by refractory tissue as in (b) and may travel on into the ventricles but also retrogradely up the fast pathway (d). Because of the short refractory period of the slow pathway the impulse may travel down the slow pathway (e) to continue the circus movement thereby generating the self-perpetuating tachycardia. The atrioventricular re-enterant tachycardia seen in Wolff–Parkinson–White (WPW) syndrome is generated in a similar manner except that the accessory pathway (bundle of Kent) is distinct from the atrioventricular node (AVN).

Bradyarrhythmias

These are due to failure of conduction from the SA node to the surrounding tissue. Second- and third-degree block becomes clinically significant. Atropine, β stimulation or pacing may be required.

Classification of Anti-Arrhythmics

Traditionally anti-arrhythmics have been classified according to the Vaughan–Williams classification (see Table 15.1). However, it does not include digoxin and more recently introduced drugs such as adenosine. In addition, individual agents do not fall neatly into one category, e.g. sotalol has class I, II and III activity.

Anti-arrhythmics may also be divided on the basis of their clinical use in the treatment of:

- **Supraventricular tachyarrhythmias (SVT)** (digoxin, adenosine, verapamil, β-blockers, quinidine)
- **Ventricular tachyarrhythmias (VT)** (lidocaine, mexiletine)
- **Both SVT and VT** (amiodarone, flecainide, procainamide, disopyramide, propafenone, sotalol)
- **Digoxin toxicity** (phenytoin).

Supraventricular Tachyarrhythmias

Digoxin

Presentation

Digoxin is a glycoside that is extracted from the leaves of the foxglove (*Digitalis lanata*) and is available as oral (tablets of 62.5–250 µg, elixir 50 µg.ml^{-1}) and intravenous (100–250 µg.ml^{-1}) preparations. The intramuscular route is associated with variable absorption, pain and tissue necrosis.

Table 15.1 Vaughan–Williams classification

Class	Mechanism	Drugs
Ia	Na$^+$ channel blockade – prolongs the refractory period of cardiac muscle	quinidine, procainamide, disopyramide
Ib	Na$^+$ channel blockade – shortens the refractory period of cardiac muscle	lidocaine, mexiletine, phenytoin
Ic	Na$^+$ channel blockade – no effect on the refractory period of cardiac muscle	flecainide, propafenone
II	β-Adrenoceptor blockade	propranolol, atenolol, esmolol
III	K$^+$ channel blockade	amiodarone, bretylium, sotalol
IV	Ca^{2+} channel blockade	verapamil, diltiazem

Uses

Digoxin is widely used in the treatment of atrial fibrillation and atrial flutter. It has been used in heart failure but the initial effects on cardiac output may not be sustained and other agents may produce a better outcome. It has only minimal activity on the normal heart. It should be avoided in patients with ventricular extrasystoles or ventricular tachycardia (VT) as it may precipitate ventricular fibrillation (VF) due to increased cardiac excitability.

Treatment starts with the administration of a loading dose of between 1.0 and 1.5 mg in divided doses over 24 hours followed by a maintenance dose of 125–500 µg per day. The therapeutic range is $1-2$ $\mu g.l^{-1}$.

Mechanism of Action

Digoxin has direct and indirect actions on the heart.

- Direct – it binds to and inhibits cardiac Na^+/K^+ ATPase leading to increased intracellular Na^+ and decreased intracellular K^+ concentrations. The raised intracellular Na^+ concentration leads to an increased exchange with extracellular Ca^{2+} resulting in increased availability of intracellular Ca^{2+}, which has a positive inotropic effect, increasing excitability and force of contraction. The refractory period of the atrioventricular (AV) node and the bundle of His is increased and the conductivity reduced.
- Indirect – the release of acetylcholine (ACh) at cardiac muscarinic receptors is enhanced. This slows conduction and further prolongs the refractory period in the AV node and the bundle of His.
- In atrial fibrillation the atrial rate is too high to allow a 1:1 ventricular response. By slowing conduction through the AV node, the rate of ventricular response is reduced. This allows for a longer period of coronary blood flow and a greater degree of ventricular filling so that cardiac output is increased.

Side Effects

Digoxin has a low therapeutic ratio and side effects are not uncommon:

- *Cardiac* – these include various arrhythmias and conduction disturbances – premature ventricular contractions, bigemini, all forms of AV block including third-degree block, junctional rhythm and atrial or ventricular tachycardia. Hypokalaemia, hypercalcaemia or altered pH may precipitate side effects. The ECG signs of prolonged PR interval, characteristic ST segment depression, T wave flattening and shortened QT interval are not signs of toxicity.
- *DC cardioversion* – severe ventricular arrhythmias may be precipitated in patients with toxic levels and it is recommended to withhold digoxin for 24 hours before elective cardioversion.
- *Non-cardiac* – anorexia, nausea and vomiting, diarrhoea and lethargy. Visual disturbances (including deranged red–green colour perception) and headache are common while gynaecomastia occurs during long-term administration. Skin rashes are rarely seen and may be accompanied by an eosinophilia.
- *Interactions* – plasma levels are increased by amiodarone, captopril, erythromycin and carbenoxolone. They are reduced by antacids, cholestyramine, phenytoin and metoclopramide. Ca^{2+} channel antagonists produce variable effects; verapamil will increase, while nifedipine and diltiazem may have no effect or produce a small rise in plasma levels.

Kinetics

The absorption of digoxin from the gut is variable depending on the specific formulation used, but the oral bioavailability is greater than 70%. It is about 25% plasma protein-bound and has a volume of distribution of 5–10 l.kg^{-1}. Its volume of distribution is significantly increased in thyrotoxicosis and decreased in hypothyroidism. It undergoes only minimal hepatic metabolism, being excreted mainly in the unchanged form by filtration at the glomerulus and active tubular secretion. The elimination half-life is approximately 35 hours but is increased significantly in the presence of renal failure.

Toxicity

Plasma concentrations exceeding 2.5 μg.l^{-1} are associated with toxicity although serious problems are unusual at levels below 10 μg.l^{-1}. Despite these figures the severity of toxicity does not correlate well with plasma levels. However, a dose of more than 30 mg is invariably associated with death unless digoxin-specific antibody fragments (Fab) are used.

Treatment of Digoxin Toxicity

Gastric lavage should be used with caution as any increase in vagal tone may precipitate further bradycardia or cardiac arrest. Owing to Na$^+$/K$^+$ ATPase inhibition, hyperkalaemia may be a feature and should be corrected. Hypokalaemia will exacerbate cardiac toxicity and should also be corrected. Where bradycardia is symptomatic, atropine or pacing is preferred to infusions of catecholamines, which may precipitate further arrhythmias. Ventricular arrhythmias may be treated with lidocaine or phenytoin.

If plasma levels rise above 20 μg.l^{-1}, there are life-threatening arrhythmias or hyperkalaemia becomes uncontrolled, digoxin-specific Fab are indicated. These are IgG fragments. Digoxin is bound more avidly by Fab than by its receptor so that it is effectively removed from its site of action. The inactive digoxin–Fab complex is removed from the circulation by the kidneys. There is a danger of hypersensitivity or anaphylaxis on re-exposure to digoxin-specific Fab.

Adenosine

Adenosine is a naturally occurring purine nucleoside consisting of adenine (the purine base) and D-ribose (the pentose sugar), which is present in all cells.

Presentation

Adenosine is presented as a colourless solution in vials containing 3 mg.ml^{-1}. It should be stored at room temperature.

Uses

Adenosine is used to differentiate between SVT, where the rate is at least transiently slowed, and VT, where the rate does not slow. Where SVT is due to re-entry circuits that involve the AV node, adenosine may convert the rhythm to sinus. Atrial fibrillation and flutter are not converted by adenosine to sinus rhythm as they are not generated by re-entry circuits involving the AV node, although its use in this setting will slow the ventricular response and aid ECG diagnosis.

Mechanism of Action

Adenosine has specific actions on the SA and AV node mediated by adenosine A_1 receptors that are not found elsewhere within the heart. These adenosine-sensitive K^+ channels are opened, causing membrane hyperpolarisation, and G_i-proteins cause a reduction in cAMP. This results in a dramatic negative chronotropic effect within the AV node.

Side Effects

Because of its short half-life its side effects are also short lived but for the patient may be very distressing.

- *Cardiac* – it may induce atrial fibrillation or flutter as it decreases the atrial refractory period. It is contraindicated in those with second- or third-degree AV block or with sick sinus syndrome.
- *Non-cardiac* – these include chest discomfort, shortness of breath and facial flushing. It should be used with caution in asthmatics as it may precipitate bronchospasm.
- *Drug interactions* – its effects may be enhanced by dipyridamole (by blocking its uptake) and antagonised by the methylxanthines, especially aminophylline.

Kinetics

Adenosine is given in incremental doses from 3 to 12 mg as an intravenous bolus, preferably via a central cannula. It is rapidly deaminated in the plasma and taken up by red blood cells so that its half-life is less than 10 seconds.

Verapamil

Verapamil is a competitive Ca^{2+} channel antagonist.

Presentation

It is presented as film-coated and modified-release tablets and as a solution for intravenous injection containing 2.5 $mg.ml^{-1}$.

Uses

Verapamil is used to treat SVT, atrial fibrillation or flutter, which it may slow or convert to a sinus rhythm. It is also used in the prophylaxis of angina and the treatment of hypertension.

Mechanism of Action

Verapamil prevents the influx of Ca^{2+} through voltage-sensitive slow (L) channels in the SA and AV node, thereby reducing their automaticity. It has a much less marked effect on the contractile tissue of the heart, but does reduce Ca^{2+} influx during the plateau phase 2. Antagonism of these Ca^{2+} channels results in a reduced rate of conduction through the AV node and coronary artery dilatation.

Side Effects

- *Cardiac* – if used to treat SVT complicating Wolff–Parkinson–White (WPW) syndrome, verapamil may precipitate VT due to increased conduction across the accessory pathway. In patients with poor left ventricular function it may precipitate cardiac failure. When administered concurrently with agents that also slow AV conduction (digoxin, β-blockers, halothane) it may precipitate serious bradycardia and AV block. It may increase the serum levels of digoxin. Grapefruit juice has been reported to increase serum levels and should be avoided during verapamil therapy. Although its effects are relatively specific to cardiac tissue it may also precipitate hypotension through vascular smooth muscle relaxation.

- *Non-cardiac* – cerebral artery vasodilatation occurs after the administration of verapamil.

Kinetics

Verapamil is used orally and intravenously. Although almost 90% is absorbed from the gut a high first-pass metabolism reduces its oral bioavailability to about 25%. Approximately 90% is bound to plasma proteins. It is metabolized in the liver to at least 12 inactive metabolites that are excreted in the urine. Its volume of distribution is 3–5 $l.kg^{-1}$. The elimination half-life of 3–7 hours is prolonged with higher doses as hepatic enzymes become saturated.

β-Blockers

The effects of catecholamines are antagonised by β-blockers. Therefore, they induce a bradycardia (by prolonging 'diastolic' depolarisation – phase 4), depress myocardial contractility and prolong AV conduction. In addition, some β-blockers exhibit a degree of membrane stabilising activity (class I) although this probably has little clinical significance. Sotalol also demonstrates class III activity by blocking K^+ channels and prolonging repolarisation.

β-Blockers are used in the treatment of hypertension, angina, myocardial infarction, tachyarrhythmias, thyrotoxicosis, anxiety states, the prophylaxis of migraine and topically in glaucoma. Their use as an anti-arrhythmic is limited to rate control in the treatment of paroxysmal SVT, AF and sinus tachycardia due to increased levels of catecholamines. They have a role following acute myocardial infarction where they may reduce arrhythmias and prevent further infarction. Owing to their negative inotropic effects they should be avoided in those with poor ventricular function for fear of precipitating cardiac failure. β-Blockers are also discussed on p. 210.

Esmolol

Esmolol is a relatively cardioselective β-blocker with a rapid onset and offset.

Presentation

It is presented as a clear liquid with either 2.5 g or 100 mg in 10 ml. The former should be diluted before administration as an infusion (dose range 50–200 $\mu g.kg^{-1}.min^{-1}$), while the latter is titrated in 10 mg boluses to effect.

Uses

Esmolol is used in the short-term management of tachycardia and hypertension in the peri-operative period, and for acute SVT. It has no intrinsic sympathomimetic activity or membrane stabilising properties.

Side Effects

Although esmolol is relatively cardioselective it does demonstrate β_2-adrenoceptor antagonism at high doses and should therefore be used with caution in asthmatics.

Like other β-blockers it may also precipitate heart failure. However, due to its short duration of action these side effects are also limited in time. It is irritant to veins and extravasation may lead to tissue necrosis.

Kinetics

Esmolol is only available intravenously and is 60% plasma protein-bound. Its volume of distribution is $3.5 \, l.kg^{-1}$. It is rapidly metabolised by red blood cell esterases to an essentially inactive acid metabolite (with a long half-life) and methyl alcohol. Its rapid metabolism ensures a short half-life of 10 minutes. The esterases responsible for its hydrolysis are distinct from plasma cholinesterase so that it does not prolong the actions of suxamethonium.

Quinidine

The use of quinidine has declined as alternative treatments have become available with improved side-effect profiles. However, it may still be used to treat SVT, including atrial fibrillation and flutter, and ventricular ectopic beats.

Mechanism of Action

Quinidine is a class Ia anti-arrhythmic and as such reduces the rate of rise of phase 0 of the action potential by blocking Na^+ channels. In addition, it raises the threshold potential and prolongs the refractory period without affecting the duration of the action potential. It also antagonises vagal tone.

Side Effects

These are common and become unacceptable in up to 30% of patients.

- *Cardiac* – quinidine may provoke other arrhythmias including heart block, sinus tachycardia (vagolytic action) and ventricular arrhythmias. The following ECG changes may be seen: prolonged PR interval, widened QRS and prolonged QT interval. When used to treat atrial fibrillation or flutter the patient should be pretreated with β-blockers, Ca^{2+} channel antagonists or digoxin to slow AV conduction, which may otherwise become enhanced leading to a ventricular rate equivalent to the atrial rate. Hypotension may result from α-blockade or direct myocardial depression, which is exacerbated by hyperkalaemia.
- *Non-cardiac* – CNS toxicity known as 'cinchonism' is characterised by tinnitus, blurred vision, impaired hearing, headache and confusion.
- *Drug interactions* – digoxin is displaced from its binding sites so that its serum concentration is increased. Phenytoin will reduce quinidine levels (hepatic enzyme induction) while cimetidine will increase quinidine levels (hepatic enzyme inhibition). The effects of depolarising and non-depolarising muscle relaxants are increased.

Kinetics

Quinidine is well absorbed from the gut and has an oral bioavailability of about 75%. It is highly protein-bound (about 90%) and is metabolised by the liver to active metabolites, which are excreted mainly in the urine. The elimination half-life is 5–9 hours.

Ventricular Tachyarrhythmias

Lidocaine

Lidocaine is a class Ib anti-arrhythmic agent.

Presentation

The 1% or 2% solutions (10–20 mg.ml^{-1}) are the preparations used in this setting.

Uses

Lidocaine is used to treat sustained ventricular tachyarrhythmias especially when associated with ischaemia (where inactivated Na^+ channels predominate) or re-entry pathways. An initial intravenous bolus of 1 mg.kg^{-1} is followed by an intravenous infusion of 1–3 mg. min^{-1} for an adult. This infusion rate should be slowed where hepatic blood flow is reduced as hepatic metabolism will also be reduced.

Mechanism of Action

Lidocaine reduces the rate of rise of phase 0 of the action potential by blocking inactivated Na^+ channels and raising the threshold potential. The duration of the action potential and the refractory period are decreased as the repolarisation phase 3 is shortened.

Side Effects

- *Cardiac* – cardiovascular toxicity becomes apparent as plasma levels exceed 10 μg. ml^{-1} and are manifest as AV block and unresponsive hypotension due to myocardial depression. Some of the cardiac effects may be due to central medullary depression.
- *Non-cardiac* – these become apparent only when the plasma levels exceed 4 μg.ml^{-1}. Initially CNS toxicity is manifest as circumoral tingling, dizziness and paraesthesia. This progresses to confusion, coma and seizures as plasma levels rise above 5 μg.ml^{-1}.

Kinetics

When used for the treatment of arrhythmias lidocaine is only given intravenously. It is 33% unionised and 70% protein-bound. It is metabolised by hepatic amidases to products that are eliminated in the urine. Its elimination half-life is about 90 minutes so that in the presence of normal hepatic function a steady state would be reached after about 6 hours in the absence of a loading dose. Its clearance is reduced in cardiac failure due to reduced hepatic blood flow.

Mexiletine

Mexiletine is an analogue of lidocaine with similar effects on ventricular tachyarrhythmias.

Presentation

It is presented as a colourless solution containing 250 mg mexiletine hydrochloride in 10 ml. The oral formulation is also available as modified release.

Uses

Mexiletine has similar indications to lidocaine, particularly when arrhythmias are associated with ischaemia or digoxin.

Mechanism of Action

Mexiletine reduces the rate of rise of phase 0 of the action potential by blocking Na^+ channels and raising the threshold potential. The duration of the action potential and the refractory period are decreased as the repolarisation phase 3 is shortened.

Side Effects

Mexiletine has a low therapeutic ratio and side effects are common.

- *Cardiac* – it may precipitate sinus bradycardia, supraventricular and ventricular tachyarrhythmias.
- *Non-cardiac* – up to 40% of patients have unacceptable nausea and vomiting and altered bowel habit. Confusion, diplopia, seizures, tremor and ataxia are also seen. Thrombocytopenia, rash and jaundice have also been reported.

Kinetics

Its oral bioavailability of 90% reflects good absorption from the upper part of the small bowel and minimal first-pass metabolism (about 10%). It is 65% plasma protein-bound and has a volume of distribution of 6–13 l.kg^{-1}. It undergoes hepatic metabolism to a number of inactive metabolites. Up to 20% is excreted unchanged in the urine.

Supraventricular and Ventricular Tachyarrhythmias

Amiodarone

Amiodarone is a benzofuran derivative.

Presentation

It is presented as tablets containing 100–200 mg and as a solution containing 150 mg per ampoule. It should be diluted in 5% dextrose before administration.

Uses

Amiodarone is used in the treatment of SVT, VT and WPW syndrome. It is a complex drug with many actions and side effects.

A loading dose of 5 mg.kg^{-1} over 1 hour followed by 15 mg.kg^{-1} over 24 hours provides a starting point for its intravenous use, which should be adjusted according to response. When used orally treatment commences with 200 mg tds for 1 week, followed by 200 mg bd for a further week and thereafter 200 mg od.

Mechanism of Action

While it has been traditionally designated a class III anti-arrhythmic, amiodarone also demonstrates class I, II and IV activity. By blocking K^+ channels it slows the rate of repolarisation thereby increasing the duration of the action potential. The refractory period is also increased.

Side Effects

The side effects of amiodarone will affect most patients if given for long enough although most are reversible if treatment is stopped.

- *Pulmonary* – patients may develop a pneumonitis, fibrosis or pleuritis. The reported incidence is 10% at 3 years with a 10% mortality rate. However, if treatment is stopped early enough the process may be reversed. There is some evidence to suggest that a high F_iO_2 may be a risk factor in the development of acute pulmonary toxicity when amiodarone is used in critically ill patients.
- *Thyroid* – both hyperthyroidism (in 0.9%) and hypothyroidism (in 6%) have been observed and both are usually reversible. It prevents the peripheral conversion of T4 to T3.
- *Hepatic* – cirrhosis, hepatitis and jaundice have all been observed. Liver function tests should be performed before and during long-term treatment.
- *Cardiac* – when large doses are given rapidly it may cause bradycardia and hypotension. It has a low arrhythmic potential. The QT interval may be prolonged.
- *Ophthalmic* – corneal microdeposits occur commonly but have little clinical significance, causing visual haloes and some mild blurring of vision. They are reversible. Ophthalmic examination is recommended annually for those on long-term treatment.
- *Gut* – during the loading dose a metallic taste may be noticed. Minor intestinal upset is seen occasionally.
- *Neurological* – peripheral neuropathy and rarely myopathy have been reported.
- *Dermatological* – the skin becomes photosensitive and may remain so for a number of months after finishing treatment. A slate-grey colour, particularly of the face, may develop.
- *Interactions* – the effects of other highly protein-bound drugs (phenytoin, warfarin) are increased and their doses should be adjusted. The plasma level of digoxin may rise when amiodarone is added due to displacement from plasma protein-binding sites and cause signs of toxicity. Caution should be exercised when used with drugs that slow AV conduction (β-blockers, verapamil) and it should not be given with other drugs that prolong the QT interval (phenothiazines, TCAs, thiazides) for fear of precipitating torsades de pointes.
- *Miscellaneous* – the intravenous preparation is irritant and should be administered via a central vein.

Kinetics

Amiodarone is poorly absorbed from the gut and has an oral bioavailability between 50% and 70%. In the plasma it is highly protein-bound (> 95%) and has a volume of distribution of $2–70 \, \text{l.kg}^{-1}$. Muscle and fat accumulate amiodarone to a considerable extent. Its elimination half-life is long, varying from 20–100 days. Hepatic metabolism produces desmethylamiodarone, which appears to have some anti-arrhythmic activity. It is excreted by the lachrymal glands, the skin and biliary tract.

Flecainide

Presentation

Flecainide is available orally or intravenously and is an amide local anaesthetic with class Ic properties. The oral dose is 100 mg bd (maximum 400 mg daily). When used intravenously the dose is 2 mg.kg^{-1} over 10–30 minutes (maximum 150 mg). This may then be followed by an infusion, initially at 1.5 mg.kg^{-1}.h^{-1}, which is then reduced to 100–250 µg.kg^{-1}.h^{-1} for up to 24 hours (maximum 24-hour dose is 600 mg).

Uses

Flecainide has powerful anti-arrhythmic effects against atrial and ventricular tachyarrhythmias including WPW syndrome.

Mechanism of Action

Flecainide prevents the fast Na$^+$ flux into cardiac tissue and prolongs phase 0 of the action potential. It has no effect on the duration of the action potential or the refractory period. Its effects are particularly pronounced on the conducting pathways.

Side Effects

- *Cardiac* – flecainide may precipitate pre-existing conduction disorders and special care is required when used in patients with SA or AV disease or with bundle branch block. A paradoxical increase in ventricular rate may be seen in atrial fibrillation or flutter. When used to suppress ventricular ectopic beats following myocardial infarction it was associated with an increased mortality. Cardiac failure may complicate its use due to its negative inotropic effects. It raises the pacing threshold.
- *Non-cardiac* – dizziness, paraesthesia and headaches may complicate its use.

Kinetics

Flecainide is well absorbed from the gut and has an oral bioavailability of 90%. It is about 50% plasma protein-bound and has a volume of distribution of 6–10 l.kg^{-1}. Hepatic metabolism produces active metabolites, which along with unchanged drug are excreted in the urine.

Procainamide

Procainamide has similar effects to quinidine but is less vagolytic.

Uses

Procainamide has been used to treat both SVT and ventricular tachyarrhythmias. It is as effective as lidocaine in terminating VT. It may be given orally or intravenously. The oral dose is up to 50 mg.kg^{-1}.day^{-1} in divided doses and the intravenous dose is 100 mg slowly up to a maximum of 1 g. This may be followed by an infusion of 2–6 mg.min^{-1}, which should subsequently be converted to oral therapy.

Mechanism of Action

Procainamide is a class Ia anti-arrhythmic and as such reduces the rate of rise of phase 0 of the action potential by blocking Na$^+$ channels. In addition, it raises the threshold potential and prolongs the refractory period without altering the duration of the action potential. It also antagonises vagal tone but to a lesser extent than quinidine.

Side Effects

These have limited its use.

- *Cardiac* – following intravenous administration it may produce hypotension, vasodilatation and a reduced cardiac output. It may also precipitate heart block. When used to treat SVT the ventricular response rate may increase. It may also prolong the QT interval and precipitate torsades de pointes.
- *Non-cardiac* – chronically a drug-induced lupus erythematosus syndrome with a positive anti-nuclear factor develops in 20–30% of patients (many of whom will be slow acetylators). Other minor effects include GI upset, fever and rash. It reduces the antimicrobial effect of sulfonamides by the production of para-aminobenzoic acid.

Kinetics

Procainamide is well absorbed from the gut and has an oral bioavailability of 75%. Its short half-life of 3 hours necessitates frequent administration or slow-release formulations. It is metabolised in the liver by amidases and by acetylation to the active N-acetyl procainamide. The latter pathway demonstrates genetic polymorphism so that patients may be grouped as slow or fast acetylators. The slow acetylators are more likely to develop side effects.

Disopyramide

Disopyramide is a class Ia anti-arrhythmic.

Presentation

It is available as tablets (including slow release) and as a solution containing 10 mg.ml^{-1}. The daily oral dose is up to 800 mg in divided doses; the intravenous dose is 2 mg.kg^{-1} over 30 minutes up to 150 mg, which is followed by an infusion of 1 mg.kg^{-1}.h^{-1} up to 800 mg.day^{-1}.

Uses

Disopyramide is used as a second-line agent in the treatment of both SVT and ventricular tachyarrhythmias. When used to treat atrial fibrillation or atrial flutter the ventricular rate should first be controlled with β-blockers or verapamil.

Mechanism of Action

Disopyramide is a class Ia anti-arrhythmic and as such reduces the rate of rise of phase 0 of the action potential by blocking Na$^+$ channels. In addition, it raises the threshold potential and prolongs the refractory period, thereby increasing the duration of the action potential. It also has anticholinergic effects.

Side Effects

- *Cardiac* – as plasma concentrations rise the QT interval is prolonged (occasionally precipitating torsades de pointes), myocardial contractility becomes depressed while ventricular excitability is increased and may predispose to re-entry arrhythmias. Cardiac failure and cardiogenic shock occur rarely.
- *Non-cardiac* – anticholinergic effects (blurred vision, dry mouth and occasionally urinary retention) often prove unacceptable.

Kinetics

Disopyramide is well absorbed from the gut and has an oral bioavailability of 75%. It is only partially metabolised in the kidney, the majority of the drug being excreted in the urine unchanged. Its elimination half-life is about 5 hours but this increases significantly in patients with renal or cardiac failure.

Propafenone

Propafenone is similar in many respects to flecainide.

Presentation

It is available only as film-coated tablets in the UK although it has been used intravenously at a dose of 1–2 mg.kg^{-1}. The oral dose is initially 600–900 mg followed by 150–300 mg bd or tds.

Uses

Propafenone is used as second-line therapy for resistant SVT, including atrial fibrillation and flutter, and also for ventricular tachyarrhythmias.

Mechanism of Action

Propafenone prevents the fast Na$^+$ flux into cardiac tissue and prolongs phase 0 of the action potential. The duration of the action potential and refractory period is prolonged, especially in the conducting tissue. The threshold potential is increased and cardiac excitability reduced by an increase in the ventricular fibrillation threshold. At higher doses it may exhibit some β-blocking properties.

Side Effects

Propafenone is generally well tolerated.

- *Cardiac* – owing to its weak β-blocking actions it should be used with caution in those with heart failure.
- *Non-cardiac* – it may produce minor nervous system effects and at higher doses GI side effects may become more prominent. It may worsen myasthenia gravis. Propafenone increases the plasma levels of concurrently administered digoxin and warfarin. It may precipitate asthma due to its β-blocking properties.

Kinetics

Absorption from the gut is nearly complete and initially oral bioavailability is 50%. However, this increases disproportionately to nearly 100% as the enzymes involved in first-pass metabolism become saturated. It is more than 95% protein-bound. Hepatic metabolism ensures that only tiny amounts are excreted unchanged. However, the enzyme responsible for its metabolism demonstrates genetic polymorphism so that affected patients may have an increased response.

Sotalol

Sotalol is a β-blocker but also has class I and III anti-arrhythmic activity.

Presentation

It is available as tablets and as a solution containing 40 mg in 4 ml. It is a racemic mixture, the D-isomer conferring the class III activity while the L-isomer has both class III and β-blocking actions.

Uses

Sotalol is used to treat ventricular tachyarrhythmias and in the prophylaxis of paroxysmal SVT. The oral dose is 80–160 mg bd and the intravenous dose is 50–100 mg over 20 minutes.

Mechanism of Action

Sotalol prolongs the duration of the action potential so that the effective refractory period is prolonged in the conducting tissue. It is also a non-selective β-blocker and is more effective at maintaining sinus rhythm following DC cardioversion for atrial fibrillation than other β-blockers. The ventricular rate is also well controlled if the rhythm degenerates back into atrial fibrillation.

Side Effects

- *Cardiac* – the most serious side effect is precipitation of torsades de pointes, which occurs in less than 2% of those being treated for sustained VT or VF. It is more common with higher doses, a prolonged QT interval and electrolyte imbalance. It may precipitate heart failure.
- *Non-cardiac* – bronchospasm, masking of symptoms of hypoglycaemia, visual disturbances and sexual dysfunction are all rare.

Kinetics

Sotalol is completely absorbed from the gut and its oral bioavailability is greater than 90%. It is not plasma protein-bound and is not metabolised. Approximately 90% is excreted unchanged in the urine while the remainder is excreted in bile. Renal impairment significantly reduces clearance.

Digoxin Toxicity

Phenytoin

Although phenytoin is mainly used for its anti-epileptic activity, it has a limited role in the treatment of arrhythmias associated with digoxin toxicity.

It depresses normal pacemaker activity while augmenting conduction through the conducting system especially when this has become depressed by digoxin. It also demonstrates class I anti-arrhythmic properties by blocking Na^+ channels.

Miscellaneous

Ivabradine

Presentation

Ivabradine is a benzazepine (comprising a benzene and azepine ring) and is available as 2.5–7.5 mg tablets.

Uses

It is used in the management of chronic stable angina and mild/severe heart failure. It appears to be most effective in those with a pre-treatment resting heart rate of > 75 bpm. The starting dose is 5 mg bd increasing to 7.5 mg bd. Its use with calcium channel blockers is contraindicated.

Mechanism of Action

Ivabradine acts by selective inhibition of the 'funny' channel pacemaker current (I_f) at the SA node. (It was described as 'funny' because it had unusual properties compared with other current systems at the time of its discovery). The inward I_f current (carried by Na^+ and K^+ ions) is central to the generation and rate of the pacemaker current, i.e. phase 4 of cardiac depolarisation. It is activated by hyperpolarisation and modulated by intracellular cAMP under the control of the autonomic nervous system (ANS). The structural subunits are therefore said to be hyperpolarisation-activated cyclic nucleotide-gated (HCN) channels. Selective blockade by ivabradine slows the heart rate while not affecting action potential duration or inotropy, unlike other agents, e.g. β-blockers or Ca^{2+} channel antagonists.

Side Effects

Ivabradine may cause luminous phenomena (a sensation of enhanced visual brightness), blurred vision, first degree heart block, headache, dizziness and uncontrolled blood pressure.

Kinetics

It has an oral bioavailability of 40%, is 70% plasma protein-bound and metabolised by hepatic CYP3A4 to an active N-desmethylated derivative which is excreted equally in bile and urine. It's use with drugs (and grapefruit juice) that strongly inhibit CYP3A4 is not recommended. Its elimination half-life is 2 hours.

Chapter 16

Vasodilators

Sodium Nitroprusside

Sodium nitroprusside (SNP) is an inorganic complex and functions as a prodrug.

Uses

Sodium nitroprusside is usually administered as a 0.005–0.02% (50–200 μg/ml) intravenous infusion, the dose of 0.5–6 $\mu g.kg^{-1}.min^{-1}$ being titrated to effect.

Mechanism of Action

Sodium nitroprusside vasodilates arteries and veins by the production of nitric oxide (NO). This activates the enzyme guanylate cyclase leading to increased levels of intracellular cyclic guanosine monophosphate (cGMP). Although Ca^{2+} influx into vascular smooth muscle is inhibited, its uptake into smooth endoplasmic reticulum is enhanced so that cytoplasmic levels fall, resulting in vasodilation.

Effects

- *Cardiovascular* – arterial vasodilation reduces the systemic vascular resistance and leads to a drop in blood pressure. Venous vasodilation increases the venous capacitance and reduces preload. Cardiac output is maintained by a reflex tachycardia. However, for those patients with heart failure the reduction in pre- and afterload will increase cardiac output with no increase in heart rate. The ventricular wall tension and myocardial oxygen consumption are reduced. It has no direct effects on contractility. Some patients develop tachyphylaxis, the exact mechanism of which is unclear.
- *Respiratory* – SNP may inhibit pulmonary hypoxic vasoconstriction and lead to increased shunt. Supplemental oxygen may help.
- *Central nervous system* – intracranial pressure is increased due to cerebral vasodilation and increased cerebral blood flow. However, cerebral autoregulation is maintained well below the normal limits during SNP infusion.

Kinetics

Sodium nitroprusside is not absorbed following oral administration. It has a short half-life and its duration of action is less than 10 minutes. However, the half-life of thiocyanate (SCN) is 2 days.

Metabolism

The metabolism of SNP is complicated (see Figure 16.1). Initially within the red blood cell it reacts with oxyhaemoglobin to form NO, five CN^- ions and methaemoglobin. The methaemoglobin may then combine with CN^- to form cyanomethaemoglobin, which is thought to be non-toxic.

The remaining CN^- is then able to escape from the red blood cell where it is converted in the liver and kidney by the mitochondrial enzyme rhodanase with the addition of a sulfhydryl group to form thiocyanate (SCN). Red blood cells contain the enzyme thiocyanate oxidase, which can convert SCN back to CN^-, but most SCN is excreted in the urine. SCN has an elimination half-life of 2 days but this may increase to 7 days in the presence of renal impairment. Alternatively CN^- combines with hydroxycobalamin (vitamin B_{12}) to form cyanocobalamin, which forms a non-toxic store of CN^- and can be excreted in the urine.

Toxicity

The major risk of toxicity comes from CN^-, although SCN is also toxic. Free CN^- can bind cytochrome oxidase and impair aerobic metabolism. In doing so a metabolic acidosis develops and the mixed venous oxygen saturation increases as tissues become unable to

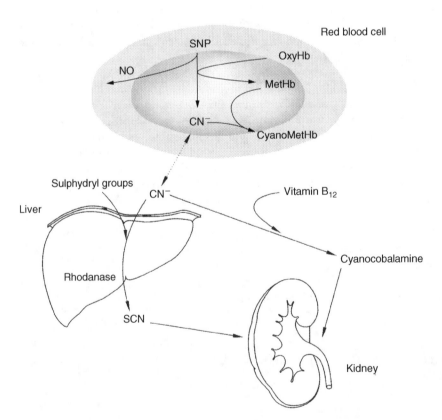

Figure 16.1 Metabolism of sodium nitroprusside (SNP). CN^-, cyanide; SCN, thiocyanate.

utilise oxygen. The management of CN⁻ toxicity involves halting the SNP infusion and optimising oxygen delivery to tissues. Three treatments are useful:

- Dicobalt edetate, which chelates CN⁻ ions.
- Sodium thiosulfate, which provides additional sulfhydryl groups to facilitate the conversion of CN⁻ to SCN. This is sometimes used as prophylaxis.
- Nitrites – either sodium nitrite or amyl nitrite will convert oxyhaemoglobin to methaemoglobin, which has a higher affinity for CN⁻ than cytochrome oxidase. While vitamin B_{12} is required to complex CN⁻ to cyanocobalamin, it is of little value in the acute setting. It is, however, sometimes used as prophylaxis.

Nitrates

Glyceryl Trinitrate

Glyceryl trinitrate (GTN) is an organic nitrate.

Presentation

Glyceryl trinitrate is prepared in the following formulations: an aerosol spray delivering 400 µg per metered dose and tablets containing 300–600 µg, both used sublingually, as required. Modified-release tablets containing 1–5 mg for buccal administration are placed between the upper lip and gum and are used at a maximum dose of 5 mg tds while the 2.6–10 mg modified-release tablets are to be swallowed and used at a maximum dose of 12.8 mg tds. The transdermal patch preparation releases 5–15 mg/24 hours, and should be resited at a different location on the chest. The clear colourless solution for injection contains 1–5 mg. ml⁻¹ and should be diluted to a 0.01% (100 µg/ml) solution before administration by an infusion pump and is used at 10–200 µg.min⁻¹. GTN is absorbed by polyvinyl chloride; therefore, special polyethylene administration sets are preferred. GTN will explode if heated so transdermal preparations should be removed before DC cardioversion.

Uses

Glyceryl trinitrate is used in the treatment and prophylaxis of angina, in left ventricular failure associated with myocardial infarction and following cardiac surgery. It has also been used in the control of intra-operative blood pressure and for oesophageal spasm.

Mechanism of Action

Glyceryl trinitrate vasodilates veins by the production of nitric oxide. This activates the enzyme guanylate cyclase leading to increased levels of intracellular cyclic GMP. Although Ca^{2+} influx into vascular smooth muscle is inhibited, its uptake into smooth endoplasmic reticulum is enhanced so that cytoplasmic levels fall resulting in vasodilation (see Figure 16.2).

Effects

- *Cardiovascular* – in contrast to SNP and despite a similar mechanism of action, GTN produces vasodilation predominantly in the capacitance vessels, that is, veins, although arteries are dilated to some extent. Consequently, it produces a reduction in preload, venous return, ventricular end-diastolic pressure and wall tension. This in turn leads to a reduction in oxygen demand and increased coronary blood flow to subendocardial

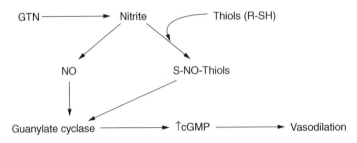

Figure 16.2 Metabolism of glyceryl trinitrate (GTN).

regions and is the underlying reason for its use in cardiac failure and ischaemic heart disease. The reduction in preload may lead to a reduction in cardiac output although patients with cardiac failure may see a rise in cardiac output. Postural hypotension may occur. At higher doses systemic vascular resistance falls and augments the fall in blood pressure which, while reducing myocardial work, will reduce coronary artery perfusion pressure and time (secondary to tachycardia). Coronary artery flow may be increased directly by coronary vasodilation. Tolerance develops within 48 hours and may be due to depletion of sulfhydryl groups within vascular smooth muscle. A daily drug-free period of a few hours prevents tolerance. It has been suggested that infusion of acetylcysteine (providing sulfhydryl groups) may prevent tolerance.

- *Central nervous system* – an increase in intracranial pressure and headache resulting from cerebral vasodilation may occur but is often only problematic at the start of treatment.
- *Gut* – GTN relaxes the GI sphincters including the sphincter of Oddi.
- *Haematological* – rarely methaemoglobinaemia is precipitated.

Kinetics

Glyceryl trinitrate is rapidly absorbed from sublingual mucosa and the GI tract although the latter is subject to extensive first-pass hepatic metabolism resulting in an oral bioavailability of less than 5%. Sublingual effects are seen within 3 minutes and last for 30–60 minutes. Hepatic nitrate reductase is responsible for the metabolism of GTN to glycerol dinitrate and nitrite (NO^{2-}) in a process that requires tissue thiols (R-SH). Nitrite is then converted to NO, which confers its mechanism of action (see above). Under certain conditions nitrite may convert oxyhaemoglobin to methaemoglobin by oxidation of the ferrous ion (Fe^{2+}) to the ferric ion (Fe^{3+}).

Isosorbide Dinitrate and Isosorbide Mononitrate

Isosorbide dinitrate (ISDN) is prepared with lactose and mannitol to reduce the risk of explosion. It is well absorbed from the gut and is subject to extensive first-pass metabolism in the liver to isosorbide 2-mononitrate and isosorbide 5-mononitrate (ISMN), both of which probably confer the majority of the activity of ISDN. ISMN has a much longer half-life (4.5 hours) and is used in its own right. It is not subject to hepatic first-pass metabolism and has an oral bioavailability of 100%. Both are used in the prophylaxis of angina.

Potassium Channel Activators

Nicorandil

Nicorandil (nicotinamidoethyl nitrate) is a potassium channel activator with a nitrate moiety and as such differs from other potassium channel activators. It has been used in Japan since 1984 and was launched in the UK in 1994.

Presentation and Uses

Nicorandil is available as tablets and the usual dose is 10–30 mg bd. It is used for the treatment and prophylaxis of angina and in the treatment of congestive heart failure and hypertension. It has been used experimentally via the intravenous route.

Mechanism of Action

ATP-sensitive K^+ channels are closed during the normal cardiac cycle but are open (activated) during periods of ischaemia when intracellular levels of ATP fall. In the open state K^+ passes down its concentration gradient out of the cell resulting in hyperpolarisation, which closes Ca^{2+} channels, resulting in less Ca^{2+} for myocardial contraction.

Nicorandil activates the ATP-sensitive K^+ channels within the heart and arterioles. In addition, nicorandil relaxes venous capacitance smooth muscle by stimulating guanylate cyclase via its nitrate moiety, leading to increased intracellular cGMP.

Effects

- *Cardiovascular* – nicorandil causes venodilation and arterial vasodilation resulting in a reduced pre- and afterload. The blood pressure falls. Left ventricular end-diastolic pressure falls and there is an improved normal and collateral coronary artery blood flow, partly induced by coronary artery vasodilation without a 'steal' phenomenon. An increase in cardiac output is seen in patients with ischaemic heart disease and cardiac failure. It is effective at suppressing torsades de pointes associated with a prolonged QT interval. High concentrations in vitro result in a shortened action potential by accelerated repolarisation. It also reduces the size of experimentally induced ischaemia, the mechanism of which is uncertain, so that an alternative, as yet undefined, cardioprotective mechanism has been postulated. Unlike nitrate therapy it is not associated with tolerance during prolonged administration. Contractility and atrioventricular conduction is not affected.
- *Central nervous system* – headaches, which usually clear with continued therapy.
- *Metabolic* – unlike other antihypertensives nicorandil has no effect on lipid profile or glucose control.
- *Haematological* – nicorandil inhibits in vitro ADP-induced platelet aggregation (in a similar manner to nitrates), which is associated with an increase of intraplatelet cGMP.
- *Miscellaneous* – giant oral apthous ulcers have been reported with its use.

Kinetics

Nicorandil is well absorbed from the gut with insignificant first-pass metabolism. The main metabolic route is denitration with 20% excreted as metabolites in the urine. The elimination half-life is 1 hour, although its actions last up to 12 hours, but neither is increased in the presence of renal impairment. It is not plasma protein-bound to any significant extent.

Calcium Channel Antagonists

Despite their disparate chemical structures (see Table 16.1), the Ca^{2+} channel antagonists are all effective in specifically blocking the entry of Ca^{2+} through L-type channels while leaving T-, N- and P-type Ca^{2+} channels unaffected. The L-type channel is widespread in the cardiovascular system and is responsible for the plateau phase (slow inward current) of the cardiac action potential. It triggers the internal release of Ca^{2+} and is regulated by cAMP-dependent protein kinase. The T-type channel is structurally similar to the L-type channel and is present mainly in cardiac cells that lack a T-tubule system, that is, sino-atrial (SA) node and certain types of vascular smooth muscle. They are not present in ventricular myocardium. N-type channels are only found in nerve cells.

Calcium channel antagonists have variable affinity for L-type channels in myocardium, nodal and vascular smooth muscle resulting in variable effects. They are all useful in the treatment of essential hypertension, although some are also particularly useful in the treatment of angina or arrhythmias.

Verapamil

Verapamil is a racemic mixture and a synthetic derivative of papaverine.

Presentation and Uses

Verapamil is available as 20–240 mg tablets, some prepared as modified release and as an oral suspension containing 40 mg/5 ml. The colourless intravenous preparation contains 2.5 mg. ml^{-1}. It is used for certain supraventricular arrhythmias (not in atrial fibrillation complicating Wolff-Parkinson-White (WPW) syndrome) and angina. It has been used to treat hypertension although its negative inotropic properties limit its usefulness in this setting.

Mechanism of Action

The L-isomer has specific Ca^{2+} channel blocking actions with a particular affinity for those at the SA node and AV node, whereas the D-isomer acts on fast Na^+ channels resulting in some local anaesthetic activity.

Effects

- *Cardiovascular* (see Table 16.2) – verapamil acts specifically to slow the conduction of the action potential at the SA and AV node resulting in a reduced heart rate. To a lesser extent it produces some negative inotropic effects and vasodilates peripheral vascular smooth muscle. It is a mild coronary artery vasodilator. Blood pressure falls. It may lead

Table 16.1 Chemical classification of calcium channel antagonists

Class I	phenylalkylamines	verapamil
Class II	dihydropyridines	nifedipine, amlodipine, nimodipine
Class III	benzothiazepines	diltiazem

Table 16.2 Main cardiovascular effects of some calcium channel antagonists

	Blood pressure	Heart rate	AV conduction time	Myocardial contractility	Peripheral and coronary artery vasodilation
Verapamil	↓	↓	↑	↓↓	↑
Nifedipine	↓	→↑	→↑	→↑	↑↑↑
Diltiazem	↓	↓	↑	↓	↑↑

to various degrees of heart block or cardiac failure in those with impaired ventricular function and ventricular fibrillation in those with WPW syndrome.
- *Central nervous system* – it vasodilates the cerebral circulation.
- *Miscellaneous* – following chronic administration it may potentiate the effects of non-depolarising and depolarising muscle relaxants.

Kinetics

Verapamil is well absorbed from the gut but an extensive first-pass hepatic metabolism reduces the oral bioavailability to 20%. Demethylation produces norverapamil, which retains significant anti-arrhythmic properties. It is 90% plasma protein-bound and is mainly excreted in the urine following metabolism, although up to 20% is excreted in bile.

Nifedipine

Presentation and Uses

Nifedipine is available as capsules containing 5–10 mg, the contents of which may be administered sublingually, and tablets containing 10–60 mg, some of which are available as sustained release. The onset of action is 15–20 minutes following oral and 5–10 minutes following sublingual administration. Swallowing the contents of an opened capsule may further reduce the onset time. It is used in the prophylaxis and treatment of angina, hypertension and in Raynaud's syndrome.

Effects

- *Cardiovascular* (see Table 16.2) – nifedipine reduces tone in peripheral and coronary arteries, resulting in a reduced systemic vascular resistance, fall in blood pressure, increased coronary artery blood flow and reflex increases in heart rate and contractility. The cardiac output is increased. Occasionally these reflex changes worsen the oxygen supply/demand ratio.

Kinetics

Nifedipine is well absorbed following oral administration although hepatic first-pass metabolism reduces its oral bioavailability to 60%. It is 95% plasma protein-bound and has an elimination half-life of 5 hours following oral administration. It is predominantly excreted as inactive metabolites in the urine (see Table 16.3).

Table 16.3 Various pharmacological properties of some calcium channel antagonists

	Absorbed (%)	Oral bioavailability (%)	Protein binding (%)	Active metabolites	Clearance	Elimination half-life (hrs)
Verapamil	95	20	90	yes	renal	6–12
Nifedipine	95	60	95	no	renal	2–5
Diltiazem	95	50	75	yes	60% hepatic, 40% renal	3–6

Nimodipine

Nimodipine is a more lipid-soluble analogue of nifedipine and as such can penetrate the blood–brain barrier. It is used in the prevention and treatment of cerebral vasospasm following subarachnoid haemorrhage and in migraine. It may be administered orally or intravenously.

Its action may be dependent on blocking a Ca^{2+}-dependent cascade of cellular processes that would otherwise lead to cell damage and destruction.

Diltiazem

Presentation and Uses

Diltiazem is available as 60–200 mg tablets, some of which are available as slow release. It is also available in combination with hydrochlorothiazide. It is used for the prophylaxis and treatment of angina and in hypertension.

Effects

- *Cardiovascular* (see Table 16.2) – diltiazem has actions both within the heart and in the peripheral circulation. It prolongs AV conduction time and reduces contractility but to a lesser extent than verapamil. It also reduces the systemic vascular resistance and the blood pressure falls although a reflex tachycardia is not usually seen. Coronary blood flow is increased due to coronary artery vasodilation.

Kinetics

Diltiazem is almost completely absorbed from the gut but hepatic first-pass metabolism reduces the oral bioavailability to 50%. Hepatic metabolism produces an active metabolite, desacetyldiltiazem, which is excreted in the urine. The urine also eliminates 40% of diltiazem in the unchanged form. Approximately 75% is plasma protein-bound.

Miscellaneous

Hydralazine

Presentation and Uses

Hydralazine is available as 25–50 mg tablets and as a powder containing 20 mg for reconstitution in water before intravenous administration (5% dextrose should be avoided as it promotes its rapid breakdown). Hydralazine is used orally in the control of chronic hypertension and severe chronic heart failure in conjunction with other agents. It is used intravenously in acute hypertension associated with pre-eclampsia at 10–20 mg. This may take up to 20 minutes to work and repeat doses may be required.

Mechanism of Action

The exact mechanism of action is uncertain but involves the activation of guanylate cyclase and an increase in intracellular cGMP. This leads to a decrease in available intracellular Ca^{2+} and vasodilation.

Effects

- *Cardiovascular* – its main effect is to reduce arteriolar tone and systemic vascular resistance, whereas the capacitance vessels are less affected. As a result postural hypotension is not usually a problem. Reflex tachycardia and an increase in cardiac output ensue but may be effectively antagonised by β-blockade.
- *Central nervous system* – cerebral artery blood flow increases as a result of cerebral artery vasodilation.
- *Renal* – despite an increase in renal blood flow, fluid retention, oedema and a reduction in urine output is often seen. This may be overcome by concurrent administration of a diuretic.
- *Gut* – nausea and vomiting are common.
- *Miscellaneous* – peripheral neuropathy and blood dyscrasias. A lupus erythematosus-type syndrome is occasionally seen after long-term use and may be more common in slow acetylators and women. It may require long-term corticosteroid therapy.

Kinetics

Hydralazine is well absorbed from the gut but is subject to a variable first-pass metabolism resulting in an oral bioavailability of 25–55% depending on the acetylator status of the individual. The plasma half-life is normally 2–3 hours but this may be shortened to 45 minutes in rapid acetylators. It is 90% protein-bound in the plasma. Up to 85% is excreted in the urine as acetylated and hydroxylated metabolites, some of which are conjugated with glucuronic acid. It crosses the placenta and may cause a fetal tachycardia.

Minoxidil

Presentation and Uses

Minoxidil is prepared as 2.5–10 mg tablets, a 2% solution for intravenous use and a 5% lotion. It is used for severe hypertension and alopecia areata.

Its mechanism of action and principal effects are essentially the same as those of hydralazine. The mechanism by which it stimulates the hair follicle is poorly understood. It may also precipitate hypertrichosis of the face and arms and breast tenderness. It does not cause a lupus erythematosus-type reaction.

Kinetics

Minoxidil is well absorbed from the gut and has an oral bioavailability of 90%. It is not protein-bound in the plasma. Its plasma half-life is only 3 hours but its hypotensive effects may last for as long as 3 days. It undergoes hepatic glucuronide conjugation and is subsequently excreted in the urine.

Diazoxide

This vasodilator is chemically related to the thiazide diuretics.

Presentation and Uses

Diazoxide is available as 50 mg tablets and as a solution for intravenous injection containing 15 $mg.ml^{-1}$. It is used intravenously to treat hypertensive emergencies associated with renal disease at $1-3$ mg.kg^{-1} up to a maximum dose of 150 mg, which may be repeated after 15 minutes. It has also been used to treat intractable hypogly-caemia and malignant islet-cell tumours.

Mechanism of Action

Its hypotensive effects are mediated through altered levels of cAMP in arterioles, producing vasodilation. It may also be due to a reduced Ca^{2+} influx. Its biochemical effects are due to inhibition of insulin secretion and increased release of catecholamines.

Effects

- *Cardiovascular* – diazoxide produces arteriolar vasodilation with little effect on capacitance vessels. As a result the blood pressure falls and there is an increase in heart rate and cardiac output. Postural hypotension is not a problem.
- *Metabolic* – it increases the levels of glucose, catecholamines, renin and aldosterone. It also causes fluid retention (despite its chemical relation to the thiazides), which may require treatment with a loop diuretic.
- *Miscellaneous* – the following effects may occur: nausea, especially at the start of treatment, extrapyramidal effects including oculogyric crisis, thrombocytopenia and hyperuricaemia.

Kinetics

Diazoxide is well absorbed from the gut with an oral bioavailability of 80%, and is extensively protein-bound in the plasma (about 90%). The hyperglycaemic effects last about 8 hours while the hypotensive effects last about 5 hours. The plasma half-life, however, may last up to 36 hours. It is partly metabolised in the liver, being excreted in the urine as unchanged drug and as inactive metabolites.

Sildenafil

Sildenafil is used in pulmonary artery hypertension and erectile dysfunction. A dose of 20 mg tds is used for pulmonary artery hypertension.

Mechanism of Action

Sildenafil is a potent cGMP type 5 inhibitor. Vascular smooth muscle in the pulmonary arteries and corpus cavernosum is relaxed as cGMP levels increase.

Kinetics

It is rapidly absorbed and has an oral bioavailability of 40%, is 95% plasma protein-bound and has a volume of distribution of 100 litres. It is metabolised by CYP3A4 (and to a lesser degree CYP2CY) to an N-demethylated active metabolite which contributes about 35% to the overall effect. Dose adjustment should be considered in the presence of CYP3A4 inducing or inhibiting enzymes. Its elimination half-life is 3–5 hours and 80% is excreted in the faeces. Significant renal impairment and hepatic impairment increase the plasma concetration-time curve.

Bosentan

Bosentan is used to treat pulmonary artery hypertension in adults and children. The adult dose is 62.5 mg bd for 4 weeks increasing to 125 mg thereafter.

Mechanism of Action

Bosentan is a dual endothelin receptor antagonist (ERA) at both A and B receptor subtypes. It decreases pulmonary and system vascular resistance without a rise in heart rate.

Kinetics

It has an oral bioavailability of 50% but plasma concentrations fall by 50% with continuous administration due to induction of its metabolising enzymes CYP2CY and CYP3A4. It is excreted in the bile.

Antihypertensives

Renin–Angiotensin–Aldosterone System

Physiology

The juxtaglomerular apparatus within the kidney consists of three distinct cell types:

- Juxtaglomerular cells form part of the afferent arteriole as it enters the glomerulus and are supplied by sympathetic nerves. They contain prorenin, which is converted to the acid protease renin before systemic release.
- The macula densa is a region of cells at the start of the distal convoluted tubule, which lie adjacent to the juxtaglomerular cells of the same nephron.
- Agranular lacis cells, which lie between the afferent and efferent arterioles adjacent to the glomerulus.

Under the following conditions the juxtaglomerular apparatus will cause the release of renin into the circulation:

- Reduced renal perfusion
- Reduced Na^+ at the macula densa
- Stimulation of the renal sympathetic fibres via β_1-adrenoceptors.

Renin (half-life 80 minutes) splits the decapeptide angiotensin I from the circulating plasma protein angiotensinogen, which is synthesised in the liver and is present in the α_2-globulin fraction of plasma proteins. Angiotensin-converting enzyme (ACE) converts angiotensin I to the active octapeptide angiotensin II, and also inactivates bradykinin. Angiotensin II is broken down in the kidney and liver to inactive metabolites and angiotensin III, which retains some activity (Figure 17.1).

Angiotensin II

Mechanism of Action

Two subtypes of angiotensin II receptor exist, AT_1 and AT_2. Angiotensin has a greater affinity for AT_1 receptors, which are G-protein-coupled.

Effects

- *Potent vasoconstriction* (about five times as potent as noradrenaline), acting directly on arterioles and indirectly via central mechanisms.
- *Blockade* of noradrenaline re-uptake (uptake 1) at sympathetic nerves and sympathetic nervous system activation.

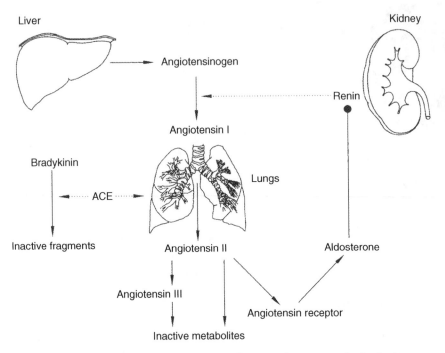

Figure 17.1 Renin–angiotensin–aldosterone system. ····▶, Enzyme action; ─●, negative feedback.

- *Central effects* – it increases thirst and the release of ADH and ACTH.
- It *stimulates* the release of aldosterone from the adrenal cortex and inhibits the release of renin from the juxtaglomerular cells.
- *Reduced* glomerular filtration rate.

ACE inhibitors and angiotensin II receptor antagonists are used widely in the treatment of hypertension. β-Blockers (see Chapter 14) reduce sympathetically mediated release of renin, which contributes to their antihypertensive effects.

Angiotensin-Converting Enzyme Inhibitors

Angiotensin-converting enzyme (ACE) inhibitors are used in all grades of heart failure and in patients with myocardial infarction with left ventricular dysfunction where it improves the prognosis. They are used in hypertension, especially in insulin-dependent diabetics with nephropathy. However, hypertension is relatively resistant to ACE inhibition in the black population where concurrent diuretic therapy may be required. While most drugs should be continued throughout the peri-operative period, ACE inhibitors and angiotensin II receptor antagonists are often omitted due to the increased frequency of peri-operative hypotension.

From a kinetic point of view ACE inhibitors may be divided into three groups:

Group 1. Captopril – an active drug that is metabolised to active metabolites.
Group 2. Enalapril, ramipril – prodrugs, which only become active following hepatic metabolism to the diacid moiety.

Group 3. Lisinopril – an active drug that is not metabolised and is excreted unchanged in the urine.

In other respects the effects of ACE inhibitors are similar and are discussed under Ramipril.

Ramipril

Presentation

Ramipril is available as 1.25–10 mg tablets. The initial dose is 1.25 mg which is then titrated up depending on its indication.

Mechanism of Action

Ramipril is converted by liver esterases to the active moiety ramiprilat, which is a competitive ACE inhibitor and therefore prevents the formation of angiotensin II and its effects. Afterload is reduced to a greater degree than preload.

Effects

- *Cardiovascular* – ramipril reduces the systemic vascular resistance significantly, resulting in a fall in blood pressure. The fall in afterload may increase the cardiac output, particularly in those with heart failure. Heart rate is usually unaffected but may increase. Baroreceptor reflexes are also unaffected. Transient hypotension may occur at the start of treatment which may be started under specialist supervision.
- *Renal* – the normal function of angiotensin II to maintain efferent arteriolar pressure (by vasoconstriction) at the glomerulus in the presence of poor renal perfusion is forfeit. Therefore renal perfusion pressure falls and renal failure may follow. As a result bilateral renal artery stenosis or unilateral renal artery stenosis to a single functioning kidney is considered a contraindication. Where normal renal perfusion is preserved, renal vasodilatation may occur leading to a natriuresis.
- *Metabolic* – reduced aldosterone release impairs the negative feedback to renin production so that renin levels become elevated. It may also lead to hyperkalaemia and raised urea and creatinine, especially in those with even mildly impaired renal function.
- *Interactions* – ramipril reduces aldosterone release, which may result in hyperkalaemia, so it should not be used with potassium-sparing diuretics. It has been associated with unexplained hypoglycaemia in type I and II diabetes. These effects usually decrease with continued treatment. Non-steroidal anti-inflammatory drugs reduce ramipril's antihypertensive effects and may precipitate renal failure.
- *Cough* – a persistent dry cough may be the result of increased levels of bradykinin, which are normally broken down by ACE.
- *Miscellaneous* – rare but serious effects may complicate its use and include angioedema (0.2%), agranulocytosis and thrombocytopenia. Less serious side effects are more common and include loss of taste, rash, pruritus, fever and aphthous ulceration. These are more common with higher doses and in patients with impaired renal function.

Kinetics

As described above ramipril is a prodrug and is almost completely metabolised to its active moiety ramiprilat. It is rapidy absorbed from the gut and the oral bioavailability of ramiprilat is 50%. It has a half-life of approximately 15 hours at high doses but longer in low doses. This is related to the saturable capacity of ACE at higher concentrations. Its excretion is essentially renal and is therefore impaired in renal failure.

Enalapril

Kinetics

Enalapril is a prodrug, which is hydrolysed in the liver and kidney to the active compound enalaprilat. It may be given orally (as enalapril) or intravenously (as enalaprilat). Its elimination half-life is 4–8 hours but increases to 11 hours in prolonged therapy. It has a duration of action of approximately 20 hours.

Angiotensin II Receptor Antagonists (ARAs)
Losartan

Losartan is a substituted imidazole compound. As its active metabolite is up to 40 times more potent at the angiotensin II receptor, it is effectively a prodrug although losartan does also have limited efficacy.

Presentation and Uses

Losartan is available as 25–50 mg tablets and in combination with hydrochlorothiazide. It is used in the treatment of hypertension where dry cough proves an unacceptable side effect of ACE inhibitor therapy.

Mechanism of Action

Losartan is a specific angiotensin II receptor (type AT_1) antagonist at all sites within the body. It blocks the negative feedback of angiotensin II on renin secretion, which therefore increases, leading to increased angiotensin II. This has little impact due to comprehensive AT_1 receptor blockade.

Effects

These are broadly similar to those of the ACE inhibitors.

- *Metabolic* – as it does not block the actions of ACE, bradykinin may be broken down in the usual manner (by ACE). As a result, bradykinin levels are not raised and the dry cough seen with ACE inhibitors does not complicate its use.

Kinetics

Losartan is well absorbed from the gut but undergoes significant first-pass metabolism to an active carboxylic acid metabolite (which acts in a non-competitive manner), and several other inactive compounds. It has an oral bioavailability of 30% and is 99% plasma protein-bound. Its elimination half-life is 2 hours while the elimination half-life of the active metabolite is 7 hours. Less than 10% is excreted unchanged in an active form in the urine. The inactive metabolites are excreted in bile and urine.

Contraindications

Like ACE inhibitors, losartan is contraindicated in bilateral renal artery stenosis and pregnancy.

Comparing ARAs to ACE inhibitors

ARA use may become more widespread for the following reasons:

1. Blockade of the AT_1-receptor is the most specific way of preventing the adverse effects of angiotensin II seen in heart failure and hypertension, especially as angiotensin II may be synthesised by alternative non-ACE pathways.
2. The AT_2-receptor is not blocked, which may possess cardioprotective properties.
3. There is a much lower incidence of cough and angioedema and therefore improved compliance.

Adrenergic Neurone Blockade

This group of drugs interferes with the release of noradrenaline from adrenergic neurones.

Physiology

Noradrenaline is synthesised from tyrosine (see Chapter 13) within the adrenergic nerve terminal. It is held in storage vesicles and subsequently released into the neuronal cleft to act on adrenoceptors. Its actions are terminated by:

- Uptake 1 – noradrenaline is taken back into the nerve terminal by a high-affinity transport system. This provides the main route for terminating its effects. Within the neurone it is recycled and returned to storage vesicles. However, while in the cytoplasm some may be deaminated by MAO.
- Uptake 2 – noradrenaline diffuses away from the nerve terminal into the circulation where it is taken up by extraneuronal tissues including the liver and metabolised by catechol-O-methyltransferase (COMT).

Guanethidine

Presentation and Uses

Guanethidine is available as tablets and as a colourless solution for injection containing 10 mg.ml^{-1}. It has been used as an antihypertensive agent but is currently used only for the control of sympathetically mediated chronic pain. The initial anti-hypertensive dose is 10 mg.day^{-1}, which is increased to a maintenance dose of 30–50 mg.day^{-1}. A dose of 20 mg is used when performing an intravenous regional block for chronic pain. Repeated blocks are usually required.

Mechanism of Action

Guanethidine gains access to the adrenergic neurone by utilising the uptake 1 transport mechanism. Following intravenous administration there is some initial hypotension by direct vasodilation of arterioles. Subsequently, it displaces noradrenaline from its binding sites, which may cause transient hypertension. Finally, guanethidine reduces the blood pressure by preventing the release of what little noradrenaline is left in the nerve terminal.

Oral administration does not produce the same triphasic response, as its onset of action is much slower. It does not alter the secretion of catecholamines by the adrenal medulla.

Effects

- *Cardiovascular* – hypotension is its main action. Postural hypotension is common as it blocks any compensatory rise in sympathetic tone. Fluid retention leading to oedema may occur.
- *Gut* – diarrhoea is common.
- *Miscellaneous* – failure to ejaculate.
- *Drug interactions* – drugs that block uptake 1 (tricyclic antidepressants, cocaine) prevent guanethidine from entering the nerve terminal and disrupting noradrenaline storage. They therefore antagonise guanethidine.

Up-regulation of adrenoceptors follows the long-term use of guanethidine so that these patients are very sensitive to direct-acting sympathomimetic amines.

Kinetics

Following oral administration, guanethidine is variably and incompletely absorbed. Hepatic first-pass metabolism results in an oral bioavailability of 50%. It is not bound by plasma proteins and does not cross the blood–brain barrier. It has an elimination half-life of several days. Elimination is by hepatic metabolism and excretion of unchanged drug and its metabolites in the urine.

Metirosine

Metirosine is a competitive inhibitor of tyrosine hydroxylase and can therefore prevent the synthesis of catecholamines. It should only be used to manage hypertension associated with phaeochromocytoma. It may cause severe diarrhoea, sedation, extrapyramidal effects and hypersensitivity reactions.

Centrally Acting

Methyldopa

Presentation and Uses

Methyldopa is available as film-coated tablets containing 125–500 mg and as an oral suspension containing 50 mg.ml^{-1}. The rarely used intravenous preparation is colourless and contains 50 mg.ml^{-1} and uses sodium metabisulfite as the preservative. It is used at 250 mg tds increasing to a maximum of 3 g.day^{-1} to control hypertension, especially that associated with pregnancy.

Mechanism of Action

Methyldopa readily crosses the blood–brain barrier where it is decarboxylated to α-methyl-noradrenaline, which is a potent α_2-agonist. It retains limited α_1-agonist properties (α_2:α_1 ratio 10:1). Stimulation of presynaptic α_2-receptors in the nucleus tractus solitarius forms a negative feedback loop for further noradrenaline release so that α-methyl-noradrenaline reduces centrally mediated sympathetic tone, leading to a reduction in blood pressure.

Effects

- *Cardiovascular* – its main effect is a reduction in systemic vascular resistance leading to a fall in blood pressure. Postural hypotension is occasionally a problem. Cardiac output is unchanged despite a relative bradycardia. Rebound hypertension may occur if treatment is stopped suddenly but this is less common than with clonidine.
- *Central nervous system* – sedation is common, while dizziness, depression, nightmares and nausea are less common. The MAC of volatile anaesthetics is reduced.
- *Haematological* – a positive direct Coombs' test is seen in 10–20% of patients taking methyldopa. Thrombocytopenia and leucopenia occur rarely.
- *Allergic* – it may precipitate an auto-immune haemolytic anaemia. Eosinophilia associated with fever sometimes occurs within the first few weeks of therapy. A hypersensitivity reaction may cause myocarditis.
- *Renal* – urine may become darker in colour when exposed to air, due to the breakdown of methyldopa or its metabolites.
- *Hepatic* – liver function may deteriorate during long-term treatment and fatal hepatic necrosis has been reported.
- *Miscellaneous* – methyldopa fluoresces at the same wavelengths as catecholamines so that assays of urinary catecholamines may be falsely high. Assays of VMA are not affected. It may cause constipation and gynaecomastia (due to suppressed prolactin release).

Kinetics

Methyldopa is erratically absorbed from the gut and has a very variable oral bioavailability and a slow onset of action. It is subject to hepatic first-pass metabolism, being converted to the O-sulfate. Less than 20% is bound to plasma proteins. Approximately 50% is excreted unchanged in the urine.

Clonidine

Clonidine is an α-agonist with an affinity for $α_2$-receptors 200 times that for $α_1$-receptors. Some studies identify it as a partial agonist.

Presentation and Uses

Clonidine is available as 25–300 µg tablets and as a colourless solution for injection containing 150 $µg.ml^{-1}$. A transdermal patch is available but this takes 48 hours to achieve therapeutic levels. It is used in the treatment of hypertension, acute and chronic pain, the suppression of symptoms of opioid withdrawal and to augment sedation during ventilation of the critically ill patient.

Mechanism of Action

The useful effects of clonidine rest on its ability to stimulate $α_2$-receptors in the lateral reticular nucleus resulting in reduced central sympathetic outflow, and in the spinal cord where they augment endogenous opiate release and modulate the descending noradrenergic pathways involved in spinal nociceptive processing. MAC appears to be reduced by stimulation of central postsynaptic $α_2$-receptors.

Transmembrane signalling of $α_2$-receptors is coupled to G_i, leading to reduced intracellular cAMP. K^+ channels are also activated.

Effects

- *Cardiovascular* – following intravenous administration the blood pressure may rise due to peripheral α_1 stimulation, but this is followed by a more prolonged fall in blood pressure. Cardiac output is well maintained despite a bradycardia. The PR interval is lengthened, atrioventricular nodal conduction depressed and the baroreceptor reflexes are sensitised by clonidine resulting in a lower heart rate for a given increase in blood pressure. The effects of clonidine on the coronary circulation are complicated as any direct vasoconstriction may be offset by a reduction in sympathetic tone and by the release of local nitric oxide. It stabilises the cardiovascular responses to peri-operative stimuli. Rebound hypertension is seen more commonly when a dose of more than 1.2 g.day^{-1} is stopped abruptly. This is due to peripheral vasoconstriction and increased plasma catecholamines and may be exacerbated by β-blockade (leaving vasoconstriction unopposed). Increasing doses have a ceiling effect and are limited by increasing α_1 stimulation.
- *Central nervous system* – clonidine produces sedation and a reduction of up to 50% in the MAC of volatile agents. It is anxiolytic at low doses but becomes anxiogenic at higher doses.
- *Analgesia* – clonidine has been used via the subarachnoid and epidural routes. It provides prolonged analgesia with no respiratory depression and appears to act synergistically with concurrently administered opioids. It does not produce motor or sensory blockade. Clonidine also appears to reduce post-operative opioid requirement when administered intravenously.
- *Renal system* – a number of mechanisms including inhibition of release of ADH have been implicated as the cause of diuresis during its use.
- *Respiratory* – in contrast to opioids it does not produce significant respiratory depression.
- *Endocrine* – the stress response to surgical stimulus is inhibited. Insulin release is inhibited although this rarely increases blood sugar levels.
- *Haematological* – despite the presence of α_2-adrenoceptors on platelets, therapeutic doses of clonidine do not promote platelet aggregation and its sympatholytic effects block adrenaline-induced platelet aggregation.

Kinetics

Clonidine is rapidly and almost completely absorbed after oral administration, achieving an oral bioavailability of nearly 100%. It is 20% plasma protein-bound and has a volume of distribution of about 2 l.kg^{-1}. The elimination half-life of clonidine is between 9 and 18 hours, with approximately 50% of the drug being metabolised in the liver to inactive metabolites, while the rest is excreted unchanged in the urine. The dose should be reduced in the presence of renal impairment.

Atipamezole

Atipamezole is a selective α_2-antagonist that crosses the blood–brain barrier to reverse the sedation and analgesia associated with clonidine and dexmedetomidine. At 2 hours its elimination half-life is similar to dexmedetomidine, with obvious clinical benefit.

The following classes of drugs are described in more detail elsewhere: diuretics (Chapter 22), adrenoreceptor antagonists (Chapter 14) and calcium channel receptor antagonists (Chapter 16).

Central Nervous System

18

Hypnotics and Anxiolytics

Physiology

γ-Aminobutyric acid (GABA) is the main inhibitory neurotransmitter within the central nervous system (CNS) and acts via two different receptor subtypes, $GABA_A$ and $GABA_B$:

- $GABA_A$ – this receptor is a **ligand-gated** Cl^- ion channel. It consists of five subunits (2α, β, δ and γ – each having a number of variants) arranged to form a central ion channel. GABA binds to and activates $GABA_A$ receptors and increases the opening frequency of its Cl^- channel, augmenting Cl^- conductance and thereby hyperpolarising the neuronal membrane. Cl^- ion conductance is potentiated by the binding of benzodiazepines (BDZs) to the α subunit of the activated receptor complex. $GABA_A$ receptors are essentially (but not exclusively) postsynaptic and are widely distributed throughout the CNS.

- $GABA_B$ – this receptor is **metabotropic** (i.e. acts via a G-protein and second messengers), and when stimulated it increases K^+ conductance, thereby hyperpolarising the neuronal membrane. $GABA_B$ receptors are located both presynaptically on nerve terminals and postsynaptically in many regions of the brain, as well as in the dorsal horn of the spinal cord. Baclofen acts only via $GABA_B$ receptors to reduce spasticity.

BDZs modulate the effects of GABA at $GABA_A$ receptors. The specific α-subunit type determines the BDZ pharmacology – anxiolytic or sedative. Two BDZ receptor subtypes have been identified: BZ_1, found in the spinal cord and cerebellum – responsible for anxiolysis; and BZ_2, found in the spinal cord, hippocampus and cerebral cortex – responsible for sedative and anticonvulsant activity.

Benzodiazepines

Uses

Benzodiazepines are used commonly in anaesthesia as premedication and to sedate patients during minor procedures. They are also used more widely as anxiolytics, hypnotics and anticonvulsants.

Structure

At its core BDZs have two ring structures. The first is a benzene ring (see p. 84); the second has seven members (five carbon and two nitrogen) and is called a di-azepine ring. However, for pharmacological activity, BDZs also have a carbonyl group at position 2 on the di-azepine ring, another benzene ring and a halogen on the first benzene ring.

Midazolam

Presentation

Midazolam is presented as a clear solution at pH 3.5. It is unique among the BDZs in that its structure is dependent on the surrounding pH. At pH 3.5 its di-azepine ring structure is open, resulting in an ionised molecule, which is therefore water-soluble. However, when its surrounding pH is greater than 4, its di-azepine ring structure closes so that it is no longer ionised and therefore becomes lipid-soluble (see Figure 18.1). Its pK_a is 6.5, so that at physiological pH 89% is present in an unionised form and available to cross lipid membranes.

As it is water-soluble it does not cause pain on injection.

Uses

Midazolam is used intravenously to sedate patients for minor procedures and has powerful amnesic properties. It is also used to sedate ventilated patients in intensive care.

Kinetics

Midazolam may be given orally (bioavailability approximately 40%), intranasally or intramuscularly as premedication. It has a short duration of action due to distribution. It is metabolised by hydroxylation to the active compound 1-α hydroxymidazolam, which is conjugated with glucuronic acid prior to renal excretion. Less than 5% is metabolised to oxazepam. It is highly protein-bound (approximately 95%) and has an elimination half-life of 1–4 hours. At 6–10 ml.kg^{-1}.min^{-1} its clearance is larger than that of diazepam and lorazepam so that its effects wear off more rapidly following infusion (see Table 18.1).

Alfentanil is metabolised by the same hepatic P450 isoenzyme (3A3/4), and when administered together their effects may be prolonged.

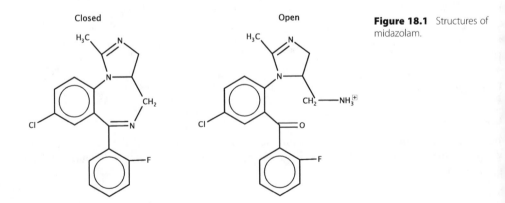

Figure 18.1 Structures of midazolam.

Table 18.1 Kinetics of some benzodiazepines

	Diazepam	Midazolam	Lorazepam
Protein binding (%)	95	95	95
Elimination half-life (h)	20–45	1–4	10–20
Volume of distribution (l.kg^{-1})	1.0–1.5	1.0–1.5	0.75–1.30
Active metabolites	yes	yes	no
Clearance (ml.kg^{-1}.min^{-1})	0.2–0.5	6–10	1.0–1.5

Diazepam

Diazepam has a high lipid solubility, which facilitates its oral absorption and its rapid central effects. It is highly protein-bound (approximately 95%) to albumin and is metabolised in the liver by oxidation to desmethyldiazepam, oxazepam and temazepam, all of which are active. It does not induce hepatic enzymes. The glucuronide derivatives are excreted in the urine. It has the lowest clearance of the BDZs discussed here and its half-life is hugely increased by its use as an infusion (see Table 18.1; see also context-sensitive half-time, p. 78).

Diazepam may cause some cardiorespiratory depression. Liver failure and cimetidine will prolong its actions by reducing its metabolism. When administered with opioids or alcohol, respiratory depression may be more pronounced. In common with other BDZs it reduces the MAC of co-administered anaesthetic agents.

Lorazepam

Lorazepam shares similar pharmacokinetics and actions to other BDZs although its metabolites are inactive. It is used for premedication as an anxiolytic and amnesic. It is first-line therapy for status epilepticus (50–100 µg.kg^{-1} intravenous, sub lingual or per rectum from 1–12 years, maximum dose 4 mg; > 12 years, 4 mg).

Lorazepam is well absorbed following oral or intramuscular administration, highly plasma protein-bound (approximately 95%) and conjugated with glucuronic acid producing inactive metabolites, which are excreted in the urine (see Figure 18.2).

Temazepam

Temazepam is used as a nighttime sedative and as an anxiolytic premedicant. It has no unique features within the BDZ family. It is well absorbed in the gut, is 75% protein-bound and has a volume of distribution of 0.8 l.kg^{-1}. Eighty per cent is excreted unchanged in the urine while glucuronidation occurs in the liver. Only a very small amount is demethylated to oxazepam. It has a half-life of about 8 hours and may result in some hangover effects.

Chlordiazepoxide

Chlordiazepoxide, the first BDZ derivative available for clinical use, is an anxiolytic sedative used to treat symptoms associated with alcohol withdrawl. When used to treat short term anxiety it is used at a dose from 5 mg tds up to 25 mg qds but this should be titrated carefully to the individual needs of the patient. It has a high oral bioavailbility and a complex metabolic

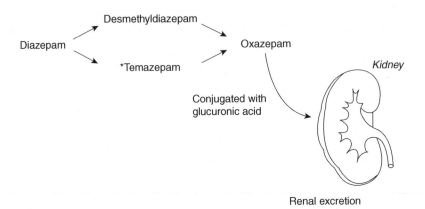

Figure 18.2 Metabolism of diazepam.*Less than 5% of temazepam is metabolised to oxazepam.

pathway into a number of active metabolites. Its elimination half life is 5–30 hours which may increase in the elderly.

Flumazenil

Flumazenil is an imidazobenzodiazepine.

Uses

Flumazenil is used to reverse the effects of BDZs, that is, excessive sedation following minor procedures or in the treatment of BDZ overdose. However, its use is cautioned in mixed drug overdose as it may precipitate fits. It is given by intravenous injection in 100 μg increments and acts within 2 minutes. Its relatively short half-life (about 1 hour) compared with many BDZs means that further doses or an infusion may be needed.

Mechanism of Action

Flumazenil is a competitive BDZ antagonist. However, it has some agonist activity as well and its ability to precipitate seizures in certain patients may be a result of inverse agonist activity.

Effects

These include nausea and vomiting. It may also precipitate anxiety, agitation and seizures especially in epileptic patients.

Kinetics

Flumazenil is 50% plasma protein-bound and undergoes significant hepatic metabolism to inactive compounds that are excreted in the urine.

α-agonists
Dexmedetomidine

Presentation and Uses

Dexmedetomidine is the S-enantiomer of medetomidine, the R- form having no pharmacological activity. It is used to produce light to moderate sedation (Richmond

Agitation-Sedation scale) for (usually ventilated) patients in ICU, but has also been used for procedural sedation (including paediatric patients) and in balanced general anaesthesia. It is presented as a colourless solution in vials containing 100 $\mu g.ml^{-1}$ and is typically diluted to a concentration of 4–8 $\mu g.ml^{-1}$ prior to use.

Dose

For sedation in ICU it is used at an initial rate of 0.7 $\mu g.kg^{-1}.hr^{-1}$ which is adjusted to effect (range of 0.2–1.4 $\mu g.kg^{-1}.hr^{-1}$). When used alone or alongside other drugs in anaesthetic practice a loading dose of 1 $\mu g.kg^{-1}.hr^{-1}$ for 10 minutes may be used followed by a maintenance infusion of 0.2–0.6 $\mu g.kg^{-1}.hr^{-1}$. Larger infusion rates (5–10 $\mu g.kg^{-1}.hr^{-1}$) are described for the uncommon use as a sole agent for general anaesthesia.

Mechanism of Action

Dexmedetomidine is highly selective for the α_2-receptor (α_2:α_1 ratio 1600:1), making it eight times more selective than clonidine. It inhibits the release of noradrenaline (NA) at the locus coeruleus of the pons which is intimately linked with the natural sleep pathways.

Effects

- *Central Nervous System* – it induces sedation and anxiolysis. The sedation is more like physiological sleep than pharmacologically induced sedation or anaesthesia and this has been supported by EEG studies. It has been associated with less delirium compared to some drug protocols. It also produces analgesia by actions in the substantia gelatinosa of the dorsal horn of the spinal cord where it reduces the release of transmitters involved in nociception.
- *Cardiovascular* – its effects here are biphasic, initially producing hypertension (mediated by α_{2B} receptors on vascular smooth muscle), and then proceeding to hypotension and bradycardia as a result of reduced central NA release. This profile is more common during the loading dose phase and has been reported to progress to asystole, albeit rarely, when administered as a sole agent. However, it should be used with extreme caution in those with conduction defects.
- *Respiratory* – it appears to have no respiratory impairment and the airway remains patent and may be especially useful during extubation. In addition, it has decongestant and antisialagogue effects which may be advantageous during sedation for fibreoptic intubation.

Kinetics

Oral absorption is unpredictable (bioavailability < 20%) but is improved when given buccally (bioavailability > 75%), but these routes do avoid the initial hypertension that parenteral administration produces. It is highly protein-bound (94%) and crosses easily into the brain. Dexmedetomidine undergoes both Phase I (hydroxylation) and Phase II (glucuronidation and methylation) hepatic metabolism and its inactive metabolites are excreted in the urine. Consequently only hepatic impairment should prompt a dose reduction. It has a distribution half-life of 6 minutes, an elimination half-life of about 2 hours, a clearance of approximately 40 $l.hr^{-1}$ and a volume of distribution of 118 litres which is increased in hypoalbuminaemia.

Non-Benzodiazepine Hypnotics (the Z Drugs)

Zopiclone, zaleplon and zolpidem are hypnotics that act via the BDZ receptor but cannot be classified as BDZs structurally. They were developed in order to try to overcome some of the side effects of the BDZs, namely dependence and next-day sedation.

Zopiclone has the longest elimination half-life of approximately 5 hours while zaleplon and zolpidem have elimination half-lives of 1 and 2 hours, respectively.

They have not had a major impact in the area of short-term hypnotics as they carry all the same side effects as the BDZs. Only where there has been a specific intolerance to a specific BDZ is switching to a Z drug recommended. Where general intolerance is a problem the patient is just as likely to experience intolerance to the Z drugs.

Antidepressants

Four groups of drugs are used to treat depression:

- **Tricyclics (TCAs)**
- **Selective serotonin reuptake inhibitors (SSRIs)**
- **Monoamine oxidase inhibitors (MAOIs)**
- **Atypical agents.**

Tricyclics (Amitriptyline, Nortriptyline, Imipramine, Dothiepin)

As its name suggests, this group of drugs was originally based on a tricyclic ring structure, although now many second-generation drugs contain different numbers of rings.

Uses

Tricyclics are used to treat depressive illness, nocturnal enuresis and as an adjunct in the treatment of chronic pain.

Mechanism of Action

They competitively block neuronal uptake (uptake 1) of noradrenaline and serotonin (5-HT). In doing so they increase the concentration of transmitter in the synapse. However, the antidepressant effects do not occur within the same time-frame, taking up to 2 weeks to work. They also block muscarinic, histaminergic and α-adrenoceptors, and have non-specific sedative effects (see Table 18.2).

Effects

- *Central nervous system* – sedation and occasionally seizures in epileptic patients.
- *Anticholinergic effects* – dry mouth, constipation, urinary retention and blurred vision.
- *Cardiovascular* – postural hypotension especially in the elderly.

Kinetics

Tricyclics are well absorbed from the gut reflecting their high lipid solubility. They are highly plasma protein-bound and have a high volume of distribution. Metabolism, which shows large interpatient variability, occurs in the liver and often produces active metabolites (e.g. imipramine to desipramine and nortriptyline).

Table 18.2 Effects of various antidepressants

	Anticholinergic effects	Sedation	Postural hypotension
TCA			
Amitriptyline	++++	++++	++
Imipramine	++	++	+++
Nortriptyline	++	++	+
Desipramine	+	+	+
SSRI			
Fluoxetine	+	nil	+

Tricyclic Overdose

This is not uncommon in depressed patients. The features of TCA overdose include a mixture of:

- *Cardiovascular effects* – sinus tachycardia is common and there is a dose-related prolongation of the QT interval and widening of the QRS complex. Ventricular arrhythmias are more likely when the QRS complex is longer than 0.16 seconds. Right bundle branch block is also seen. The blood pressure may be high or low but in serious overdose hypotension may be refractory to treatment and culminate in pulseless electrical activity.
- *Central effects* – excitation, seizures (correlating with a QRS duration of more than 0.1 seconds) and then depression. Mydriasis is a feature, as is hyperthermia.
- *Anticholinergic effects.*

Treatment

This includes gastric lavage followed by activated charcoal. Supportive care may require supplementation with specific treatment. Seizures may be treated with BDZs or phenytoin and ventricular arrhythmias with phenytoin or lidocaine. Inotropes should be avoided where possible as this may precipitate arrhythmias. Intravascular volume expansion is usually sufficient to correct hypotension. The anticholinergic effects may be reversed by an anticholinesterase, but this is not recommended as it may precipitate seizures, brady-cardia and heart failure.

Selective Serotonin Reuptake Inhibitors (Fluoxetine, Paroxetine, Sertraline, Venlafaxine)

As their name suggests, selective serotonin reuptake inhibitors (SSRIs) selectively inhibit the neuronal re-uptake of 5-HT. They are no more effective than standard antidepressants but do not have their associated side-effect profile. SSRIs are less sedative, have fewer anticholinergic effects and appear less cardiotoxic in overdose although they are associated with GI side effects (nausea and constipation). There is some evidence that they inhibit 5-HT uptake in platelets, impairing their function. This may become significant in the presence of other antiplatelet agents.

Despite their side-effect profile, when combinations of serotonergic drugs are used the potentially fatal serotonergic syndrome may result, which is characterised by hyper-reflexia, agitation, clonus and hyperthermia. The commonest combination is a monoamine oxidase inhibitor (MAOI) and SSRI – however, the phenylpiperidine opioids (particularly pethidine) have weak serotonin re-uptake inhibitor properties and can also precipitate the syndrome.

Fluoxetine is an effective antidepressant causing minimal sedation. It is a 50:50 mix of two isomers that are equally active. It is well absorbed and metabolised in the liver by cytochrome P450 enzymes. In addition, there are non-saturable enzymes that prevent an unchecked rise in levels. However, the dose should be reduced in renal failure as accumulation may result. Side effects include nausea and vomiting, headache, insomnia, reduced libido and mania or hypomania in up to 1%.

Venlafaxine appears to block the re-uptake of both noradrenaline and 5-HT (and to a lesser extent dopamine) while having little effect on muscarinic, histaminergic or α-adrenoceptors.

Monoamine Oxidase Inhibitors

The MAOI group of drugs is administered orally for the treatment of resistant depression, obsessive compulsive disorders, chronic pain syndromes and migraine.

MAO is present as a variety of isoenzymes within presynaptic neurones and is responsible for the deamination of amine neurotransmitters. They have been classified as types A and B. Following their inhibition there is an increase in the level of amine neurotransmitters, which is thought to be the basis of their central activity. MAO-A preferentially deaminates 5-HT and catecholamines, while MAO-B preferentially deaminates tyramine and phenylethylamine.

There are now two generations of MAOIs. The original generation inhibit MAO irreversibly and non-selectively (i.e. MAO-A and -B) while the new generation selectively and reversibly inhibit only MAO-A (RIMA). Neither group is used as first-line therapy because of the potential for serious side effects and hepatic toxicity.

Non-Selective Irreversible Monoamine Oxidase Inhibitors (Phenelzine, Isocarboxazid, Tranylcypromine)

Phenelzine and isocarboxazid are hydrazines while tranylcypromine is a nonhydrazine compound. Tranylcypromine is potentially the most dangerous as it possesses stimulant activity.

Effects

In addition to controlling depression they also produce sedation, blurred vision, orthostatic hypotension and hypertensive crises following tyramine-rich foods (cheese, pickled herring, chicken liver, Bovril and chocolate) and indirectly acting sympathomimetics. Hepatic enzymes are inhibited and the hydrazine compounds may cause hepatotoxicity. Interaction with pethidine may precipitate cerebral irritability, hyperpyrexia and cardiovascular instability. Interaction with fentanyl has also been reported.

Selective Reversible Inhibitors of Monoamine Oxidase-A

Moclobemide causes less potentiation of tyramine than the older generation MAOIs and in general patients do not need the same level of dietary restriction. However, some patients are especially sensitive to tyramine and so all patients should be advised to avoid tyramine-rich foods and indirect-acting sympathomimetic amines.

Moclobemide is completely absorbed from the gut but undergoes significant first-pass metabolism resulting in an oral bioavailability of 60–80%. It is metabolised in the liver by cytochrome P450 and up to 2% of the Caucasian and 15% of the Asian population have been shown to be slow metabolisers. The metabolites are excreted in the urine.

Linezolid is an antibiotic indicated for methicillin-resistant *Staphylococcus aureus* and vancomycin-resistant enterococci. It is also a MAOI and as such has the typical range of cautions and contraindications.

Monoamine Oxidase Inhibitors and General Anaesthesia

Those patients receiving MAOIs and presenting for emergency surgery should not be given pethidine or any indirectly acting sympathomimetic amines (e.g. ephedrine). If cardiovascular support is indicated, direct-acting agents should be used but with extreme caution as they may also precipitate exaggerated hypertension. The elective case presents potential difficulties. If MAOI therapy is withdrawn for the required 14–21 days before surgery, the patient may suffer a relapse of their depression with potentially disastrous consequences. However, the newer agents may control depression more effectively and reduce the chance of a serious peri-operative drug interaction.

Indirectly acting sympathomimetic amines are heavily dependent on MAO for their metabolism and therefore may produce exaggerated hypertension and arrhythmias when administered with an MAOI. The directly acting sympathomimetic amines should also be used with caution although they are also metabolised by COMT and therefore are not subject to the same degree of exaggerated response.

MAOIs should be stopped for 2 weeks before starting alternative antidepressant therapy and 2 weeks should have elapsed from the end of TCA therapy to the start of MAOI therapy.

Atypical Agents

Mianserin

Mianserin is a tetracyclic compound used in depressive illness, especially where sedation is required. It does not block the neuronal re-uptake of transmitters, in contrast to the TCAs. It does, however, block presynaptic α_2-adrenoceptors, which reduces their negative feedback, resulting in increased synaptic concentrations of neurotransmitters.

It has very little ability to block muscarinic and peripheral α-adrenoceptors and as such causes less in the way of antimuscarinic effects or postural hypotension.

Its important side effects are agranulocytosis and aplastic anaemia, which are more common in the elderly.

Lithium Carbonate

Lithium is used in the treatment of bipolar depression, mania and recurrent affective disorders. It has a narrow therapeutic index and plasma levels should be maintained at 0.5–1.5 mmol.l^{-1}. In excitable cells, lithium imitates Na^+ and decreases the release of neurotransmitters.

It may increase generalised muscle tone and lower the seizure threshold in epileptics. Many patients develop polyuria and polydipsia due to antidiuretic hormone antagonism. It may also produce raised serum levels of Na^+, Mg^{2+} and Ca^{2+}. Lithium prolongs neuromuscular blockade and may decrease anaesthetic requirements as it blocks brain stem release of noradrenaline and dopamine.

The thyroid gland may become enlarged and underactive and the patient may experience weight gain and tremor. Above the therapeutic level patients suffer with vomiting, abdominal pain, ataxia, convulsions, arrhythmias and death.

Anticonvulsants

Where possible a single agent should be used to treat epilepsy as it avoids the potential for drug interaction. In addition patients rarely improve with a second agent.

Phenytoin

Uses

Phenytoin has been used widely for many years in the treatment of grand mal and partial seizures, trigeminal neuralgia and ventricular arrhythmias following TCA overdose. It may be given orally or intravenously but the dose must be tailored to the individual patient as wide interpatient variation exists (about 9% of the population are slow hydroxylators) and blood assays are useful in this regard. It is incompatible with 5% dextrose, in which it becomes gelatinous. The normal therapeutic level is 10–20 μg.ml^{-1}.

Mechanism of Action

The action of phenytoin is probably dependent on its ability to bind to and stabilise inactivated Na^+ channels. This prevents the further generation of action potentials that are central to seizure activity. It may also reduce Ca^{2+} entry into neurones, blocking transmitter release and enhancing the actions of GABA.

Effects

- *Idiosyncratic* – acne, coarsening of facial features, hirsutism, gum hyperplasia, folate-dependent megaloblastic anaemia, aplastic anaemia, various skin rashes and peripheral neuropathy.
- *Dose-related* – ataxia, nystagmus, paraesthesia, vertigo and slurred speech. Rapid undiluted intravenous administration is associated with hypotension and heart block.
- *Teratogenicity* – it causes craniofacial abnormalities, growth retardation, limb and cardiac defects and mental retardation.
- *Drug interactions* – as phenytoin induces the hepatic mixed function oxidases it increases the metabolism of warfarin, BDZs and the oral contraceptive pill. Its metabolism may be inhibited by metronidazole, chloramphenicol and isoniazid leading

to toxic levels. Furthermore phenytoin's metabolism may be induced by carbamazepine or alcohol resulting in reduced plasma levels.

Kinetics

The oral bioavailability is approximately 90% and it is highly plasma protein-bound (90%). It undergoes saturable hepatic hydroxylation resulting in zero-order kinetics just above the therapeutic range. It can induce its own metabolism and that of other drugs. Its major metabolite is excreted in the urine.

Carbamazepine

Carbamazepine is also used in the treatment of trigeminal neuralgia. Its mode of action is similar to that of phenytoin. It may be given orally or rectally.

Effects

- *Central nervous system* – mild neurotoxic effects including headache, diplopia, ataxia, vomiting and drowsiness are common and often limit its use.
- *Metabolic* – it may produce an antidiuretic effect leading to water retention.
- *Miscellaneous* – drug-induced hepatitis, rashes in 5–10% and rarely agranulocytosis.
- *Teratogenicity* – it causes facial abnormalities, intrauterine growth retardation, microcephaly and mental retardation. The incidence increases with dose. Overall incidence is about 1/300–2000 live births.
- *Drug interactions* – as carbamazepine induces hepatic enzymes, it demonstrates many of the interactions seen with phenytoin. Levels of concurrently administered phenytoin may be elevated or reduced. Erythromycin can increase serum levels of carbamazepine.

Kinetics

Carbamazepine is well absorbed from the gut with a high oral bioavailability. It is approximately 75% plasma protein-bound and undergoes extensive hepatic metabolism to carbamazepine 10,11-epoxide, which retains about 30% of carbamazepine's anticonvulsant properties. It powerfully induces hepatic enzymes and induces its own metabolism. Its excretion is almost entirely in the urine as unconjugated metabolites.

Sodium Valproate

Uses

Sodium valproate is used in the treatment of various forms of epilepsy including absence (petit mal) seizures and in the treatment of trigeminal neuralgia.

Mechanism of Action

Sodium valproate appears to act by stabilising inactive Na^+ channels and also by stimulating central GABA-ergic inhibitory pathways. It is generally well tolerated.

Effects

- *Abdominal* – it may cause nausea and gastric irritation. Pancreatitis and potentially fatal hepatotoxicity are recognised following its use.

- *Haematological* – thrombocytopenia and reduced platelet aggregation.
- *Miscellaneous* – transient hair loss.
- *Teratogenicity* – it causes neural tube defects.

Kinetics

Sodium valproate is well absorbed orally, highly protein-bound (approximately 90%) and undergoes hepatic metabolism to products (some of which are active), which are excreted in the urine.

Phenobarbital

Phenobarbital is an effective anticonvulsant but its use is associated with significant sedation, which limits its use. It is a long-acting barbiturate that induces hepatic enzymes and interacts with other agents (warfarin, oral contraceptives, other anticonvulsants).

Benzodiazepines

Benzodiazepines (see above) are widely used in the emergency treatment of status epilepticus and act by enhancing the chloride-gating function of GABA.

Lamotrigine

Lamotrigine is an adjunct therapy that is used in a range of seizure types in adults and children down to 2 years of age. It is also used in bipolar disorder and as a mood stabiliser.

Mechanism of Action

It is chemically unrelated to other anticonvulsants and works by inactivation of voltage-sensitive sodium channels on neurones that produce the excitatory neurotransmitters glutamate and aspartate. It may have other actions as it has additional effects not seen with more classic sodium channel blocking anticonvulsants, such as phenytoin.

Effects

- *Abdominal* – it may cause hepatotoxicity, pancreatitis and nausea.
- *Dermatological* – it has been associated with life-threatening skin reactions.
- *Neurological* – a few cases of neuroleptic malignant syndrome have been reported.

Kinetics

It has a half-life of 14 hours and has an oral bioavailability of 98%. It is conjugated to an inactive metabolite.

Gabapentin

Gabapentin is a drug used to treat focal seizures at a dose of 900–1200 mg.day^{-1} and neuropathic pain at a dose of 1800 mg.day^{-1}. The dose should be titrated up and down at the start and end of therapy. It has been used as premedication in an attempt to reduce post-operative pain.

Mechanism of Action

It acts on the presynaptic $\alpha_2\delta$ subunit of voltage-gated calcium channels in cortical neurones and increases the synaptic concentration of GABA. It may also have some NMDA antagonist activity.

Effects

- *Infective* – viral infections are common.
- *Neurological* – a range of psychiatric symptoms may develop as well as ataxia, dizziness, fatigue and fever.

Kinetics

Gabapentin has an oral bioavailability of about 60% which decreases with increasing doses. It is not bound by plasma proteins and is not metabolised, which makes use with other anticonvulsants simpler. It is eliminated solely by the kidneys and has an elimination half-life of 6 hours.

Vigabatrin

Vigabatrin is used as an adjunct with other anti-epileptic agents for complex partial seizures at a maximum dose of 1.5 g bd.

Mechanism of Action

This is thought to be by irreversible inhibition of GABA-transaminase, the enzyme responsible for the breakdown of GABA. Its duration of action is 24 hours.

Kinetics

It is excreted unchanged in the urine and interacts with phenytoin by an unknown mechanism, reducing its concentration by up to 25%. It has an elimination half-life of 6 hours.

Pregabalin

Pregabalin is used as an adjunct for partial seizures in adults and is also used in anxiety. It was specifically designed to be a successor to gabapentin.

Mechanism of Action

It binds to the $\alpha_2\delta$ subunit of voltage-gated calcium channels in cortical neurones in a manner similar to gabapentin. However it does not appear to alter synaptic GABA concentration.

Effects

Central – it commonly causes dizziness and drowsiness and a wide range of other unpleasant effects such as weight gain, confusion, ataxia, GI upset and erectile dysfunction.

Kinetics

It is rapidly absorbed and has an oral bioavailability of 90% which is unaffected by dose, but is delayed by food. It is not bound to plasma proteins and is not metabolised, being eliminated in the urine.

Chapter 19

Antiemetics and Related Drugs

Nausea and vomiting has many causes including drugs, motion sickness, fear, pregnancy, vestibular disease and migraine. In previous decades anaesthesia was almost synonymous with vomiting, but with the advent of new anaesthetic agents and more aggressive treatment the incidence of vomiting has decreased. However, even the latest agents have failed to eradicate this troublesome symptom encountered in the perioperative period.

Physiology

The vomiting centre (VC) coordinates vomiting. It has no discrete anatomical site but may be considered as a collection of effector neurones situated in the medulla. This collection projects to the vagus and phrenic nerves and also to the spinal motor neurones supplying the abdominal muscles, which when acting together bring about the vomiting reflex.

The VC has important input from the chemoreceptor trigger zone (CTZ), which lies in the area postrema on the floor of the fourth ventricle but is functionally outside the blood–brain barrier. The CTZ is rich in dopamine (D_2) receptors and also serotonin (5-HT) receptors. Acetylcholine (ACh) is important in neural transmission from the vestibular apparatus. Other input is summarised in Figure 19.1.

The treatment of nausea and vomiting is aimed at reducing the afferent supply to the VC. While the administration of antiemetics forms a vital part of treatment, attention should also be given to minimising the administration of opioids by the use of non-steroidal anti-inflammatory drugs and avoiding unnecessary anticholinesterase administration. When propofol is used to maintain anaesthesia for minor surgery, where the use of opioids is limited, it may reduce the incidence of post-operative nausea and vomiting (PONV).

The following types of agents have been used:

- **Dopamine antagonists**
- **Anticholinergics**
- **Antihistamines**
- **5-HT$_3$ antagonists**
- **Neurokinin (NK) antagonists**
- **Miscellaneous.**

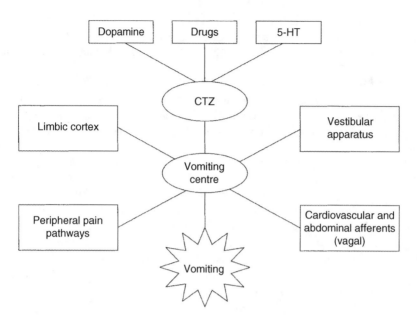

Figure 19.1 Summary of the various neural inputs that result in vomiting.

Table 19.1 Groups of phenothiazines

Group	Drug
Propylamine	Chlorpromazine
Piperidine	Thioridazine
Piperazine	Prochlorperazine, perphenazine

Dopamine Antagonists

Phenothiazines

Phenothiazines are the main group of anti-psychotic drugs (neuroleptics) and have only a limited role in the treatment of vomiting. They are divided into three groups on the basis of structure, which confers typical pharmacological characteristics (see Table 19.1).

Chlorpromazine

Chlorpromazine's proprietary name 'Largactil' hints at the widespread effects of this drug.

Uses

Chlorpromazine is used in schizophrenia for its sedative properties and to correct altered thought. Its effects on central neural pathways are complicated but are thought to involve isolating the reticular activating system from its afferent connections. This results in sedation, disregard of external stimuli and a reduction in motor activity (neurolepsy). It is sometimes used to control vomiting or pain in terminal care where other agents have been unsuccessful. It has also been shown to be effective in preventing PONV. It is occasionally used to treat hiccup.

Mechanism of Action

Chlorpromazine antagonises the following receptor types: dopaminergic (D_2), muscarinic, noradrenergic (α_1 and α_2), histaminergic (H_1) and serotonergic (5-HT). It also has membrane stabilising properties and prevents noradrenaline uptake into sympathetic nerves (uptake 1).

Effects

- *Central nervous system* – extrapyramidal effects are due to central dopamine antagonism. The neuroleptic malignant syndrome occurs rarely. It has variable effects on hypothalamic function, reducing the secretion of growth hormone while increasing the release of prolactin (dopamine functions as prolactin release inhibitory factor). Temperature regulation is altered and may result in hypothermia.
- *Cardiovascular* – it antagonises α-adrenoceptors resulting in peripheral vasodilation, hypotension and increased heat loss.
- *Anticholinergic* – it has moderate anticholinergic effects.
- *Gut* – appetite is increased and patients tend to gain weight (exacerbated by inactivity). While it has been shown to be an adequate antiemetic, its other effects have limited this role.
- *Miscellaneous* – contact sensitisation. Direct contact should be avoided unless actually taking chlorpromazine. Cholestatic jaundice, agranulocytosis, leucopenia, leucocytosis and haemolytic anaemia are all recognised.

Kinetics

Absorption from the gut is good but, due to a large hepatic first-pass metabolism (limiting its oral bioavailability to about 30%), it is often given parenterally. The large number of hepatic metabolites is excreted in the urine or bile, while a variable but small fraction is excreted unchanged in the urine.

Prochlorperazine

Uses

Prochlorperazine is effective in the prevention and treatment of PONV and vertigo, as well as in schizophrenia and other psychoses.

Effects

- *Central nervous system* – extrapyramidal effects are seen more commonly in this class of phenothiazine (Table 19.2). Acute dystonias and akathisia seem to be the most commonly encountered effects. Children and young adults are the most affected groups. When used peri-operatively it produces only mild sedation and may prolong the recovery time but the effects are not marked.
- *Group specific* – in common with other phenothiazines, prochlorperazine may cause cholestatic jaundice, haematological abnormalities, skin sensitisation, hyperprolactinaemia and rarely the neuroleptic malignant syndrome.

Table 19.2 Effects of some dopamine antagonists

	Sedation	Anticholinergic effects	Extrapyramidal effects
Chlorpromazine	+++	++	++
Droperidol	+	0	++
Metoclopramide	+	0	++
Domperidone	+	0	0
Prochlorperazine	+	+	+++

Kinetics

Absorption by the oral route is erratic and the oral bioavailability is very low due to an extensive hepatic first-pass metabolism. It may be given by suppository, intravenous or intramuscular injection.

Perphenazine has similar indications and kinetics to prochlorperazine, and has been shown to be effective in the prevention and treatment of PONV. It is associated with a higher incidence of extrapyramidal effects and increased post-operative sedation than prochlorperazine.

Butyrophenones
Droperidol

Droperidol is the only butyrophenone that is used in anaesthetic practice.

Uses

Droperidol has been shown to be effective in the prevention and treatment of PONV at doses from 0.25–5 mg, although the incidence of side effects increases with dose. It is also used in neurolept analgesia and in the control of mania.

Mechanism of Action

Droperidol antagonises central dopamine (D$_2$) receptors at the CTZ.

Effects

These are similar to those seen with phenothiazines.

- *Central nervous system* – sedation is more pronounced compared to the phenothiazines. The true incidence of extrapyramidal effects is unknown but increases with higher doses. They may develop more than 12 hours after administration and up to 25% of patients may experience anxiety up to 48 hours after administration. In sufficient dose it induces neurolepsis.
- *Metabolic* – it may cause hyperprolactinaemia.
- *Cardiovascular* – hypotension resulting from peripheral α-adrenoceptor blockade may occur. It was withdrawn for a while over concerns of QT prolongation and VT, but has now regained its UK licence for low-dose (0.625–1.25 mg) treatment of PONV.

Kinetics

Droperidol is usually given intravenously although it is absorbed readily after intramuscular injection. It is highly plasma protein-bound (approximately 90%) and extensively metabolised in the liver to products that are excreted in the urine, only 1% as unchanged drug.

Domperidone

This D_2 antagonist is less likely to cause extrapyramidal effects as it does not cross the blood–brain barrier. Its use in children is limited to nausea and vomiting following chemotherapy or radiotherapy. It also increases prolactin levels and may cause galactorrhoea and gynaecomastia. The intravenous preparation was withdrawn following serious arrhythmias during the administration of large doses. It is only available as tablets or suppositories.

Benzamides
Metoclopramide

Uses

Metoclopramide is used as an antiemetic and a prokinetic. Approximately half of the clinical studies have demonstrated placebo to be as effective as metoclopramide as an antiemetic. However, metoclopramide appears to be most effective when 20 mg is given at the end of anaesthesia rather than at induction.

Mechanism of Action

Metoclopramide exerts its antiemetic actions primarily through dopamine (D_2) receptor antagonism at the CTZ, although it does have prokinetic effects on the stomach (see Chapter 20). It also blocks $5\text{-}HT_3$ receptors, which may account for some of its antiemetic properties.

Effects

- *Central nervous system* – metoclopramide crosses the blood–brain barrier and may precipitate extrapyramidal effects up to 72 hours after administration. Such effects are more common in young females (1 in 5000). Rarely it may precipitate the neuroleptic malignant syndrome. Sedation is seen more commonly during long-term administration. Agitation is occasionally seen following intramuscular premedication with 10–20 mg.
- *Cardiovascular* – hypotension, tachy- and bradycardias have been reported following rapid intravenous administration.

Kinetics

Metoclopramide is well absorbed from the gut although first-pass metabolism varies significantly, producing a wide range in oral bioavailability (30–90%). It may be given intravenously. It is conjugated in the liver and excreted along with unchanged drug in the urine.

Anticholinergics

While so-called 'anticholinergic' agents are effective antagonists at muscarinic receptors, they have very little activity at nicotinic receptors and may therefore be thought of as essentially selective agents at normal doses.

The naturally occurring tertiary amines, atropine and hyoscine, are esters formed by the combination of tropic acid and an organic base (tropine or scopine) and are able to cross the blood–brain barrier. Their central effects include sedation, amnesia, antiemesis and the central anticholinergic syndrome. Glycopyrrolate is a synthetic quaternary amine (therefore charged) with no central effects as it is unable to cross the blood–brain barrier.

Hyoscine

Hyoscine is a racemic mixture, but only l-hyoscine is active.

Uses

Hyoscine has traditionally been given with an intramuscular opioid as premedication, and in this setting has been shown to reduce PONV. It has also been used as a sedative and amnesic agent.

Effects

While hyoscine's main uses are derived from its central antimuscarinic effects, it also has peripheral antimuscarinic effects some of which can be useful and are summarised in Table 19.3.

- *Other central effects* – it may precipitate a central anticholinergic syndrome, which is characterised by excitement, ataxia, hallucinations, behavioural abnormalities and drowsiness.

Kinetics

Its absorption is variable and its oral bioavailability lies between 10–50%. Transdermal administration is effective in reducing PONV and motion sickness despite very low plasma levels. It is extensively metabolised by liver esterases and only a small fraction is excreted unchanged in the urine. Its duration of action is shorter than that of atropine.

Atropine

Atropine is a racemic mixture, but only l-atropine is active.

Table 19.3 Effects of some anticholinergics

	Hyoscine	Atropine	Glycopyrrolate
Antiemetic potency	++	+	0
Sedation/amnesia	+++	+	0
Anti-sialagogue	+++	+	++
Mydriasis	+++	+	0
Placental transfer	++	++	0
Bronchodilation	+	++	++
Heart rate	+	+++	++

Uses

Atropine is used to treat bradycardia and as an anti-sialogogue. It is also used to antagonise the muscarinic side effects of anticholinesterases. It is not used to treat PONV because of its cardiovascular effects.

Effects

- *Central nervous system* – it is less likely to cause a central cholinergic crisis than hyoscine and is less sedative.
- *Cardiovascular* – it may cause an initial bradycardia following a small intravenous dose. This may be due to its effects centrally on the vagal nucleus or reflect a partial agonist effect at cardiac muscarinic receptors.
- *Respiratory system* – bronchodilation is more marked than with hyoscine, leading to an increase in dead space. Bronchial secretions are reduced.
- *Gut* – it is a less effective anti-sialogogue than hyoscine. The tone of the lower oesophageal sphincter is decreased and there is a small decrease in gastric acid secretion.
- *Miscellaneous* – sweating is inhibited and this may provoke a pyrexia in paediatric patients. When administered topically it may increase intra-ocular pressure, which may be critical for patients with glaucoma.

Kinetics

Intestinal absorption is rapid but unpredictable. It is 50% plasma protein-bound and extensively metabolised by liver esterases. It is excreted in the urine, only a tiny fraction unchanged.

Glycopyrrolate

Gylcopyrrolate is indicated for anti-sialogogue premedication, the treatment of bradycardias and to protect against the unwanted effects of anticholinesterases. Its charged quaternary structure gives it a different set of characteristics compared to the tertiary amines. Intestinal absorption is negligible and the oral bioavailability is consequently less than 5%. It does not cross the blood–brain barrier and so it is devoid of central effects. It is minimally metabolised and 80% is excreted in the urine unchanged.

Antihistamines

Cyclizine

Cyclizine is a piperazine derivative. The parenteral preparation is prepared with lactic acid at pH 3.2. Consequently intramuscular and intravenous injection may be particularly painful.

Uses

Cyclizine is used as an antiemetic in motion sickness, radiotherapy, PONV and emesis induced by opioids. It is also used to control the symptoms of Ménière's disease.

Mechanism of Action

Cyclizine is a histamine (H_1) antagonist, but also has anticholinergic properties that may contribute significantly to its antiemetic actions.

Effects

- *Gut* – it increases lower oesophageal sphincter tone.
- *Anticholinergic* – these are mild although it may cause an increase in heart rate following intravenous injection.
- *Extrapyramidal effects* and *sedation* do rarely complicate its use.

Kinetics

Cyclizine is well absorbed orally and has a high oral bioavailability (approximately 75%). Surprisingly little is known regarding the rest of the kinetics of this drug.

5-HT₃ Antagonists

Ondansetron

Ondansetron is a carbazole.

Presentation

Ondansetron is available as tablets (4–8 mg), a strawberry-flavoured lyophilisate (4–8 mg) to dissolve on the tongue, a suppository (16 mg) and as a clear solution containing 2 mg. ml^{-1} for slow intravenous injection.

Uses

Ondansetron is indicated for the treatment of nausea and vomiting associated with chemo- or radiotherapy and in the peri-operative period. It is ineffective for vomiting induced by motion sickness or dopamine agonists. It is licensed for children above 2 years of age. It should be used immediately prior to emergence from anaesthesia.

Mechanism of Action

The activation of 5-HT_3 receptors peripherally and centrally appears to induce vomiting. Chemo- and radiotherapy may cause the release of 5-HT from enterochromaffin cells. Peripheral 5-HT_3 receptors in the gut are then activated and stimulate vagal afferent neurones that connect to the VC, again via 5-HT_3 receptors. Thus ondansetron may antagonise 5-HT_3 both peripherally and centrally.

Effects

Ondansetron is well tolerated and its other effects are limited to headache, flushing, constipation and bradycardia following rapid intravenous administration.

Kinetics

Ondansetron is well absorbed from the gut with an oral bioavailability of about 60%. It is 75% protein-bound and undergoes significant hepatic metabolism by hydroxylation and subsequent glucuronide conjugation to inactive metabolites. Its half-life is 3 hours. The dose should be reduced in hepatic impairment.

Neurokinin 1 Receptor Antagonists

Aprepitant and Fosaprepitant

Neurokinin 1 (NK_1) receptor antagonists block the actions of substance P in the brainstem nuclei of the dorsal vagal complex which is central to the regulation of vomiting. They appear most useful in the control of delayed chemotherapy-induced nausea and vomiting (CINV).

Aprepitant

Aprepitant is an oral NK_1 receptor antagonist, fosaprepitant is its intravenous prodrug preparation.

They are used for CINV and PONV and appear to potentiate the effects of other antiemetics (ondansetron and dexamethasone).

Kinetics

Its oral bioavailability is about 60% and is 97% plasma protein-bound. It is metabolised by CYP3A4 to a number of weakly active metabolites which are excreted in the urine and faeces.

Miscellaneous

Steroids

Dexamethasone is a synthetic glucocorticoid with an established role in the prevention of post-operative nausea and vomiting when given at the start of anaesthesia. It is not effective in established vomiting. Low-dose regimes (3.3 mg) appear to be as effective as higher doses. The mechanism of action is not well understood but may involve prostaglandin antagonism or the release of endorphins, resulting in elevated mood and appetite stimulation. Its anti-inflammatory effects may also reduce 5-HT release within the gut. Single low-dose administration is not associated with the common side effects seen with chronic glucocorticoid use.

Cannabinoids

Nabilone acts at the VC and has been used as an antiemetic following chemotherapy.

Benzodiazepines

Lorazepam is used as an antiemetic during chemotherapy. It has amnesic and sedative properties. Its mode of action as an antiemetic is uncertain but it may modify central connections to the VC and prevent the anticipatory nausea that is seen with repeated doses of chemotherapy.

Acupuncture

Several studies have demonstrated the effectiveness of acupuncture in the prevention of PONV. The acupuncture point lies between the tendons of flexor carpi radialis and palmaris longus about 4 cm from the distal wrist skin crease. It should be performed on the awake patient and is free from side effects.

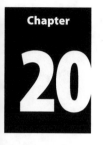

Drugs Acting on the Gut

Antacids

Antacids neutralise gastric acidity. They are used to relieve the symptoms of dyspepsia and gastro-oesophageal reflux. They promote ulcer healing but less effectively than other therapies.

Aluminium- and Magnesium-Containing Antacids

Neither is absorbed from the gut significantly and due to their relatively low water solubility they are long-acting providing that they remain in the stomach. Aluminium-containing antacids have a slower action and produce constipation, while magnesium-containing antacids produce diarrhoea. Aluminium ions form complexes with some drugs (e.g. tetracycline) and reduce their absorption.

Sodium Bicarbonate and Sodium Citrate

These antacids are water-soluble and their onset of action is faster than the aluminium- and magnesium-containing antacids. They are absorbed into the systemic circulation and may cause a metabolic alkalosis if taken in excess. Sodium bicarbonate releases carbon dioxide as it reacts with gastric acid, resulting in belching. Thirty millilitres of 0.3 M sodium citrate is often used with ranitidine to reduce gastric acidity before caesarean section. It should be given less than 10 minutes before the start of surgery due to its limited duration of action.

Drugs Influencing Gastric Secretion

Physiology

Gastrin and acetylcholine (ACh) stimulate parietal cells (via gastrin and muscarinic receptors) to secrete H^+ into the gastric lumen. ACh is released from parasympathetic postganglionic fibres while gastrin is released from G-cells in the antral mucosa. However, the main stimulus for parietal cell acid secretion is via histamine receptor activation. Gastrin and ACh also stimulate the adjacent paracrine cells to produce and release histamine, which acts on the parietal cell, increasing cAMP and therefore acid secretion.

H_2 Receptor Antagonists
Cimetidine

Cimetidine is the only H_2 receptor antagonist with an imidazole structure.

Uses

It is used in peptic ulcer disease, reflux oesophagitis, Zollinger–Ellison syndrome and pre-operatively in those at risk of aspiration. It has not been shown to be of benefit in active haematemesis.

Mechanism of Action

Cimetidine is a competitive and specific antagonist of H_2 receptors at parietal cells.

Effects

- *Gut* – the gastric pH is raised and the volume of secretions reduced, while there is no change in gastric emptying time or lower oesophageal sphincter tone.
- *Cardiovascular* – bradycardia and hypotension follow rapid intravenous administration.
- *Central nervous system* – confusion, hallucinations and seizures are usually only seen when impaired renal function leads to high plasma levels.
- *Respiratory system* – low-grade aspiration of gastric content that has been stripped of its acidic, antibacterial environment will result in increased nosocomial pulmonary infections in critically ill ventilated patients.
- *Endocrine* – gynaecomastia, impotence and a fall in sperm count are seen in men due to the anti-androgenic effects of cimetidine.
- *Metabolic* – it inhibits hepatic cytochrome P450 and will slow the metabolism of the following drugs: lidocaine, propranolol, diazepam, phenytoin, tricyclic antidepressants, warfarin and aminophylline.

Kinetics

Cimetidine is well absorbed from the small bowel (oral bioavailability approximately 60%), poorly plasma protein-bound (20%), partially metabolised (up to 60% if administered orally) in the liver by cytochrome P450 and approximately 50% excreted unchanged in the urine.

Ranitidine

Ranitidine is more potent than cimetidine.

Uses

Ranitidine has similar uses to cimetidine. However, because it does not inhibit hepatic cytochrome P450, it is often preferred to cimetidine. It is used in combination with antibiotics to eradicate *H. pylori*. It is also used widely in labour with apparently no deleterious effects on the fetus or progress of labour.

Mechanism of Action

Similar to that of cimetidine.

Effects

- *Gut* – similar to that of cimetidine.
- *Cardiovascular* – it may produce cardiac arrhythmias during rapid intravenous administration.
- *Metabolic* – it should be avoided in porphyria, although reports detailing this interaction are inconclusive. It has no anti-androgenic effects.

- *Miscellaneous* – rarely it may cause thrombocytopenia, leucopenia, reversible abnormalities of liver function and anaphylaxis.

Kinetics

Ranitidine is well absorbed from the gut, poorly protein-bound (15%) and partially metabolised in the liver. It undergoes a greater degree of first-pass metabolism than cimetidine (oral bioavailability approximately 50%), while 50% of an administered dose is excreted unchanged in the urine.

Nizatidine and famotidine are newer H_2 antagonists with increased potency. Like ranitidine they do not inhibit hepatic cytochrome P450.

Proton Pump Inhibitors

Omeprazole

Omeprazole has a chiral centre and is administered as a racemic mixture of the *R*- and *S*-enantiomers or as the enantiopure preparation esomeprazole, which contains only the *S*-enantiomer.

Uses

Omeprazole is used for similar indications to that of ranitidine but also in cases where H_2 blockade is insufficient. It may be given orally or intravenously.

Mechanism of Action

A proton pump (K^+/H^+ ATPase) in the membrane of the parietal cell mediates the final common pathway of gastric acid secretion. Omeprazole irreversibly blocks the proton pump and so achieves complete achlorhydria.

Effects

- *Gut* – the acidity and volume of gastric secretions is reduced, while no change is seen in lower oesophageal sphincter tone or gastric emptying.
- *Metabolic* – inhibition of hepatic cytochrome P450. This is limited, and although close monitoring is recommended with concurrent use of warfarin and phenytoin, their effects are rarely potentiated. The effects of diazepam may be increased via a similar mechanism.
- *Miscellaneous* – rashes and gastrointestinal upset are rare.

Kinetics

Omeprazole is degraded in gastric acid and so is prepared as a capsule with enteric-coated granules so that absorption occurs in the small intestine. It is a prodrug, becoming active within the parietal cell. It undergoes complete hepatic metabolism by cytochrome CYP2C19 (and to a lesser extent CYP3A4) to inactive metabolites, which are excreted in the urine (80%) and bile (20%). CYP2C19 is subject to genetic polymorphism with ultrarapid metabolisers (CYP2C19*17, which may result in ineffective treatment) and poor metabolisers (CYP2C19*3, with markedly reduced or absent enzyme activity in up to 20% of Asians).

Omeprazole is the most potent inhibitor of CYP2C19 of all the PPIs and may interfere with the metabolism of the prodrug to the active form of clopidogrel, thereby reducing its antiplatelet effect. Pantoprazole and esomeprazole may be considered as an alternative to omeprazole.

Drugs Influencing Gastric Motility

Metoclopramide

Metoclopramide is a dopamine antagonist with structural similarities to procainamide although it has no local anaesthetic properties.

Uses

Metoclopramide is used as a prokinetic and an antiemetic (see Chapter 19).

Mechanism of Action

Its prokinetic actions are mediated by antagonism of peripheral dopaminergic (D_2) receptors and selective stimulation of gastric muscarinic receptors (which can be blocked by atropine).

Effects

- *Central nervous system* – extrapyramidal effects, the most common manifestations of which are akinesia and oculogyric crisis, are only seen when metoclopramide is given in high doses, in renal impairment, and to the elderly and the young. They can be treated with the anticholinergic agent procyclidine. Metoclopramide may cause some sedation and enhance the actions of antidepressants. The neuroleptic malignant syndrome may also be triggered. Its central effects on the chemoreceptor trigger zone are discussed in Chapter 19.
- *Gut* – its peripheral actions result in an increased lower oesophageal sphincter tone and relaxation of the pylorus. It has no effect on gastric secretion.
- *Cardiovascular* – acute conduction abnormalities follow rapid intravenous administration, and acute hypertension occurs in phaeochromocytoma.
- *Metabolic* – it may precipitate hyperprolactinaemia and galactorrhoea, and should be avoided in porphyria. It inhibits plasma cholinesterase activity in vitro and may therefore prolong the effects of drugs metabolised by this enzyme.

Kinetics

Metoclopramide is well absorbed from the gut although first-pass metabolism varies significantly, producing a wide range in oral bioavailability (30–90%). It may be given intravenously. It is conjugated in the liver and excreted along with unchanged drug in the urine.

Domperidone

This dopamine antagonist is less likely to cause extrapyramidal effects as it does not cross the blood–brain barrier. Its use in children is limited to nausea and vomiting following chemotherapy or radiotherapy. It also increases prolactin levels and may cause galactorrhoea and gynaecomastia. The intravenous preparation was withdrawn following serious arrhythmias during administration of large doses. It is only available as tablets or suppositories.

Mucosal Protectors

Sucralfate

Sucralfate exerts a generalised cytoprotective effect by forming a barrier over the gut lumen. It protects ulcerated regions specifically. It does not alter gastric pH, motility or lower oesophageal sphincter tone, although it has been reported to have bacteriostatic effects.

Its actions are due to its local effects and virtually none is absorbed from the gut. Consequently it has no effect on the central nervous or cardiorespiratory systems.

Effects

- *Gut* – minor gastric disturbances. Enhanced aluminium absorption in patients with renal dysfunction or on dialysis. It may reduce the absorption of certain drugs (ciprofloxacin, warfarin, phenytoin and H_2 antagonists) by direct binding.

Prostaglandin Analogues

Misoprostil

Misoprostil is a synthetic analogue of prostaglandin E_1.

Uses

It is used for the prevention and treatment of non-steroidal anti-inflammatory induced ulcers.

Mechanism of Action

It inhibits gastric acid secretion and increases mucous secretion thereby protecting the gastric mucosa.

Effects

- *Endocrine* – it increases uterine tone and may precipitate miscarriage. Menorrhagia and vaginal bleeding have been reported.
- *Gut* – severe diarrhoea and other intestinal upset.
- *Cardiovascular* – at normal doses it is unlikely to produce hypotension but its use is cautioned where hypotension could precipitate severe complications (i.e. in cerebrovascular or cardiovascular disease).

Kinetics

Misoprostil is rapidly absorbed from the gut. Metabolism is by fatty-acid-oxidising systems throughout the body and no alteration in dose is required in renal or hepatic impairment.

Intravenous Fluids, Minerals and Nutrition

Body Fluid Compartments

Total body water represents approximately 60% of body weight (45 litres in a 75 kg male). Sixty-six per cent is intracellular water (30 litres), 33% is extracellular (15 litres). The extracellular fluid volume is 25% intravascular (3 litres) and 75% extravascular (interstitial) (12 litres). Total intravascular volume combines intravascular extracellular fluid (3 litres) and cellular components (2 litres).

Intracellular

The composition of the intracellular volume is maintained by a metabolically active cellular membrane. It has a low sodium concentration (10 mmol.l^{-1}) and a high potassium (150 mmol.l^{-1}) concentration.

Interstitial (Extravascular)

The interstitial volume is that part of the extracellular volume that is not present in the plasma. It has an electrolyte composition that is similar to plasma with a high sodium concentration (140 mmol.l^{-1}) and a low potassium concentration (4 mmol.l^{-1}). It has less protein than the plasma and therefore a lower oncotic pressure.

Intravascular

The intravascular compartment has a composition similar to the interstitial space. The plasma has a number of key functions, which include providing the fluid volume necessary to suspend the red cells, clotting and immunological functions.

Movement between Compartments

Traditionally, fluid moves between compartments via osmotic and hydrostatic gradients, as predicted by the Starling equation:

$$Jv \propto [(Pc - Pi) - \sigma(\pi c - \pi i)]$$

Capillary hydrostatic pressure (Pc) is affected by circulating volume and intravenous fluid administration.

Interstitial hydrostatic pressure (Pi) is affected by interstitial volume.

The reflection coefficient (σ) is altered in states of acute inflammation, trauma, surgery or illness resulting in loss of barrier function and increase in transcapillary flux (Jv). Chronic ill health and poor nutritional status result in hypoalbuminemia and subsequent reduction in capillary oncotic pressure and tissue oedema.

πi represents interstitial oncotic pressure.

Traditionally, net Jv is out of the capillary into the interstitium at the arteriolar end but the direction of Jv reverses at the venous end to be into the capillary. Thus, fluid is lost from the capillary at the arteriolar end and reabsorbed at the venous end. According to Starling, intravenous infusion of artificial colloids increases the capillary oncotic pressure (πc) and promotes fluid reabsorption into the capillaries.

However, an alternative 'revised' Starling equation has been suggested, in which no fluid reabsorption takes place within the capillary, even at the venous end (the 'no absorption rule'). Consequently, Jv out of the capillary occurs all along its length, with fluid not being reabsorbed directly into the capillaries at all, but rather being returned to the circulation via the lymphatics. This is based on the relatively recent discovery of an endothelial glycocalyx layer (glycocalyx), an endoluminal web of membrane bound proteoglycans, glycoproteins and glycosaminoglycans which is present in capillaries, arterioles and venules.

The glycocalyx separates plasma from a 'protected' region of the sub-glycocalyx space which is almost protein free. The sub-glycocalyx space contains non-circulating plasma volume and has a colloid oncotic pressure of approximately 70% of the capillary lumen. The sub-glycocalyx colloid oncotic pressure (πsg) replaces the interstitial colloid oncotic pressure πi as a major determinant of transcapillary flow along oncotic gradients. Jv is therefore proportional to πc – πsg. Jv out of the capillary depends entirely on Pc when the πc – πsg difference is maximal (as is usual in health) therefore in a euvolaemic patient infusion of colloid (or crystalloid) increases the Pc and fluid moves out of the capillary despite the potential increase in πc (seen with colloid) .

The volume status of the patient and subsequent Pc is the most important determinant of fluid movement out of the capillaries, more so than the colloid oncotic effect of the infused fluid, in contrast to traditional Starling physiology.

In hypovolaemia or vasodilation, Pc is low. Infusion of crystalloid or colloid does not increase Pc above the oncotic pressure gradient πc – πsg, and as a result, Jv remains close to zero. The important role played by Pc in Jv is especially in evidence where the capillary hydrostatic pressure falls with the induction of anaesthesia.

In inflammatory states there is a reduction in plasma albumin (an important contributor to πc) and trans-capillary escape of albumin to the tissues. Administering albumin does not seem to improve flow back into the tissues due to the no absorption rule. An increase in capillary porosity, such as might occur in severe inflammation, sepsis or trauma, increases the Jv out of the vasculature for any given Pc.

Volume Kinetics

It is possible to apply a two-compartment model to intravenous fluids with two functional, rather than anatomical compartments, V1 and V2 (see Figure 21.1). V1 corresponds to plasma volume and V2 represents the interstitial fluid volume that can be expanded by fluid moving out of the plasma after intravenous infusion. V2 is smaller than the total interstitial volume because not all of the interstitial fluid volume can be expanded (e.g. that contained inside the skull or long bones).

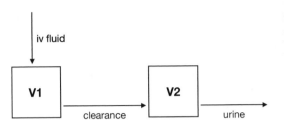

Figure 21.1 Diagram showing the movement of intravenous fluids through the functional volumes, V1 and V2, and subsequent elimination via the urine.

Crystalloids are reported to expand the plasma volume by 20%, but this is an understatement in patients undergoing general anaesthesia who are vasodilated and where the plasma volume expanding effects are greater and longer lasting. This is because there is a dramatic fall in fluid movement from V1 to V2 under general anaesthesia. The pattern is such that at the onset of general or spinal anaesthesia fluid movement falls to such an extent (temporarily) that fluid transfer out of the vascular space (equivalent to Jv) might stop completely depending on the fall in mean arterial pressure.

Fluid and Mineral Requirements

The following are normal daily fluid and electrolyte requirements.

25–30 ml.kg^{-1}.day^{-1} water

1 mmol.kg^{-1} per day sodium, potassium and chloride

50–100 g.day^{-1} glucose

Intravenous Fluids

Intravenous fluids may broadly be classified into crystalloid and colloid solutions.

Crystalloid Solutions

Solutions of inorganic ions and small organic molecules dissolved in water are referred to as crystalloids. The main solute is either glucose or sodium chloride (or both), and the solutions may be isotonic, hypotonic, or hypertonic with respect to plasma. Table 21.1 lists the contents of common intravenous crystalloid solutions.

0.9% Sodium Chloride

First used in the late 1800s, 0.9% saline is a solution of sodium and chloride. The 154 mmol.l^{-1} sodium and 154 mmol.l^{-1} of chloride maintains electrochemical neutrality. It is difficult to describe it as 'normal' when the chloride content is nearly 50% greater than plasma. There is a plethora of evidence from a variety of patient and volunteer studies that use of 0.9% saline causes unwanted and potentially undesirable physiological effects. Infusion of 0.9% saline in healthy volunteers has been shown to cause the following effects; metabolic acidosis (hyperchloraemic), renal vasoconstriction, reduced renal blood flow, reduced glomerular filtration rate, abdominal pain, tiredness and difficulty thinking.

Table 21.1 Composition of crystalloids

	Na⁺ mmol.l⁻¹	Cl⁻ mmol.l⁻¹	K⁺ mmol.l⁻¹	HCO₃⁻ precursor mmol.l⁻¹	Ca²⁺ mmol.l⁻¹	Mg²⁺ mmol.l⁻¹	Glucose mmol.l⁻¹	pH	Osmolarity mOsm.l⁻¹	Osmolality mOsm.kg⁻¹ (tonicity)
Plasma	134–145	95–105	3.5–5.3	24–32	2.2–2.6	0.8–1.2	3.5–5.5	7.35–7.45		275–295
0.9% NaCl	154	154	0	0	0	0	0	4.5–7.0	308	286
0.18% NaCl & 4% glucose	31	31	0	0	0	0	222	4.5	284	52
0.45% NaCl & 4% glucose	77	77	0	0	0	0	222		432	134
5% glucose	0	0	0	0	0	0	278	3.5–5.5	278	0
0.9% NaCl in 5% glucose	154	154	0	0	0	0	278		586	286
Hartmanns	131	111	5	29 (lactate)	2	0	0	5.0–7.0	278	256
Lactated Ringers	130	109	4	28 (lactate)	1	1	0	6.0–7.5	273	256
Plasma-lyte	140	98	5	27 (acetate) 23 (gluconate)	0	1.5	0	7.4	295	271
8.4% sodium bicarbonate	1000	0	0	1000	0	0	0		2000	0

Balanced Solutions

To address the problems with 0.9% sodium chloride, balanced solutions have been developed that provide an ion content similar to that of plasma by avoiding the excess chloride. One potential option with which to substitute chloride in balanced solutions (to maintain overall electrochemical neutrality) is bicarbonate. However, difficulties with storage and poor solubility of bicarbonate salts has led to the use of bicarbonate precursors. The most common bicarbonate precursors are the organic anions lactate, acetate or gluconate.

Balanced Solutions with Lactate

Ringer's solution appeared in the 1800s and was probably the first balanced crystalloid that contained sodium chloride, potassium chloride and calcium chloride. The solution as we know it today is Lactated Ringer's, after sodium lactate was added by Alexis Hartmann in the 1930s. The exact composition and marketing name of Lactated Ringer's varies slightly between different manufacturers. Commercial solutions available include Hartmann's solution and compound sodium Lactate.

The advantages of lactate are that it can be metabolised at high rates (up to 100 mmol.hr^{-1}) in patients with normal liver function so that up to 4 litres can be given quickly to a healthy adult patient weighing 70 kg without any lactate accumulation. Metabolism is to carbon dioxide (CO_2) or via gluconeogenesis. A potential disadvantage in the peri-operative use of lactate-balanced solutions is the need for a functioning liver and the increased oxygen consumption due to its metabolism. Accumulation of lactate from balanced solutions might confound the use of lactate as a marker of tissue hypoperfusion, but there is no associated acidaemia because these solutions contain lactate not lactic acid.

Other Anions

Other balanced solutions use acetate or gluconate as the anion to maintain electrochemical neutrality. Plasma-lyte^{TM}, Normosol^{TM} and Ringer's acetate are examples of these solutions. As with Lactated Ringer's solution the exact composition varies between manufacturers.

The advantages of acetate are solubility of its salts and metabolism within and outside the liver up to 300 mmol.hr^{-1} (three times faster than L-Lactate) in health and experimental shock states. It is rapidly metabolised to bicarbonate and therefore fluids containing acetate have an alkalising effect. Acetate in haemodialysis solutions has been associated with haemodynamic instability through pro-inflammatory and cardiotoxic effects. It has been removed from haemodialysis fluids in Australia because of this although there is little evidence this effect occurs in peri-operative or intensive care unit (ICU) practice in commonly administered volumes.

Less is known about the fate of gluconate in the body. Although it is labelled as a bicarbonate precursor it appears that most of the gluconate is excreted unchanged in the urine and may act as an osmotic diuretic. The clinical implications of this are unclear.

Glucose-Containing Solutions

A wide variety of solutions containing glucose with or without sodium chloride are available. Traditionally they are used to give water to treat dehydration because the glucose is rapidly metabolised leaving the remaining water to diffuse throughout the entire total body water volume. The glucose is added to prevent lysis of cells on infusion into the blood stream. Various percentages are available from 5%, 10%, 20% and 50%. Twenty per cent and 50% are extremely irritant to veins and should only be given centrally.

Solutions Containing Crystalloid and Glucose

There are a wide variety of solutions available that contain glucose and some electrolytes. 0.18% sodium chloride with 4% glucose has been associated with severe hyponatraemia in infants and children and is not recommended in this group. Five per cent glucose is usually combined with sodium chloride 0.45% or 0.9% in paediatric practice. Glucose is also available in combination with Lactated Ringer's and Hartmann's solution although this is not widely available.

Osmolality and Tonicity

Water moves across cell membranes and between compartments due to osmotic gradients. An intravenous solution with the same osmolality as plasma is likely to stay in the extra-cellular fluid compartment. Solutions with an osmolality below that of plasma are likely to move along osmotic gradients and therefore spread through the intracellular compartment as well as the extracellular compartment.

Osmolarity describes the number of osmoles per litre of solution. Osmolality describes the number of osmoles per kilogram of solvent. The product literature quotes osmolarity. The osmotic pressure applied across a semipermeable membrane in vivo is osmolality. Tonicity is used in a medical context to mean the *effective* osmolality and is equal to the sum of the concentrations of the solutes which have the capacity to exert an osmotic force across the membrane. Osmolality is a property of a solution and is independent of any membrane. Tonicity is a property of a solution in reference to a membrane.

This difference is important because the osmolarity of intravenous solutions as calculated in the laboratory from the sum of the osmotically active particles is very different to the effective 'in vivo' value once infused. This difference is due to rapid metabolism of glucose (if present) and incomplete dissociation of ions in solution. For example, the calculated osmolarity of 0.9% sodium chloride is 308 $mOsm.L^{-1}$ whereas the effective osmolality is 286 $mOsm.kg^{-1}(H_2O)$ (plasma 275–295 $mOsm.kg^{-1}(H_2O)$).

One can see from the above example that the traditional description of 0.9% sodium chloride as 'hypertonic' is incorrect. It is isotonic in vivo.

It is also important to note that although the calculated osmolarity of the 'balanced solutions' is within the normal range for plasma, their effective osmolality in vivo is lower, making them hypotonic in vivo. This has implications for several clinical situations includ-ing the brain-injured patient and those undergoing neurosurgery where infusion of hypo-tonic solutions can result in cerebral oedema.

Other Problems with Balanced Solutions

Some balanced solutions contain calcium which, if used in the same giving set or line as blood components preserved in citrate-based solutions results in coagulation.

Outcomes

It is not known if balanced solutions have an outcome benefit compared to unbalanced (0.9% sodium chloride) crystalloids in peri-operative or ICU practice (excluding neurosurgery and neurological injury). Equally there is no evidence of an outcome benefit comparing use of one balanced crystalloid compared to another.

Colloids

A colloid is a homogeneous non-crystalline substance consisting of large molecules or microscopic particles of one substance dispersed through a second substance. The particles do not settle and cannot be separated out by ordinary filtering or centrifuging as can those of a suspension such as blood. Colloid solutions are divided into the semisynthetic colloids (gelatins, dextrans (no longer used intravenously), and hydroxyethyl starches (HES)) and the naturally occurring human plasma derivatives (human albumin solutions, plasma protein fraction, fresh frozen plasma, and immunoglobulin solution). Most colloid solutions are presented with the colloid molecules dissolved in 0.9% sodium chloride (see Table 21.2), but glucose or balanced solutions are also used.

Gelatins

Gelatins are large molecular weight proteins. Those in use today are manufactured from bovine gelatin, which is heated, allowing the protein to denature, and cooled, allowing new inter-chain bonds to form. These bonds are either succinylated (Gelofusine™) or urea cross-linked (Hemaccel™) depending on the chemical conditions during cooling. The resultant product has a range of molecular weights, which is quoted in one of two ways: the weight average or the number average. The number average best reflects the mean osmotically active particle weight of a colloid and is the total weight of all the molecules divided by the total number of all the molecules. The weight average is a more complicated calculation, usually larger and usually quoted by the manufacturer.

Kinetics

More than 95% of infused gelatin is excreted unchanged in the urine. Unlike hydroxyethyl starches, gelatins are not stored in the reticulo-endothelial system. Due to the 'no absorption rule' and the complex interplay between all the components of the revised Starling equation their plasma volume expansion effect is often very similar to crystalloids.

Side Effects

The only significant side effect is anaphylactic and anaphylactoid reactions, which occur in approximately 6.2 per 100,000 administrations (similar incidence to rocuronium). The evidence on disturbances of coagulation is inconclusive. Because of the significant calcium content of Hemaccel™, blood should not be infused through a giving set that has been previously used for this product. European guidelines recommend that gelatins are avoided in patients with severe sepsis, those at risk of acute kidney injury, and patients with head injury or those who are potential organ donors.

Table 21.2 Composition of colloids

	Na$^+$ mmol.l^{-1}	Cl$^-$ mmol.l^{-1}	K$^+$ mmol.l^{-1}	Ca^{++} mmol.l^{-1}	Mg^{++} mmol.l^{-1}	Misc	pH
Gelofusine	154	125	0.4	0.4	0.4	Gelatin 40 g	7.4
Haemaccel 3.5%	145	145	5.1	6.25	0	Gelatin 35 g	7.3
Hespan 6%	154	154	0	0	0	Starch 60 g	5.5
Human albumin solution 4.5%	100–160	100–160	< 2	0	0	Albumin 45 g, citrate < 15	6.9 +/− 0.5
Human albumin solution 20%	50–120	< 40	< 10	0	0	Albumin 200 g	6.9 +/− 0.5

Hydroxyethyl Starches

Hydroxyethyl starch (HES) is a derivative of amylopectin, a highly branched starch compound. When anhydroglucose residues are substituted with hydroxyethyl groups two important changes occur: first, increased solubility and second, reduced metabolism, which increases its half-life. There are many more preparations of HES than there are of gelatins. The types of preparation are based around concentration, molecular weights, the degree of substitution as described above and the C2:C6 ratio, which reflects the position of the substitution.

Kinetics

The high molecular weight HES solutions provide the longest plasma-volume-expanding effect but are also associated with unwanted effects. The low molecular weight HES solutions only have very limited duration of action, whereas the medium molecular weight HES solutions provide the best balance.

Side Effects

- *Renal* – HES has been demonstrated to increase acute kidney injury in all patient groups.
- *Coagulation* – the effects on coagulation are variable and depend on the molecular weight and degree of substitution of the HES.
- *Accumulation* – the reticuloendothelial system takes up HES and stores it, causing pruritus.
- *Anaphylaxis* – the incidence is in the order of 1 in 20,000.

In 2018 the marketing authorisations for HES were suspended across the European Union because of the risk of death and acute kidney injury in certain patient populations including critically ill patients and those with sepsis, renal failure or undergoing cardiac surgery.

Albumin

Albumin accounts for approximately 50% of the five available plasma proteins, the other 50% comprising α_1-, α_2-, β-globulin and γ-globulin. It is made up of 585 amino acids, has a molecular weight of 69,000 Da and is folded into a series of α helices, which form three domains each with a hydrophobic core and a polar outer exterior.

Functions

Albumin exerts a greater colloid osmotic effect than its molecular weight alone might suggest due to its high negative charge. It is the major contributor to colloid oncotic pressure.

Albumin binds and transports drugs and endogenous molecules in the plasma. Acidic drugs (warfarin, aspirin, furosemide and amiodarone) tend to bind to albumin while basic drugs bind to α_1-acid glycoprotein. Reductions in albumin concentration can increase the effects of drugs such as warfarin by increasing the free fraction. Albumin carries bilirubin, fatty acids, calcium and magnesium. Despite a low binding affinity, a significant amount of steroid is carried by albumin due to its abundance.

Kinetics

Albumin is synthesised in the liver ($10-15$ g.day^{-1}) in response to changes in plasma oncotic pressure and has a half-life of 20 days. Just under 50% is intravascular, the remainder being present in the skin and muscle with lesser amounts in the gut, liver and subcutaneous tissue. In health, albumin synthesis is balanced to match metabolism. Where metabolism or loss (renal or gastrointestinal) are significantly increased synthesis may not be able to keep up and hypoalbuminaemia ensues.

Intravenous Albumin Infusions

Intravenous infusions of albumin are used in the treatment of pancreatitis, burns and as part of plasma exchange. Human albumin solutions (HAS) have an established role in patients with ascites who require large volume paracentesis, those who have developed hepatorenal syndrome or have spontaneous bacterial peritonitis. It is also used in some paediatric patients with nephrotic syndrome. It is associated with worse outcome when used in head injuries. HAS preparations are traditionally available in 4.5%, 5% and 20%. The 4.5% and 5% solution have the same oncotic pressure as plasma and their uses are quite different from the hyper-oncotic 20% solution. The manufacturing process involves use of plasma from many (up to thousands) of donors. There are multiple steps taken to purify the albumin and eradicate transmissible viruses and other pathogens (cold ethanol fractionation or chromatographic purification processes, followed by pasteurisation). The resultant mixture is typically over 99% albumin. In the UK all plasma derivatives are sourced from imported plasma to reduce the risk of variant CJD transmission. No two HAS products will be identical, and there are currently eight UK manufacturers.

Bicarbonate

In vivo bicarbonate forms part of the bicarbonate-carbonic acid buffering system, the major extracellular buffering system. It is in equilibrium with carbonic acid which rapidly dissociates to dissolved CO_2 and water. The ratio of dissolved CO_2 to bicarbonate is 20:1. The bicarbonate-carbonic acid buffering system becomes more effective as pH falls below normal.

Kinetics

Sodium bicarbonate is presented as a crystalloid solution in several different strengths. 1.26% and 1.4% are effectively isotonic or mildly hypo-tonic crystalloid solutions that can be used for maintenance fluids (attractive due to the lack of chloride).

Hypertonic 4.2% and 8.4% solutions are also available. It should be noted that these solutions are highly irritant and should only be infused into a central vein. They also have a significant sodium load. 1.26% contains (150 mmol.l^{-1} Na$^+$ and 150 mmol.l^{-1} HCO$_3^-$). 8.4% preparation contains (1000 mmol.l^{-1} Na$^+$ and 1000 mmol.l^{-1} HCO$_3^-$).

Uses

- Severe inorganic metabolic acidosis, pH < 7.1
- Forced alkaline diuresis
- Management of hyperkalaemia
- Dysrhythmias or QT prolongation in tricyclic antidepressant overdose
- Restores plasma [H$^+$] towards concentrations at which enzyme activity is usually most efficient.
- To restore cardiovascular stability in severe metabolic acidosis pending resolution of the underlying cause (when given slowly). Restoration of pH to more than 7.1 is thought to

reverse the myocardial depression and poor catecholamine sensitivity that occurs when the pH is less than 7.1
- As a buffer in dialysate fluids.

Side Effects
- Hypokalaemia
- Hypernatraemia
- Decreased ionised calcium with excessive doses causing impaired myocardial activity and dysrhythmias.
- Impaired oxygen release from haemoglobin (left shift)
- Hypercarbia in ventilated patients if ventilation is not temporarily increased during administration
- Intracellular acidosis can worsen as the dissolved CO_2 moves readily across the cell membrane while bicarbonate moves much less so, which could impair myocardial contractility.

The effect of bicarbonate on cardiovascular performance is complex depending on the predominant effect (restoration of pH and subsequent optimisation of enzyme kinetics, intracellular acidosis or hypocalcaemia). Administration should be slow to maximise the beneficial effects while having minimal negative effect on ionised calcium.

Minerals

Magnesium

Magnesium is the second most abundant intracellular cation after potassium and 99% is intracellular. Magnesium is an essential cofactor in multiple enzymatic reactions. It is required for ATP function. It plays a key role in neurotransmission and neuromuscular excitability. Magnesium sulfate ($MgSO_4$) is presented as either a 20% or 50% solution. A 10 ml vial of 50% contains 5 g or 20 mmol. The normal serum range is $0.7-1.0$ mmol.l^{-1}.

Uses
- Asthma: intravenous magnesium sulfate 2 g over 20 minutes is used as a bronchodilator in acute severe asthma. The mechanism of action is thought to be smooth muscle relaxation, however, there is limited evidence of benefit.
- Pre-eclampsia and eclampsia. Magnesium is indicated to treat eclamptic seizures and to prevent seizures in those with severe pre-eclampsia. A loading dose of 4 g should be given intravenously over 5 to 15 minutes, followed by an infusion of 1 g per hour maintained for 24 hours. If the woman has had an eclamptic fit, the infusion should be continued for 24 hours after the last fit. Recurrent fits should be treated with a further dose of 2-4 g given intravenously over 5-15 minutes.
- Arrhythmias. Magnesium is indicated specifically in the treatment of torsades de pointes and other ventricular and supraventricular tachycardias.
- It has been used as an adjunct for analgesia and may reduce opiate requirements.

Cautions

Hypermagnesaemia is defined as a serum concentration of greater than 1.05 mmol.l^{-1}. It is usually due to excess parenteral administration. Rapid, or excessive intravenous dosing can cause flushing, hypotension, weakness, bradycardia and ultimately severe cardiovascular suppression.

Management is by use of intravenous calcium because the two minerals are physiological antagonists of each other.

Adverse Effects

These relate to the plasma concentration.

- > 4 mmol.l^{-1} – nausea, hyporeflexia, slurred speech
- > 6 mmol.l^{-1} – muscle weakness, respiratory depression and bradycardia
- > 10 mmol.l^{-1} – cardiac arrest.

Calcium

Calcium is a widespread cation with a central role in muscle contraction, excitable tissue and messenger functions. There are many calcium preparations available, but calcium gluconate and calcium chloride are the key intravenous preparations. Calcium chloride contains three times the amount of Ca^{2+} per gram due to the additional mass associated with gluconate. It is used to treat hypocalcaemic tetany or acute hyperkalaemia. 10 ml calcium chloride 10% (centrally) or 30 ml 10% calcium gluconate are indicated to stabilise the myocardium in hyperkalaemia.

Phosphorus

Most of the phosphorus in the body is found in bone. Only a small component exists in tissues and extracellular fluid. Within cells it forms a vital part of the various intracellular messenger and other molecules (ATP, cAMP, 2,3-DPG).

Serum phosphate levels are regulated by intake and renal reabsorption controlled by parathyroid hormone. The normal serum range is 0.8–1.4 mmol.l^{-1}.

Uses

Intravenous phosphate is used to treat symptomatic or severe hypophosphataemia. Common causes of hypophosphataemia include redistribution into cells (refeeding syndrome, severe respiratory alkalosis, sepsis, insulin, adrenaline and glucose use – therefore it is seen commonly in diabetic hyperglycaemic disorders during treatment). Increased urinary excretion and decreased intestinal absorption are also causes. Clinical features include arrythmias, respiratory failure due to muscle weakness (in particular the diaphragm), seizures, confusion and paraesthesia.

Intravenous phosphate comes in a variety of preparations and is indicated for severe or symptomatic disease. Intravenous preparations may cause thrombophlebitis or hypocalcaemia with rapid administration and are therefore given as a prolonged infusion.

Nutrition

Parenteral Nutrition

Parenteral nutrition (PN) support refers to the provision of calories (lipid and carbohydrate), nitrogen (amino acids), electrolytes, vitamins, minerals, trace elements, and water via a parenteral route. The macronutrients are in their elemental forms and do not require digestion as they bypass the gastrointestinal tract. Generally, the infusion is contained within an 'all-in-one' bag. Most solutions have a high osmolality and are irritant to veins therefore require infusion via a central venous access device. It is possible to use peripheral veins if low osmolarity solutions are used. Standard bags often contain no vitamins or trace elements which therefore need to be added in a sterile pharmacy preparation area.

Energy requirements are often based on body weight. In the acute phase of critical illness, the recommended dose is 20–25 $kcal.kg^{-1}.day^{-1}$ rising to 25–30 $kcal.kg^{-1}.day^{-1}$ in the recovery phase. For those at risk of refeeding syndrome, the dose should be reduced to 10 $kcal.kg^{-1}.day^{-1}$ or even 5 $kcal.kg^{-1}.day^{-1}$. Overfeeding has negative consequences in terms of metabolic dysfunction even in those without refeeding syndrome.

The main calorie source in parenteral nutrition is glucose which provides up to 60% of non-protein calories. Up to 40% of non-protein calories are provided as lipid. In health the predominant lipid in the diet is triglycerides (containing three fatty acid chains). A variety of intravenous lipid emulsions have been developed based on soybean oil (the most common), fish oil and olive oil containing mostly long chain triglycerides as well as some phospholipids (essential for membrane synthesis) and essential fatty acids. Advanced mixtures have medium-chain triglycerides added. The theoretical advantage of medium-chain triglycerides are that they are hydrolysed faster by lipases, are not incorporated into chylomicrons therefore go directly to the liver (avoiding the lymphatics) and passively cross the mitochondrial membrane.

Nitrogen is given as mixtures of essential and non-essential amino acids. 0.8–1.5 g protein (0.13–0.24 g nitrogen).$kg^{-1}.day^{-1}$ is the recommended dose, and this should be reduced to 50% in patients at risk of refeeding syndrome.

Complications of parenteral nutrition relate to the vascular access device and the metabolic complications (refeeding syndrome, fatty liver, abnormal LFTs, hyperglycaemia and micronutrient deficiencies). To avoid trace element deficiencies these must be measured regularly and added to the bag as required. It is recommended that zinc, selenium, manganese, ferritin, folate and vitamins B12 and D are measured on starting parenteral nutrition and after six weeks use.

Refeeding Syndrome

The refeeding syndrome is defined as the clinical complications that can occur as a result of fluid and electrolyte shifts during aggressive nutritional rehabilitation of malnourished patients. These complications are potentially fatal when not detected or treated early. Common manifestations of the refeeding syndrome are:

- Hypophosphatemia
- Hypokalaemia
- Congestive heart failure
- Peripheral oedema

- Rhabdomyolysis
- Seizures.

Early and frequent measurement of electrolytes with aggressive replacement of deficiencies is required, along with high doses of B vitamins.

Enteral Nutrition

Enteral nutrition support refers to the provision of calories, protein, electrolytes, vitamins, minerals, trace elements, and fluids via an intestinal route, usually via some form of gastric or jejunal tube. A wide variety of enteral feeding formulations exist. They vary by osmolarity, density of calories, protein content and the form that these macronutrients take (predigested or not). Most preparations contain the daily required amounts of vitamins and minerals.

Typically, about half of calories come from carbohydrate, 30% from lipid and the rest from protein. A variety of high/low macronutrient combinations are available.

There are three overall categories:

- Polymeric (whole protein): these contain protein in the form in which it is normally within the diet i.e. as whole protein.
- Pre-digested (peptide/semi-elemental/elemental): these contain protein as smaller molecules i.e. short peptides, or even free amino acids. Pre-digestion of components aims to improve nutrient absorption in the presence of malabsorption. Pre-digested feeds may be useful in patients with digestive defects (e.g. malabsorptive syndromes that are unresponsive to supplementation of pancreatic enzymes) or a failure to tolerate standard enteral nutrition, such as persistent diarrhoea.
- Disease-specific or immune-enhancing feeds include omega-3, arginine and antioxidants. Evidence of benefit is lacking.

The 'standard' enteral feed has a calorie density of 1 $kcal.ml^{-1}$, is lactose free, isotonic and contains simple and complex carbohydrates as well as fatty acids. For patients who are volume restricted concentrated feeds can be used (up to 2 $kcal.ml^{-1}$). The result is that they are hyperosmolar and may contribute to the development of diarrhoea. A variety of other feeds are available containing low sodium, low potassium and even additional fibre.

Thiamine

Vitamin B1 (thiamine) deficiency is common in those who abuse alcohol, or who are malnourished for another reason. As well as peripheral neuropathy and cardiomyopathy, one feared complication is the Wernicke-Korsakoff's syndrome which can progress to Korsakoff's psychosis. To prevent this, it is recommended that those who drink alcohol regularly take 100 $mg.day^{-1}$ of thiamine. When starting any form of calorie input or nutrition in a patient deplete in B vitamins it can result in a precipitation of Wernicke's syndrome. As a precaution it is recommended when starting parenteral nutrition that intravenous B vitamins should be given for 3 days. This is commonly given as Pabrinex.

Pabrinex is a mixture of vitamin B substances and ascorbic acid (vitamin c). It is unusual in that it is presented as a pair of ampules labelled 1 and 2. Ampule 1 contains thiamine, riboflavin and pyridoxine. Ampule 2 contains ascorbic acid, nicotinamide, and glucose. Dosing is expressed as the number of pairs of ampules. For the treatment of suspected or established Wernicke's encephalopathy the dose is high, at 2–3 pairs, tds. It can be given intravenously or intramuscularly and may also be used to treat vitamin B and C deficiency.

Chapter 22

Diuretics

The kidney is a complex organ maintaining fluid, electrolyte and acid–base balance. It also serves an endocrine function by secreting renin and erythropoietin. Diuretics are drugs that act on the kidney (see Figure 22.1) to increase urine production and can be divided into the following groups:

- **Thiazides**
- **Loop diuretics**
- **Potassium sparing**
- **Aldosterone antagonists**
- **Osmotic**
- **Carbonic anhydrase inhibitors.**

Thiazides

Bendroflumethiazide, Chlorothiazide, Metolazone

Thiazides (which are chemically related to the sulfonamides) are widely used in the treatment of mild heart failure and hypertension, alone or in combination with other drugs. They have also been used in diabetes insipidus where they act by a complex (not fully understood) mechanism, initially causing a diuresis by decreasing Na^+ and water reabsorption in the *distal* convoluted tubule which in turn reduces glomerular filtration, thereby enhancing Na^+ and water absorption in the *proximal* tubule. In addition, they have been used in renal tubular acidosis. The main difference among the drugs is their rate of absorption from the gut due to differences in lipid solubility and rate of onset and duration of action due to differences in handling by the renal tubule.

Mechanism of Action

Thiazides are moderately potent and act mainly on the early segment of the distal tubule by inhibiting Na^+ and Cl^- reabsorption. This leads to increased Na^+ and Cl^- excretion and therefore increased water excretion. The increased Na^+ load reaching the distal tubule stimulates an exchange with K^+ and H^+ so that thiazides tend to precipitate a hypokalaemic, hypochloraemic alkalosis. Thiazides also reduce carbonic anhydrase activity resulting in an increased bicarbonate excretion; however, this effect is small and of little clinical significance.

Metolazone has very powerful synergistic effects when combined with a loop diuretic and is useful in cases of severe oedema.

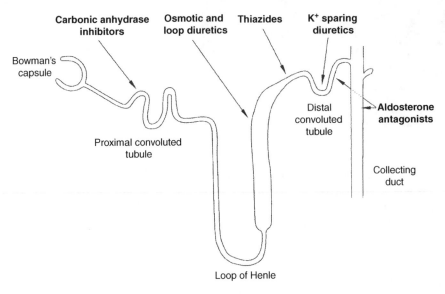

Figure 22.1 Main sites of action of the diuretics.

Effects

- *Cardiovascular* – thiazides appear to produce their antihypertensive effect by a reduction in plasma volume and systemic vascular resistance, which is maximally achieved at low dose.
- *Renal* – they reduce renal blood flow and may cause a reduction in glomerular filtration rate.
- *Biochemical* – their actions on the kidney lead to various biochemical imbalances. Hypokalaemia may provoke dangerous arrhythmias in those patients taking digoxin concurrently, although oral K^+ supplements usually maintain plasma levels within normal limits. Combination with a K^+ sparing diuretic may help to control plasma K^+. Hypercalcaemia may result from reduced renal Ca^{2+} excretion. Thiazides may also precipitate a hypochloraemic alkalosis, hyponatraemia and hypomagnesaemia. Thiazides and uric acid are secreted by the same mechanism within the renal tubules. This competition leads to reduced uric acid excretion and a rise in plasma levels, which may precipitate gout.
- *Metabolic* – reduced glycogenesis and insulin secretion coupled with enhanced glycogenolysis tends to raise plasma glucose levels. These effects are most noticeable in diabetic patients. Thiazides increase plasma cholesterol and triglyceride levels.
- *Haematological* – various blood dyscrasias are occasionally seen and include aplastic and haemolytic anaemia, leucopenia, agranulocytosis and thrombocytopenia.
- *Miscellaneous* – impotence, rash and photosensitivity occur rarely. Bendroflumethiazide may precipitate pancreatitis.
- *Interactions* – the hypokalaemia produced by thiazides may prolong the duration of action of non-depolarising muscle relaxants. Non-steroidal anti-inflammatory drugs antagonise the effects of thiazides.

Kinetics

Bendroflumethiazide is well absorbed from the gut in contrast with chlorothiazide, which is incompletely and variably absorbed. They both produce effects within 90 minutes of oral administration although bendroflumethiazide has twice the duration of action at 18–24 hours. The lower lipid solubility of chlorothiazide results in elimination solely via the kidney – none being metabolised, unlike bendroflumethiazide, which is 70% metabolised in the liver to active metabolites, the rest being eliminated unchanged in the urine.

Loop Diuretics

Furosemide, Bumetanide

Loop diuretics (carboxylic acid derivatives) are used in severe heart failure to reduce peripheral and pulmonary oedema. They are also used in chronic and acute renal failure.

Mechanism of Action

Loop diuretics inhibit Na^+ and Cl^- reabsorption in the thick ascending limb of the loop of Henle and to a lesser extent in the early part of the distal tubule. This impairs the action of the counter-current multiplier system and reduces the hypertonicity of the medulla, which reduces reabsorption of water in the collecting system. The thick ascending part of the loop of Henle has a large capacity for NaCl reabsorption, so when ion reabsorption is blocked the effects are marked.

Effects

- *Cardiovascular* – like thiazides they produce arteriolar vasodilatation which reduces systemic vascular resistance. In acute pulmonary oedema the preload is also reduced (and dyspnoea) ahead of any change that could be attributed to a diuresis.
- *Renal* – in contrast with the thiazides an increase in renal blood flow is seen with blood being diverted from the juxtaglomerular region to the outer cortex.
- *Biochemical* – the disturbances seen are similar to those induced by the thiazides and include hyponatraemia, hypokalaemia, hypomagnesaemia and a hypochloraemic alkalosis. In contrast with the thiazides the loop diuretics may precipitate hypocalcaemia due to increased Ca^{2+} excretion. Hyperuricaemia is sometimes seen and occasionally precipitates gout.
- *Metabolic* – hyperglycaemia is less common than with thiazides. Loop diuretics increase plasma cholesterol and triglyceride levels although these usually return to normal during long-term treatment.
- *Miscellaneous* – deafness occasionally follows rapid administration of a large dose and is more common in patients with renal failure, and those on aminoglycoside therapy. Bumetanide is less ototoxic than furosemide but may also cause myalgia.
- *Interactions* – lithium levels may rise when given with loop diuretics.

Kinetics

Both furosemide and bumetanide are well absorbed from the gut although their oral bioavailability is different (65% and 95%, respectively). Both drugs are highly plasma protein-bound (> 95%) and excreted largely unchanged in the urine.

Potassium Sparing

Amiloride

Amiloride is a weak diuretic that is frequently used in combination with loop diuretics to prevent hypokalaemia.

Mechanism of Action

At the distal convoluted tubule it blocks Na^+/K^+ exchange, creating a diuresis, and decreasing K^+ excretion.

Effects

- *Metabolic* – hyperkalaemia may sometimes follow its use. The hypokalaemic, hypochloraemic metabolic alkalosis seen with thiazide and loop diuretics is not a feature of K^+ sparing diuretics.

Kinetics

Amiloride is poorly absorbed from the gut, minimally protein-bound and not metabolised.

Aldosterone Antagonists

Spironolactone

Spironolactone is only available as an oral preparation. Potassium canrenoate is available parenterally and is metabolised to canrenone, which is also a metabolite of spironolactone.

Owing to its mode of action its effects take a few days to become established. It is used to treat ascites, nephrotic syndrome and primary hyperaldosteronism (Conn's syndrome).

Mechanism of Action

Spironolactone is a competitive aldosterone antagonist. Normally aldosterone stimulates the reabsorption of Na^+ in the distal tubule, which provides the driving force for the excretion of K^+. When aldosterone is antagonised, K^+ excretion is significantly reduced while increased Na^+ excretion produces a diuresis. The diuresis produced is limited as only 2% of Na^+ reabsorption is under the control of aldosterone.

Effects

- *Biochemical* – hyperkalaemia is most common in patients with renal impairment. Angiotensin-converting enzyme (ACE) inhibitors also predispose to hyperkalaemia because they reduce aldosterone secretion. It may also produce hyponatraemia.
- *Hormonal* – gynaecomastia in men and menstrual irregularity in women are seen due to spironolactone's anti-androgenic effects. It is contraindicated in Addison's disease.

Kinetics

Spironolactone is incompletely absorbed from the gut and highly protein-bound. It is rapidly metabolised and excreted in the urine.

Osmotic

Mannitol

The carbohydrate derivative mannitol is a polyhydric alcohol. Mannitol is used to reduce intracranial pressure (ICP) in the presence of cerebral oedema or during neurosurgery. It is also used to preserve peri-operative renal function in the jaundiced patient and those undergoing major vascular surgery. It is prepared in water as a 10% or 20% solution. For the treatment of raised ICP, the initial dose is 1 g.kg^{-1}, which is then reduced to 0.1–0.2 g.kg^{-1}. However, if the serum osmolality rises above 320 mOsm.kg^{-1}, further doses of mannitol should not be given due to an increased risk of renal failure.

Mechanism of Action

Mannitol is freely filtered at the glomerulus but not reabsorbed in the tubules. It increases the osmolality of the filtrate so that by an osmotic effect the volume of urine is increased. It is unable to pass through an intact blood–brain barrier and by virtue of an increased plasma osmolality it draws extracellular brain water into the plasma. However, a head injury may give rise to a damaged blood–brain barrier. In this situation mannitol traverses the blood–brain barrier and will drag water with it, thereby increasing cerebral oedema.

Effects

- *Cardiovascular* – initially circulating volume is increased producing an increased preload and cardiac output. In susceptible patients this may precipitate heart failure.
- *Renal* – it produces an osmotic diuresis and increased renal blood flow that may result in a reduced intravascular volume.
- *Central nervous system* – it produces an acute reduction in ICP, which is not sustained during prolonged administration. It may also reduce the rate of formation of cerebrospinal fluid.
- *Allergic* – these responses occur rarely.

Kinetics

Mannitol is minimally absorbed from the gut. Following intravenous administration mannitol is distributed throughout the extracellular fluid space. It is freely filtered at the glomerulus and not reabsorbed, resulting in an elimination half-life of 100 minutes. It is not metabolised to any significant extent.

Carbonic Anhydrase Inhibitors

Acetazolamide

Acetazolamide is a weak diuretic that is more commonly used as prophylaxis against mountain sickness. When used as eye drops it inhibits aqueous humour production and is useful in the treatment of glaucoma.

Mechanism of Action

Acetazolamide inhibits (non-competitively) carbonic anhydrase, which catalyses the formation of H^+ and HCO_3^- from CO_2 and H_2O via H_2CO_3 in the proximal tubule. As a result fewer H^+ ions are available for excretion resulting in a metabolic acidosis, counteracting the respiratory alkalosis associated with mountain sickness.

Effects

*   *Biochemical* – H^+ excretion is inhibited and HCO_3^- is not reabsorbed, leading to an alkaline urine. Na^+ and water excretion are slightly increased providing an increased drive for K^+ secretion. Therefore, it produces an alkaline urine in the presence of a hyperchloraemic acidosis.

Kinetics

Acetazolamide has an oral bioavailability of more than 95%, is highly protein-bound and is excreted unchanged in the urine.

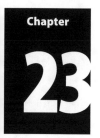

Antimicrobials

Antimicrobial agents are used to kill or suppress the growth of microorganisms and are used widely both to treat and prevent infection. In order to understand how antimicrobial drugs work it is necessary to understand the anatomy and structure of microorganisms.

Structure and Classification

Microorganisms capable of causing disease in humans consist of five main classes:

- Bacteria
- Viruses
- Fungi
- Protozoa
- Algae.

When considering the cellular structure of macro and microorganisms there are two broad types, eukaryotes and prokaryotes (see Table 23.1). Cells making up animals, plants, fungi, protozoa and algae are eukaryotic. Characteristics of eukaryotic cells are that they are larger, more complex and have larger internal volumes. Prokaryotic cells are smaller, simpler and of a smaller internal volume. Bacteria are prokaryotes. The differences between mammalian cells and those of microorganisms are important for identifying therapeutic targets. These are important so that antimicrobial agents offer selective toxicity (toxicity to microorganisms without toxicity to host cells).

Bacteria

- Morphology
- Staining properties
- Aerobic or anaerobic metabolism.

Bacteria have peptidoglycan cell walls. Bacteria are described in terms of their morphology (cocci, rods etc.) and formation of colonies (clusters, chains etc.). They are also classified by the staining pattern of their cell walls into three separate groups. This is directly relevant to the antimicrobial prescriber because the cell wall staining pattern guides the choice of antibiotic. The gram staining system relies on the differing staining properties of cell walls.

1. **Gram-positive** bacteria retain the initial dye crystal violet and appear purple under the microscope. They have a thick peptidoglycan cell wall with no additional outer membrane covering it (see Figure 23.1).

Table 23.1 Some characteristics of eukaryotes and prokaryotes

	Eukaryotes	Prokaryotes
Cell membrane	Phospholipid bilayer with sterols	Phospholipid bilayer with *no* sterols
Ribosomes	60S and 40S	30S and 50S
Cell wall	Some have cell walls (plants, algae, fungi) but these never contain peptidoglycan Animal (including human) cells have no cell walls	All have cell walls containing peptidoglycan
Membrane bound organelles	Contain membrane-bound organelles, including a nucleus	Do not contain a nucleus or any other membrane-bound organelle

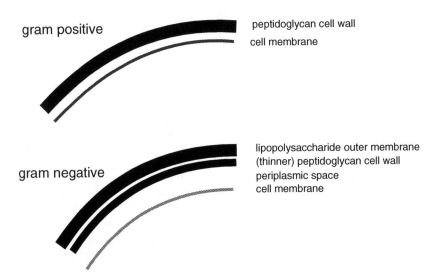

Figure 23.1. Simplified diagram to show the major structural differences between gram-positive and gram-negative bacteria.

2. **Gram-negative** bacteria have a thin peptidoglycan cell wall, covered by an additional outer membrane rich in lipopolysaccharides (LPS), therefore they do not retain crystal violet dye. Gram-negative cells stain pink with the counter stain sufenin. When gram-negative bacteria break down upon death, they release large quantities of LPS into the circulation provoking an extreme cytokine response. LPS is also known as endotoxin.
3. **Acid fast bacilli** resist decolouration with the above stains. They retain red dye after contact with an acid/alcohol mixture.

Aerobic bacteria require oxygen to survive. Anaerobic bacteria do not. The aerobic or anaerobic nature, combined with the gram staining properties above, can be used to classify virtually all bacteria (see Table 23.2).

Table 23.2 Classification of the most commonly encountered bacterial pathogens

	Gram-positive Cocci (spheres)	Bacilli (rods)	Gram-negative Cocci (spheres)	Bacilli (rods)
Aerobic	Staphylococcus *S. aureus*; *S. epidermidis* Streptococcus *S. pneumoniae* Enterococcus *E. faecalis*	Bacillus *B. anthracis*	Neisseria *N. gonorrhoeae*, *N. meningitidis* Moraxella *M. catarrhalis*	Haemophilus *H. influenzae* Klebsiella Pseudomonas *P. aeruginosa* Enterobacter Campylobacter, Salmonella, Legionella, Proteus, Citrobacter, Serratia Mycobacteria *M. tuberculosis, M. avium* Yersinia *Y. pestis*
Anaerobic	*Streptococcus viridians*	Actinomyces Clostridium *C. difficile*, *C. perfringens* Lactobacillus Listeria		Bacteroides Escherichia *E. coli*

Antibiotics and Antimicrobial Chemotherapeutic Agents

Antibiotics are naturally occurring substances produced by one microorganism that act against another microorganism. Antimicrobial chemotherapeutic agents are synthetic substances that act against microorganisms but, for the purposes of this chapter when acting against bacteria, will be called by the common name, antibiotics.

Antibiotics can be classified by their:

- mechanism of action (or more simply by whether they kill [bactericidal] or inhibit growth [bacteriostatic] of bacteria), or
- pharmacological structure.

Therapeutic Targets for Antibiotics

Antibiotics target four different aspects of the microorganism in order to achieve their goal (see Figure 23.2).

1. **Inhibition of cell wall synthesis**
- β-lactams
- Glycopeptides

   Gram-positive bacteria rely on their thick cell walls for cellular integrity. They have no protective outer membrane or lipopolysaccharide layer; therefore, they are more susceptible to drugs affecting cell wall synthesis than Gram-negative bacteria.

2. **Inhibition of protein synthesis**
- Aminoglycosides
- Tetracyclines
- Macrolides
- Oxazolidinones.

3. **Disruption of the cytoplasmic cellular membrane**
- Polymyxins
- Colistins
- Daptomycin.

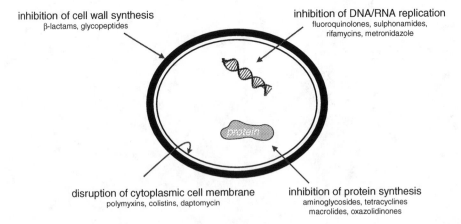

inhibition of cell wall synthesis
β-lactams, glycopeptides

inhibition of DNA/RNA replication
fluoroquinolones, sulphonamides,
rifamycins, metronidazole

disruption of cytoplasmic cell membrane
polymyxins, colistins, daptomycin

inhibition of protein synthesis
aminoglycosides, tetracyclines
macrolides, oxazolidinones

Figure 23.2 Summary of the mechanism of action of antibiotics.

4. **Inhibition of normal nucleic acid replication**
   - Fluroquinolones
   - Sulphonamides
   - Rifampicin
   - Metronidazole.

Pharmacokinetics of Antibiotics

In order to be effective, antibiotics must reach the site of infection which often involves passing across the capillary membrane and out of the circulation. Their ability to penetrate the infected tissue depends on local factors such as tissue perfusion and the nature of the barrier (e.g. blood brain barrier) and the properties of the antibiotic itself such as protein binding, lipid solubility and pKa. The organs with the greatest perfusion are the brain, kidney, liver, and heart and it would be expected that drug concentrations would increase most rapidly in these organs. Conversely, tissues with inherently poor blood flow (tendons) or caused by disease (e.g. distal diabetic osteomyelitis) are difficult to achieve therapeutic concentrations of antibiotics.

Passive diffusion across capillaries is the most common mechanism of tissue penetration but the blood-brain barrier has non-fenestrated capillaries reducing the ability of some antibiotics to pass. Lipophilic antibiotics such as metronidazole have an advantage in this situation over water-soluble antibiotics such as β-lactams, although increasing the dose of the latter can overcome these difficulties. Despite meningeal inflammation reducing the effectiveness of the blood-brain barrier, higher doses of β-lactams are used for suspected central nervous system (CNS) infections than for infections elsewhere.

Only the unbound (free) drug is active. The total serum concentration of a drug might be well above the concentration required to kill bacteria, however, if it is highly protein-bound, the unbound portion of the drug is likely to be less than the concentration required to kill bacteria.

Once in the infected tissues, there are several local factors that play a role:

- Infected tissues tend to have a low pH which renders some antibiotics ineffective (e.g. gentamicin and erythromycin).
- Local hypoxia. Penetration of the cell wall by aminoglycosides is by an oxygen-dependent reaction, therefore activity may be reduced in an anaerobic environment.
- Presence of antimicrobial defences. Some bacteria produce substances that inactivate antibiotics (e.g. β-lactams).
- Calcium ion concentration. This can adversely affect activity of some drugs (e.g. gentamicin).
- Biofilm formation. A biofilm is a complex structure consisting of a variety of microorganisms and associated secreted substances. The resulting biofilm resists attack from host cells and antibiotics as well as adhering to foreign bodies.

After an intravenous bolus of drug, the serum concentration declines due to the initial distribution into tissues and then by elimination (metabolism and excretion). The elimination of antibiotics involves the hepatic and renal routes which can be to the clinician's advantage but may also present a challenge in multi-organ failure.

β-lactams are excreted by glomerular filtration and tubular secretion. As described in earlier chapters, competition can occur between these secretion systems. Probenecid can be used to reduce excretion of penicillins, cephalosporins and some other β-lactams by competitively inhibiting the secretion of these substances via the active transport secretion mechanisms.

Gentamicin is concentrated in the urine by glomerular filtration. The concentration of gentamicin achieved in the urine may be high enough to treat an organism that is considered 'resistant' to concentrations achievable in other body tissues.

Erythromycin, azithromycin, moxifloxacin, clindamycin and rifampicin are mainly excreted by the liver into the bile.

Pharmacodynamics of Antibiotics

Appropriate treatment regimens are critical for antibiotic prescribing not just to maximise the success rate, but also to prevent the increasingly important issue of resistance.

Bacteriostatic antibiotics inhibit bacterial growth and subsequently allow host defences to kill the bacteria. Host defences are ineffective in states of generalised immunodeficiency or at certain anatomical sites in the early stages of certain infections e.g. the cerebrospinal fluid (CSF). Conversely bactericidal antibiotics actively kill the bacteria and are independent of host defences.

The minimum inhibitory concentration (MIC) is defined as the lowest concentration of antibiotic that prevents a defined number of bacteria in suspension becoming turbid after overnight incubation in vitro in standard conditions. It is therefore a measure of potency. Different samples of the same species will have different MICs (sensitive isolates will have low MICs and resistant isolates will have high MICs). The minimum bactericidal concentration (MBC) is the lowest concentration of antibiotic required to cause bacterial death. For bactericidal antibiotics, the MBC is similar to the MIC. For bacteriostatic drugs the MBC is many times greater than the MIC. The 'cut-off' MIC that decides whether a bacterial isolate is sensitive or resistant is called the 'breakthrough MIC'. The MIC is measured after overnight aerobic incubation of a standard inoculum of bacteria in a low protein liquid medium at pH 7.2 at a standard temperature, and at a defined number of bacteria – all of which vary significantly from the actual site of infection.

It must be remembered that the MIC is an in vitro measurement and that the antibiotic concentration achieved in the various body cavities will vary widely. Areas with low antibiotic concentrations include abscess cavities and areas with poor blood flow. Areas with high concentrations include the bile and urine, due to active concentration of drug in these areas.

When an antibiotic is administered, the number of bacteria will decline due to bacterial death whilst the concentration of the unbound antibiotic is greater than the MBC. When antibiotic concentration falls below the MBC (but still are above the MIC) the bacterial count may remain stable or continue to decline as a result of killing by host defences.

Once the antibiotic concentration falls below the MIC, some suppression of bacterial growth can still occur. Several mechanisms are responsible for this:

- The post antibiotic effect (PAE). The suppression of bacterial growth after short exposure to antibiotic even without a contribution from host defences.
- The post antibiotic leukocyte enhancement (PALE). After exposure to an antibiotic, bacteria are more susceptible to attack by host defences.
- Minimal antibacterial concentration (MAC). Antibiotic drug concentrations less than the MIC can alter morphology, slow rate of growth and prolong the PAE. Concentrations above the MAC but below the MIC cause this effect.

As antibiotic levels fall, eventually bacteria start to resume growth. This rate of growth depends on the activity of the host defences and the species of bacterium. Rapidly growing bacteria in immunocompromised individuals or at certain anatomical sites can double their numbers every 20 minutes. The next dose of antibiotic needs to be given before significant regrowth occurs, and there are three main pharmacodynamic classes.

1. **Drugs with time-dependent bactericidal action.** Slow bactericidal drugs that require levels to be above the MIC for as much time as possible. The magnitude of the concentration above the MIC has little relevance (i.e. more killing does not occur at higher concentrations). They have minimal post-antibiotic effect. These drugs need to be given frequently so that levels remain above the MIC as much as possible. Larger doses only work by increasing the duration of time the drug concentration is above the MIC. Giving multiple daily doses increases the time spent above the MIC. The drug concentration needs to be above the MIC for at least 50% of the dosing interval. Examples are penicillins and vancomycin. As a result, these drugs are very amenable to continuous infusions (following a loading dose) and this is currently being investigated although at the time of writing there is little evidence outcomes are better. For vancomycin and teicoplanin, in clinical practice, maintenance of trough serum levels of free drug that are greater than the MIC is most commonly recommended.

2. **Drugs with a concentration-dependent bactericidal action.** These drugs kill more bacteria the higher the concentrations they achieve (in contrast to above). They have significant and prolonged post-antibiotic effects. Efficacy depends on the maximum concentration achieved and the time spent above the MIC. The amount of drug rather than the frequency of dosing determines efficacy. Examples include aminoglycosides, fluoroquinolones, daptomycin, colistin, and metronidazole. Maximising serum concentrations of drugs that exhibit concentration-dependent bactericidal activity by increasing the dose will maximise the rate and extent of bactericidal activity, if adverse effects are not also concentration-dependent.

3. **Drugs with predominately bacteriostatic actions.** These have prolonged PAEs. Efficacy is determined by the time spent above MIC.

Antibiotic Combinations

Adding an aminoglycoside to a drug with a relatively slow rate of bactericidal activity (e.g. β-lactams or glycopeptides) can improve antimicrobial action. For example, a penicillin is slowly bactericidal, and an aminoglycoside alone at concentrations achieved in serum after standard dosing exhibits only bacteriostatic activity, but the combination of the penicillin with an aminoglycoside results in rapid bactericidal activity. The presence of a drug that affects cell wall synthesis (penicillin) enhances the penetration of the aminoglycoside.

However, this type of interaction between antibiotics can also be antagonistic. Penicillin is bactericidal and inhibits cell wall synthesis, weakening the wall and eventually causing cell lysis as it grows. Penicillin requires the organisms to be growing. Tetracycline prevents cell growth therefore reducing the susceptibility of some bacteria to penicillin.

1. Specific Antibiotics that Affect Cell Wall Synthesis
β-lactams

β-lactam antibiotics are subdivided into the following classes:

- Penicillins
- Cephalosporins

Table 23.3 Classification of penicillins

Type	Examples	Indications
Narrow-spectrum, naturally occurring	benzylpenicillin (Penicillin G); phenoxymethylpenicillin (Penicillin V)	G+ve coccii (meningococcal infections)
Narrow-spectrum, semisynthetic	flucloxacillin	penicillinase producing staphylococcal infections
Narrow-spectrum, staphylococcal β-lactamase resistant	temocillin	G-ve lactamase-producinig bacteria (not pseudomonas)
Broad-spectrum penicillins	ampicillin, amoxycillin, co-amoxiclav	G+ve and some G-ve cover. Ampicillin and amoxicillin are increasingly less effective due to resistance. Co-amoxiclav has increased activity by combining amoxicillin with clavulanic acid, a β-lactamase inhibitor.
Antipseudomonal penicillins	piperacillin, ticarcillin	Broad spectrum of activity against Gram+ve and G-ve bacteria and anerobes.

- Carbapenems
- Monobactams.

Penicillins

Structure

Penicillins contain a β-lactam ring fused with a thiazolidine ring (see Figure 23.3). Structurally they differ in the type of acyl side-chain attached to the β-lactam ring, which determines both susceptibility to acid degradation in the stomach and spectrum of activity. Only penicillin V (acid resistant) and penicillin G (acid sensitive) are produced naturally, the others are semisynthetic (see Table 23.3). An intact β-lactam ring is essential for activity.

Uses

Penicillins are used widely against a variety of infections and are most effective against Gram-positive bacteria.

Mechanism of Action

Penicillins are bactericidal antibiotics that inhibit cell wall synthesis by preventing peptidoglycan cross-linkage, resulting in weakening of the cell wall. The β-lactam ring resembles the natural substrate D-ala-D-ala on the side-chain of the peptidoglycan where cross-linkage occurs. Penicillins bind to several penicillin-binding proteins (PBP) in the cell wall that act as

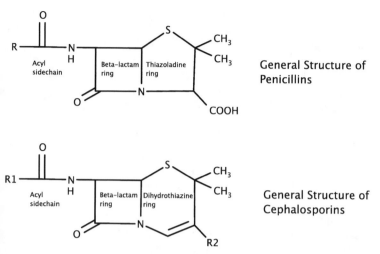

Figure 23.3 Structures of penicillins and cephalosporins. R, variable groups on the β-lactam ring in penicillins; R1, R2, variable groups on the cepham ring structure.

transpeptidase enzymes responsible for forming cross-links. On binding, the β-lactam structure is ruptured to form a bond with the active serine site on the PBP resulting in irreversible inactivation of the transpeptidase enzyme. Penicillin activity is lost in the presence of β-lactamase, which hydrolyses the β-lactam ring. β-lactamases are encoded on bacterial chromosomes and plasmids, which may be disseminated and lead to acquired resistance.

When Gram-positive bacteria are exposed to β-lactams, growth continues but with reduced cross-linkage of peptidoglycan until the cell wall becomes weakened and lysis is inevitable. The use of β-lactams against susceptible Gram-positive cocci rarely results in complete eradication of bacteria, a significant number of β-lactam sensitive cells, known as persistors, will remain dormant until the antibiotic is removed. Complete eradication can be achieved by the addition of a synergistic antibiotic, such as the aminoglycoside gentamicin, the potency of which is enhanced by cell-wall damage allowing better intracellular access.

The cell walls of Gram-negative bacilli are different and damage to the thin peptidoglycan layer only weakens it, since the thicker lipopolysaccharide outer layer remains intact. However, internal hydrostatic pressure forces the bacteria to become spherical (spheroplasts) which may lead to cell lysis. In some bacilli, such as *Haemophilus influenzae*, intracellular osmolality is so low that lysis rarely occurs. When the antibiotic is removed, peptidoglycan integrity is restored, their normal rod-like shape returns and they continue to divide normally.

Pharmacology

Penicillins are drugs with time-dependent bactericidal action. In order for bacteria to be killed the concentration of the drug must be above the MIC for as much time as possible.

Intestinal absorption depends on whether the type of penicillin is susceptible to acid-induced degradation in the stomach; amoxicillin is absorbed more readily than ampicillin. Some penicillins, such as benzylpenicillin (penicillin G), are so susceptible to acid hydrolysis that they are available only for parenteral administration. Plasma half-lives are short (benzylpenicillin, 30 minutes; ampicillin, 2 hours). Tissue penetration is generally good although inflammation is necessary for penicillins to pass into bone and through the blood–brain barrier. Penicillins are excreted by the kidneys unchanged (60–90%), mainly by renal tubular secretion, but they are also excreted in bile (10%) and up to 20% is metabolised.

Clavulanic acid and tazobactam are β-lactamase inhibitors. The combination of a penicillin with one of these agents can restore sensitivity in bacteria producing a β-lactamase enzyme. Amoxicillin is combined with clavulanic acid in co-amoxiclav and piperacillin with tazobactam. Clavulanic acid itself has weak antibacterial activity whereas tazobactam does not.

Side Effects and Special Points

- Hypersensitivity – allergy to penicillins occurs in up to 10% of the population and anaphylaxis in 0.01% (1 in 10,000). Cross-reactivity exists between penicillins, cephalosporins and carbapenems and is discussed below.
- Encephalopathy – benzylpenicillin is the most pro-convulsant β-lactam. Toxic CSF levels can be reached by intrathecal injection, using large intravenous doses in meningitis patients with renal impairment, and concomitant probenecid use.
- Diarrhoea is common during oral therapy. Ampicillin is associated with a low risk of pseudomembranous colitis (0.3–0.7%).
- Miscellaneous – ampicillin produces a maculopapular rash in 10% of all patients.

Cephalosporins

Structure

Cephalosporins possess a similar structure to penicillins but the β-lactam ring is fused with a dihydrothiazine ring (see Figure 23.3) to produce the cephem nucleus. The cephalosporins are less sensitive to β-lactamases and are extended-spectrum bactericidal antimicrobials classified by generation (see Table 23.4). With each generation Gram-positive cover is maintained but Gram-negative cover is steadily improved.

Uses

A wide range of Gram-positive infections.

Table 23.4 Classification of cephalosporins. Fourth-generation agents are not available in the UK

Generation	Examples	Features
First	Cefaclor; cefalexin; cefradine	Narrow-spectrum, G+ve cocci
Second	Cefuroxime; cefaclor; cefoxitin	Narrow-spectrum, G+ve cocci; cefuroxime also effective against *H. influenzae*
Third	Cefotaxime; ceftazidime; ceftriaxone	Broader spectrum; enhanced resistance to β-lactamase; less potent against G+ve; Pseudomonas sensitive; cross BBB
(Fourth)	Cefepime; cefpirome	Active against Enterobacter and Pseudomonas
Fifth	Ceftaroline; ceftobripole	Also active against multi-drug resistant *S. aureus* (MRSA, VISA, VRSA)

Mechanism of Action

Cephalosporins are bactericidal and, like penicillins, disrupt peptidoglycan cell wall integrity. The modified β-lactam ring in cephalosporins is more stable than that in penicillins, making it less susceptible to β-lactamase.

Pharmacology

Cephalosporins distribute widely in the body, readily crossing the placenta. CSF penetration of first- and second-generation agents is poor. Penetration improves with third-generation agents such as ceftriaxone and cefotaxime, especially if the meninges are inflamed, as seen in bacterial meningitis. Plasma half-lives are short (1–1.5 hours) with the exception of ceftriaxone, which has a half-life of 5.5–11 hours allowing once-daily dosing. Cefradine, cefuroxime and ceftazidime are not metabolised and are excreted unchanged in the urine. Cefotaxime is metabolised by the liver (the activity of the metabolites being 10% that of the parent compound) with only 50% appearing unchanged in the urine. Renal excretion is due to both filtration and tubular secretion; probenecid increases peak concentration and plasma half-life but to a lesser extent than with penicillins.

Side Effects and Special Points

- Hypersensitivity – cross-reactivity with penicillins (see 'Allergy to Penicillins and Related Drugs' below).
- Gastrointestinal (GI) – antibiotic-associated colitis, especially with third-generation agents.

Carbapenems

Structure

Carbapenems are part of the β-lactam group of antibiotics. Due to subtle modification of the β-lactam ring some groups are changed and the ring is fused resulting in significant resistance to most β-lactamases. Carbapenem-hydrolysing β-lactamases have been increasingly isolated from gram-negative organisms and may limit therapy with these agents in these circumstances.

Uses

Carbapenems have a very broad spectrum of activity covering Gram-positive and Gram-negative aerobic (particularly *Pseudomonas aeruginosa)* and anaerobic organisms. They do not affect Methicillin-resistant *Staphlococcus aureus* (MRSA) or *Enterococcus faecalis* and, if used in isolation, allow development of *Pseudomonas* resistance.

Mechanism of Action

As a member of the β-lactam family they are bactericidal drugs that disrupt cell wall synthesis.

Pharmacology

All carbapenems need dose reduction in renal dysfunction.

Special Points

- Imipenem is resistant to β-lactamase but is only moderately effective against *Clostridium perfringens*. Imipenem induces β-lactamase expression in *Pseudomonas*, which reduces the effectiveness of other β-lactam antibiotics. It is metabolised by renal dehydropeptidase so is often combined with the inhibitor cilastatin. Very high doses are associated with neurotoxicity especially in the presence of inflamed meninges, limiting its use in meningitis.

- Meropenem is similar to imipenem but is not metabolised by renal dehydropeptidase and is not combined with cilastatin. It appears to be less neurotoxic making it suitable therapy for bacterial meningitis.
- Ertapenem has a narrower spectrum of activity than meropenem or irtapenem, with less activity against pseudomonas and some Gram-positive bacteria. Ertapenem has a long half-life allowing for once daily dosing.

Monobactams

Aztreonam is a monocyclic β-lactam (monobactam) antimicrobial with a spectrum of activity limited to Gram-negative aerobic bacteria. Both *Enterobacter* and *Pseudomonas* are sensitive although it is often combined with gentamicin when treating severe pseudomonal infections. Aztreonam can be given by nebuliser for treatment of chronic *Pseudomonas* infections in cystic fibrosis. It can be used in patients who are allergic to penicillin.

Allergy to Penicillin and Related Drugs

Penicillin allergy is reported commonly by patients, however, it is widely known that more than 90% of patients with a reported penicillin allergy do not have IgE-mediated sensitivity when skin testing is performed. There are many reasons for this including inappropriate labelling of patients, incorrect diagnosis of other side effects or less commonly because they had an earlier allergy that resolved with time. That said, penicillins are one of the most widespread causes of anaphylaxis in anaesthesia and intensive care practice. There are multiple parts of the penicillin (or related drug) molecule that are antigenic and there is a degree of cross reactivity between groups.

The appropriate strategy is to take a history of the reaction and decide if this was an Ig-E mediated anaphylactic reaction, another type of severe reaction such as Stevens Johnsons syndrome or misreporting of a side effect (nausea, diarrhoea). Ideally allergy testing should be performed. Up to 10% of patients with a true allergy to penicillins will have a similar reaction if given a cephalosporin. Figures suggest that 99% of those with a positive skin prick test to a penicillin will tolerate carbapenems. Aztreonam is the only monobactam available for clinical use. There is no evidence of immunologic cross-reactivity between penicillins and monobactams, and penicillin-allergic patients may receive aztreonam normally.

Glycopeptides

Structure

Vancomycin and Teicoplanin are naturally occurring first generation glycopeptide antibiotics. They are glycosylated non-ribosomal heptapeptides that do not contain a β-lactam ring. Semi-synthetic glycopeptide antibiotics (second generation) have been developed as Dalbavancin and Telavancin.

Uses

Glycopeptide antibiotics have bactericidal activity against aerobic and anaerobic Gram-positive bacteria. Vancomycin is used intravenously for the treatment of serious Gram-positive infections such as endocarditis. It has activity against MRSA. Bacterial strains resistant to vancomycin are occurring, particularly vancomycin resistant *Enterococci* (VRE). Vancomycin is used via the oral route for treatment of *clostridium* colitis due to its minimal systemic absorption. Teicoplanin has a similar spectrum of activity to vancomycin but with a longer duration of action and a greater potency. This allows for once daily dosing. Bone and CSF penetration are more reliable than with vancomycin (where it is poor). Usual dosing regimens for teicoplanin include a twice daily loading dose for two days then once daily dosing.

Mechanism of Action

Glycopeptides have a time-dependent bactericidal action. The efficacy is related to the time spent above the MIC. They inhibit cell wall synthesis by binding to subunits of the peptidoglycan preventing addition of new molecules and cell wall synthesis. This is similar to the mechanism by which β-lactams are bactericidal but there is no competition between penicillins and glycopeptides for the active binding site.

Pharmacology

Vancomycin is not absorbed from healthy intestine and when treating infections elsewhere needs to be given intravenously. Intravenous vancomycin is excreted mostly unchanged in the urine. Peak levels are governed predominantly by initial dose and trough levels governed by initial dose and dosing interval. Measuring and maintaining trough levels between 10 and 20 $mg.l^{-1}$ are important due to its relatively short duration of action, minimal post antibiotic effect, and efficacy being related to the time spent above the MIC. Teicoplanin has a longer half-life and the manufacturer does not advise monitoring of trough levels after completion of the loading dose but does advise during ongoing therapy.

Side Effects and Special Points

- Red man syndrome is a histamine-mediated flushing of mainly the face and neck but can include the whole body, during or immediately following infusion of vancomycin and is related to an over rapid infusion rate or an excessive dose. It is rarely fatal but easily confused with a true hypersensitivity reaction.
- Vancomycin has been associated with renal and ototoxicity.
- Teicoplanin has fewer side effects than vancomycin and causes less renal toxicity. It can be used in patients who have previously suffered from red man syndrome due to vancomycin, although reports of red man syndrome with teicoplanin also exist.
- Teicoplanin is used widely for surgical prophylaxis and in a recent national audit in the UK it was found to be 17 times more likely to cause anaphylaxis compared to alternatives.

2. Antibiotics that Inhibit Protein Synthesis
Aminoglycosides

Structure

The aminoglycoside group contains a large number of naturally occurring and synthetic drugs including gentamicin, amikacin, neomycin, streptomycin and tobramycin. Aminoglycosides are characterised by a core structure of amino sugars connected via glycosidic linkages to a dibasic aminocyclitol.

Uses

They are bactericidal against a wide range of Gram-negative enterobacteria and have Gram-positive cover that includes *Staphylococcus* and to a limited extent *Streptococcus*. Amikacin, gentamicin and tobramycin are also active against *Pseudomonas*. Aminoglycosides have no anaerobic activity but are synergistic with β-lactams and vancomycin.

Gentamicin is the aminoglycoside most used in the UK, however, cases of resistance to gentamicin are increasing. Amikacin is less resistant to enzyme inactivation than gentamicin and is used where there is gentamicin resistance for serious Gram-negative infections. Tobramycin has similar activity to gentamicin but can be given via the nebulised route and this is used in chronic *Pseudomonas* infection affecting patients with cystic fibrosis. Streptomycin is active against *Mycobacterium tuberculosis* and is used only in this setting. Neomycin is too toxic for parenteral therapy and is only used orally for decontamination of the GI tract or topically on the skin or mucus membranes.

Mechanism of Action

Aminoglycosides are bactericidal antimicrobials that block protein synthesis by binding irreversibly to the bacterial 30S ribosomal subunit. Once bound, aminoglycosides interfere with tRNA attachment and mRNA is either not transcribed or misread depending on aminoglycoside concentration. Inhibition of protein synthesis and mistranslation of proteins occurs once aminoglycoside molecules access the cytoplasm. These mistranslated proteins insert into and cause damage to the bacterial membrane, increasing the ability for further aminoglycoside antibiotics to enter the cytoplasm, eventually causing cell death. There are several established mechanisms by which resistance occurs, with the same resistant species often having multiple mechanisms. Enzymes from bacteria can modify the structure of the antibiotic, the target site can be modified preventing binding, or the bacteria may develop mechanisms to remove the antibiotic from the cell after it has entered.

Pharmacology

Aminoglycosides are not lipid soluble and are not absorbed from the GI tract except in cases of severe inflammatory bowel disease and liver failure and are therefore given by injection. They have low protein binding, distribute predominantly in extracellular fluid and penetrate cells, CSF and sputum poorly. They are large polar molecules that need active transportation to enter bacterial cells. This transportation is inhibited by the divalent cations calcium and magnesium, acidosis and low oxygen tension. They are not metabolised and are excreted unchanged in the urine by filtration, making them ideal agents for infections of the urinary tract. Their narrow therapeutic index requires monitoring of blood levels to determine the most appropriate dose and the adequacy of clearance. Dosage must be reduced in renal impairment.

It is widely accepted that extended interval dosing (administering larger doses of aminoglycosides less frequently) may be associated with improved outcomes and less toxicity compared with providing the same total daily dose in a multiple daily injection regime. Aminoglycosides are suitable for extended interval dosing because of three features common to the class; concentration-dependent killing, rapid elimination, and a prolonged post-antibiotic effect. Larger doses are thought to increase target body site concentrations (concentration-dependent killing), while minimising potential toxicity by allowing sufficient dosing intervals for drug concentrations to fall. The post antibiotic effect properties of the class allow for an extended period of killing after the drug is cleared from the body and before the next dose is administered. Therapeutic drug monitoring of levels also helps to reduce toxicity, by ensuring low drug levels between doses and avoiding early administration before levels fall.

Side Effects and Special Points

Ototoxicity and nephrotoxicity are the major side effects and are dose dependent. Renal function must be checked before starting therapy.

- Nephrotoxicity. Aminoglycosides are freely filtered across the glomerulus but up to 10% of the intravenous dose is taken up into the cells lining the proximal convoluted tubule. The drug is concentrated here, and intracellular concentrations can considerably exceed the serum concentration. The affinity of the drug for the membrane of the proximal tubular cells correlates with nephrotoxicity. Neomycin has the highest affinity and therefore the highest nephrotoxicity whereas amikacin has the lowest. Nephrotoxicity can be reduced by choosing the least toxic drug (gentamicin is more nephrotoxic than amikacin), correcting hypokalaemia and hypomagnesaemia (to reduce uptake), optimising intravascular volume status prior to administration, suspending other nephrotoxic drugs, extended interval dosing, limiting duration, reducing the size of individual doses and therapeutic drug monitoring. Even when aminoglycosides are given as a single dose (with no repeat dosing), regardless of indication, many patients will have a transient rise in serum creatinine. This is also the case in single dose use for surgical prophylaxis where the dose should be reduced if indicated. However, the proximal convoluted tubules can regenerate so that renal function usually recovers after aminoglycoside-induced nephrotoxicity.
- Ototoxicity. Aminoglycosides are associated with cochlear and vestibular toxicity in a substantial proportion of patients receiving the drug for prolonged periods. The mechanism of aminoglycoside-induced ototoxicity with hearing loss is less understood than nephrotoxicity. There is a genetic component to risk as well as sustained use or excessive serum concentrations, but this is not absolute. The risk of ototoxicity is increased in renal failure and with simultaneous use of furosemide or other ototoxic drugs.
- Muscle weakness. Aminoglycosides decrease the pre-junctional release of acetylcholine (ACh), reduce post-junctional sensitivity to ACh and increase non-depolarising muscle relaxant potency. They should be avoided in myasthenia gravis.

Chloramphenicol

Structure

Chloramphenicol is an amphenicol.

Uses

While first used in 1948 it fell out of favour due to side effects but has made a reappearance recently after emergence of strains resistant to other antibiotics. It is used for Gram-positive and Gram-negative infections especially via the topical route for the eye and ear as well as the intravenous route for soft tissue infections, pneumonia and meningitis.

Mechanism of Action

Chloramphenicol is bacteriostatic by inhibiting protein synthesis. It binds to residues of the 50S ribosomal subunit preventing peptide bond formation and subsequent protein synthesis.

Pharmacology and Special Points

Rare but serious complications are aplastic anaemia and agranulocytosis. The full blood count should be monitored frequently in these patients and repeated dosing avoided. Topical use has a much lower risk.

Tetracyclines

Structure

This group of drugs is based on a linear fused tetracyclic nucleus with differing side-chains giving specific drugs (Doxycycline, Tetracycline, Lymecycline, Tigecycline and Demeclocycline) their individual characteristics.

Uses

Tetracyclines are broad spectrum antibiotics with action against aerobic Gram-positive, Gram-negative and atypical bacteria. While they remain the drug of choice for *Chlamydia trachomatis* and Lyme disease, as well as acne and dental infections, their overall usefulness is decreasing in the wake of increased bacterial resistance.

Mechanism of Action

Tetracyclines enter the bacterial cell wall via passive diffusion and an active transport system. They bind reversibly to the 30S ribosomal subunit at a position that inhibits the attachment of the tRNA–amino acid complex to the ribosome, inhibiting codon–anticodon interaction and inhibition of protein synthesis. They are bacteriostatic and efficacy is determined by the time spent above the MIC.

Pharmacology

They can be given intravenously or orally. Oral bioavailability is variable but highest (95%) with doxycycline within three hours of a dose. Absorption occurs in the stomach and small intestine. Tetracyclines are chelated by milk and should not be co-administered orally with calcium- or magnesium-containing salts nor with antacids. Co-administration of penicillin (bactericidal) reduces the susceptibility of some bacteria to treatment and is seen as an antagonistic combination. All tetracyclines penetrate body tissues well. Routes of elimination vary but with doxycycline it is mostly via the intestine.

Side Effects and Special Points

- Tetracyclines can increase muscle weakness in myasthenia gravis and exacerbate systemic lupus erythematosus.
- The most common side effect is GI upset.
- Children. Tetracyclines have been associated with permanent tooth discolouration in young children if used repeatedly or for long courses. Doxycycline binds less readily to calcium therefore is safer in this respect.
- Pregnancy. Tetracyclines cross the placenta and concentrations in the foetus are significantly higher than in the mother. Most tetracyclines are contraindicated in pregnancy (especially the second and third trimester) because of the significant concentration found in fetal bone and teeth that can lead to transient inhibition of bone growth and permanent discolouration of teeth. Doxycycline binds less readily to calcium and is therefore the tetracycline of choice in pregnancy, if there are no alternatives.

Macrolides

Structure

Macrolides are derived from erythromycin and have a lactone ring at their centre. Newer agents have different groups attached to the lactone ring resulting in improved oral tolerance.

Uses

Macrolides have a range of activity similar to penicillin and may be used as alternative therapy in penicillin allergy. They cover most Gram-positive organisms and are active against Gram-negative anaerobes. In addition, the Gram-negative aerobes *Mycoplasma pneumoniae* and *Legionella pneumophilia* are sensitive. Erythromycin represents the parent member of this group. Clarithromycin causes less GI upset and gives better cover against *Streptococci*, *Listeria monocytogenes* and *Legionella pneumophilia*. Azithromycin provides better Gram-negative cover against *Moraxella catarrhalis*, *Neisseria meningitidis* and *Haemophilus influenzae* with improved bioavailability and longer half-life than erythromycin.

Mechanism of Action

Macrolides enter the bacteria and bind to the 50S subunit of the bacterial ribosome resulting in impaired protein synthesis. Depending on concentration and bacterial species, its actions are either bactericidal or bacteriostatic. Resistance is a growing problem with bacteria modifying the subunit binding site to prevent attachment or developing mechanisms to remove the macrolide from the cell.

Pharmacology

Macrolides can be administered orally or parenterally. CSF penetration is poor even with inflamed meninges, but sputum and lung penetration are good. Macrolides are frequently concentrated in leukocytes facilitating transport to the site of infection. They may also have immunomodulatory properties separate to their antimicrobial action which can be useful in certain diseases such as cystic fibrosis. Macrolides are metabolised and excreted mainly via the liver. Erythromycin and clarithromycin are strong inhibitors of hepatic cytochrome CYP3A4 and p-glycoprotein (PGP), the transport protein responsible for limiting enteral uptake of many drugs.

Side Effects and Special Points

- *Interactions.* The macrolides have a variety of drug interactions, many of which are mediated by inhibition of hepatic cytochrome CYP3A4 enzymes. Simvastatin, warfarin and carbamazepine levels are all increased in the presence of clarithromycin. Azithromycin has less effect on hepatic enzymes but does have other important interactions discussed below.

- *Cardiovascular.* All macrolides have been associated with QT interval prolongation but particular attention has been drawn to clarithromycin and azithromycin and their potential for causing fatal torsades de pointes. This is made worse in combination with other drugs that also affect the QT interval, such as cetirizine, cisapride, quinidine or terfenadine.

- *Gastrointestinal.* Nausea, vomiting and diarrhoea occur frequently, especially following intravenous injection due to its prokinetic effect. Erythromycin should be avoided in porphyria.

Oxazolidinones

Structure

The oxazolidinones were originally developed as antidepressant monoamine oxidase inhibitors but now form a class of synthetic antibiotics unrelated to other classes. Currently available drugs in the UK include linezolid and tedizolid.

Uses

They are active against Gram-positive bacteria including MRSA and glycopeptide resistant enterococci. They are not effective against Gram-negative organisms. They are used in pneumonia and complicated soft tissue infections (in combination with other antibiotics).

Mechanism of Action

Oxazolidinones inhibit bacterial protein synthesis by binding to bacterial 50S subunit. Linezolid is bacteriostatic against enterococci and *Staphylococci* and bactericidal against most strains of *Streptococci*.

Side Effects and Special Points

- Severe optic neuropathy and haemopoietic disorders have been reported requiring regular monitoring of blood counts weekly and regular vision checks.

Lincosamides

Uses

Clindamycin is the only lincosamide currently available in the UK. It is active against Gram-positive cocci including those that are penicillin resistant, as well as many anaerobic bacteria. Clindamycin is able to achieve high concentrations in phagocytic cells, bile and bone. It is used for osteomyelitis and severe soft tissue infections. It has little activity against Gram-negative aerobic organisms despite anaerobic rods being highly susceptible. It is also active against most MRSA and the protozoal *Plasmodium falciparum* but not *Plasmodium vivax*.

Mechanism of Action

Clindamycin binds to the 50S ribosomal subunit and disrupts protein synthesis. It competes for the same 50S binding site as macrolide antibiotics. It can be bacteriostatic or bactericidal depending on concentration and the organism being treated. In some bacteria it can have a prolonged post-antibiotic effect. Resistance is inducible in Gram-positive organisms that are normally sensitive and when present often imparts resistance to macrolides.

Clindamycin is particularly useful in staphylococcal toxic shock syndrome because it significantly inhibits the production of alpha toxin (in contrast to β-lactams).

Side Effects and Special Points

Clindamycin is generally well tolerated but one significant disadvantage is the high risk of antibiotic associated diarrhoea and *Clostridium difficile* colitis.

3. Antibiotics that Disrupt the Cytoplasmic Cellular Membrane

Polymyxins

Uses

Only two polymyxins are in clinical use and both have very similar chemical structures. Polymyxin B and polymyxin E (colistin) are bactericidal antibiotics that have recently been brought back into clinical practice to treat highly resistant, often hospital-acquired, Gram-negative bacterial infections such as *Pseudomonas* and *Acinetobacter*.

Mechanism of Action

Polymyxins bind to lipopolysaccharides (LPS) and phospholipids in the outer cell membrane of Gram-negative bacteria leading to disruption of the outer cellular membrane and cell death. Helpfully, polymyxins can bind to LPS and reduce their adverse effects. Polymyxins have concentration-dependent killing against bacteria but no post-antibiotic effect thus they require frequent dosing.

Pharmacology

Their pharmacology is not completely understood. Colistin is excreted via the urine making it useful in urinary tract infection but necessitating dose adjustment in renal impairment. This contrasts with polymyxin B which is not excreted via the urine so not indicated in urinary infections or needing dose adjustment in renal impairment. Routes of administration include intravenous, intrathecal and inhalational and dosing often needs consultation with specialists.

Side Effects and Special Points

Polymyxins should be avoided in myasthenia gravis. There is a high rate of nephrotoxicity and acute tubular necrosis.

Lipodepsipeptides

Structure

Cyclic lipodepsipeptides are molecules that are frequently expressed by bacteria and consist of a lipid joined to a peptide. The base structures are being used to develop a variety of new antibiotics.

Uses

The most well-known of these is daptomycin which is used for complicated skin and soft tissue infections caused by highly resistant, Gram-positive bacteria.

Mechanism of Action

Daptomycin binds to components of the cell membrane of susceptible organisms and causes rapid depolarisation. It is bactericidal and activity increases in a concentration-dependent manner.

Side Effects and Special Points

A wide range of side effects have been reported including eosinophilic pneumonia and rhabdomyolysis.

4. Inhibition of Normal Nucleic Acid Replication (DNA and Transcription to RNA)
Fluoroquinolones

Structure

The basic chemical structure is a bicyclic ring with a fluorine atom at position C-6.

Uses

Fluoroquinolones are broad-spectrum antibiotics with extensive activity against aerobic Gram-negative bacteria. Some of the class also have activity against *Pseudomonas*, some Gram-positives, anaerobes and mycobacteria. Ciprofloxacin is the most commonly used fluoroquinolone and has a broad spectrum of activity, being particularly active against Gram-negative bacteria such as *Salmonella*, *Neisseria* and *Pseudomonas*. It is also first-line treatment for anthrax and pneumonic plague infections. Moxifloxacin has greater pneumococcal activity than ciprofloxacin and is used in the treatment of sinusitis and community-acquired pneumonias.

Mechanism of Action

Fluoroquinolones are bactericidal antibiotics that inhibit bacterial DNA synthesis, by blocking topoisomerase enzymes, which are essential for supercoiling, replication and separation of the circular bacterial DNA. This results in a reduction in bacterial DNA production and cell death.

Pharmacology

Fluoroquinolones are well absorbed from the gut, are widely distributed and have excellent CSF and tissue penetration. They undergo limited metabolism with excretion in urine and faeces mainly in the unchanged form.

Side Effects and Special Points

- Certain bacteria (*Neisseria gonorrhoeae* and *Pseudomonas*) are developing widespread resistance so that fluoroquinolones as a class have only limited use.
- GI side effects are the most common. The broad-spectrum nature of fluoroquinolones has been associated with a higher risk of *Clostridium difficile* colitis and prescribing has been discouraged.
- Fluoroquinolones should be used with caution in patients with epilepsy (especially in the presence of non-steroidal anti-inflammatory drugs (NSAIDs)) as they can precipitate seizures. Peripheral neuropathy is common with long-term use. Fluoroquinolones have neuromuscular-blocking activity and may exacerbate muscle weakness in individuals with myasthenia gravis.

- Cardiovascular system – fluoroquinolones can prolong the QT interval and must not be used with drugs that have similar effects.
- Tendinopathy. Fluoroquinolone use has been associated with a broad range of tendinopathies such as tendon rupture.

Sulphonamides

Structure

The term sulphonamide is employed as a generic name for the derivatives of para amino benzene sulphonamides. A broad group of different drugs with antimicrobial, hypoglycaemic (oral sulphonylurea diabetic drugs), diuretic (acetazolamide) and anti-convulsant (topiramate) activity. The sulphonamide antibiotics such as sulfadiazine are rarely used now following the development of modern agents. The exception is sulfamethoxazole which is combined with trimethoprim in a synergistic combination as co-trimoxazole.

Uses

Co-trimoxazole has activity against a wide variety of aerobic Gram-positive and Gram-negative bacteria. It is used for hospital-acquired pneumonia, other susceptible infections and *Pneumocystis jerovicii*.

Mechanism of Action

p-Amino benzoic acid (PABA) is required for the synthesis of folic acid, which in turn is needed for the synthesis of DNA and RNA. Due to the structural resemblance of suphonamides with PABA, sulphonamides competitively inhibit PABA. This causes folic acid deficiency, resulting in arrest of bacterial growth and cell division. Trimethoprim inhibits folic acid reduction to tetrahydrofolate by reversible inhibition of dihydrofolate reductase, inhibiting bacterial synthesis of nucleic acids and proteins.

Side Effects and Special Points

Co-trimoxazole is contraindicated in acute porphyria. The most common adverse effects are GI disturbance and skin rash. Life-threatening effects include agranulocytosis and Stevens-Johnson syndrome.

Fusidanes

Fusidic acid is a naturally occurring bactericidal antibiotic that exhibits activity against Gram-positive bacteria *Staphylococcus aureus*, MRSA and *Staphylococcus epidermidis,* but *Streptococci* and pneumococci are relatively resistant. Some Gram-negative organisms are sensitive although bacilli are highly resistant.

Mechanism of Action

Fusidic acid does not bind to bacterial ribosome but forms a complex with elongation factor and GTP. This complex is involved in protein translocation and will allow the incorporation of one amino acid residue before blocking further chain elongation. Consequently, protein synthesis is inhibited and cell death follows.

Kinetics

Fusidic acid is well distributed and penetrates cerebral abscesses well but is not active in the CSF. Bone penetration is good and fusidic acid is often used to treat staphylococcal bone and joint sepsis. The drug is concentrated and excreted unchanged in the bile but little active drug appears in faeces. Similarly, little drug activity is detected in urine and renal failure has little effect on plasma levels.

Side Effects

Fusidic acid is well tolerated with only occasional reports of rash or GI symptoms.

Rifamycins

Uses

Several rifamycins are in clinical use. Rifampicin is a semi-synthetic antimicrobial with potent activity against Gram-positive bacteria. *Legionella, Neisseria* and *Haemophilus influenzae* are susceptible but other Gram-negative organisms remain resistant. Most mycobacteria, including *Mycobacterium tuberculosis*, are sensitive to rifampicin but *Mycobacterium avium* tends to be resistant. It is a key element in tuberculosis therapy and should always be used unless there is a specific contraindication. It is well tolerated with few side effects Other rifamycins include rifabutin for non-tuberculous mycobacterial disease, and rifaximin for reduction in recurrence of hepatic encephalopathy (taking advantage of its very poor absorption from the GI tract).

Mechanism of Action

Rifampicin is bactericidal and binds to the β-subunit of DNA-dependent RNA polymerase, preventing DNA transcription to RNA. Resistance is readily inducible with rifampicin and this antimicrobial should not be used as a single agent. Combination therapy needs careful consideration as some antimicrobials (e.g. ciprofloxacin) are antagonised by rifampicin.

Pharmacology

Rifampicin is very lipid-soluble, penetrating CSF, abscesses and heart valves. It is metabolised by liver microsomes and excreted into the bile. Active transport of the drug into bile can become saturated and remaining drug will be excreted unchanged in the urine, where it imparts the characteristic red colour.

Side Effects and Special Points

Rifampicin is a potent inducer of hepatic CYP450 enzymes, reducing plasma concentration of many drugs including anticonvulsants, oral contraceptives and warfarin. Plasma levels are unaffected by renal failure.

Nitroimidazole

Structure

Metronidazole and tinidazole are nitroimidazole antibiotics.

Uses

Metronidazole is a potent inhibitor of obligate anaerobes and protozoa such as *Trichomonas vaginalis, Clostridium difficile, Bacteroides biacutis, Treponema pallidum* and *Campylobacter jejuni* are all sensitive whilst anaerobic *Streptococci* and *Lactobacilli* are resistant. Despite extensive use worldwide, resistance remains rare.

Mechanism of Action

Metronidazole can enter bacterial cells by passive diffusion. Metronidazole is reduced by the pyruvate-ferredoxin oxidoreductase system in obligate anaerobes. The nitro group of reduced metronidazole acts as an electron sink, capturing electrons that would usually be transferred to hydrogen ions in the metabolic cycle. As a result, cytotoxic inter-mediates accumulate along with free radicals that induce DNA strand breakage and cell death follows.

Pharmacology

Metronidazole has almost 100% bioavailability, distributes widely in CSF, cerebral abscesses, prostate and pleural fluid and has a half-life of 8 hours. It is completely metabo-lised in the liver with an active hydroxy metabolite that is eliminated slowly from plasma. Metabolites are excreted through the kidney.

Side Effects and Special Points

Metronidazole is generally well tolerated. The most common side effects are nausea or a metallic taste being most often described. It should not be combined with alcohol as a severe disulfiram-like reaction occurs with nausea, vomiting, severe headache, flushing and hypotension.

Mechanisms of Resistance

Bacterial resistance to antibiotics is a complex topic, a full discussion of which is beyond the scope of this book. There are however several broad mechanisms that are important to understand (see Figure 23.4).

- **Modification of the antimicrobial molecule.** Some bacteria are able to modify antibiotics and reduce their activity, e.g. aminoglycosides are subject to subtle changes by 'aminoglycoside-modifying enzymes' and rifampicin can be inactivated by glycosylation.
- **Destruction of the antimicrobial molecule** is the main mechanism of β-lactam resistance. β-lactamases destroy the amide bond within the β-lactam ring and render the antimicrobial ineffective. Extended spectrum β-lactamase enzyme (ESBL) producing Gram-negative bacteria such as *Klebsiella pneumoniae* and *Escherichia coli* are a serious problem. Carbapenemase producing *Enterobacteriaceae* (CPE) have evolved to render carbapenems ineffective.
- **Prevention of the antibiotic reaching the intracellular target** by either reducing penetration (which is common in Gram-negative bacteria with an outer membrane), or active extrusion of the antibiotic after it has entered the cell. A common mechanism of *Pseudomonas* resistance to carbapenems is a reduction in the amount of porin, the drug's primary portal of entry. Actively extruding the antibiotic via an efflux pump is a common mechanism of tetracycline and fluroquinolone resistance.
- **Changes to target sites**, e.g. the changing of the peptidoglycan precursors target of glycopeptides to significantly reduce affinity. Vancomycin resistant *Enterococci* (VRE)

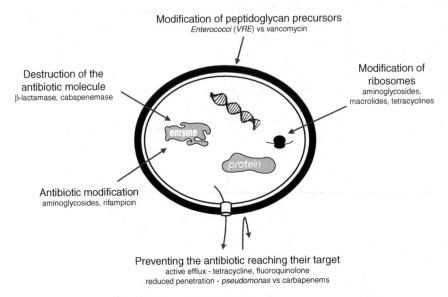

Figure 23.4 Summary of mechanisms of antibiotic resistance.

are an example of bacteria with resistance by this mechanism. Modification of ribosome subunits provides resistance to macrolides, tetracyclines, and aminoglycosides.

Viruses and Antiviral Drugs

Viruses are microscopic pathogens that are smaller than bacteria. They are unable to survive (although may remain dormant for long periods) or reproduce without a host. Viruses are parasites that need to enter host cells to then exploit host cell enzymes. Internal cellular machinery including protein synthesis is exploited for replication and subsequent shedding of new virus particles. Cell damage and death occurs as a result of a variety of mechanisms such as the diversion of the cells energy away from vital functions, competition for protein synthesis mechanisms, integration of the viral genome, induction of mutations in the host genome, inflammation, and the host immune response towards the infected cell.

Viral replication exploits host cell enzymes, they are obligate intracellular parasites, making it difficult to target replication of the virus without causing damage to the host cell. Viruses can be broadly classified into DNA and RNA viruses (see Figure 23.5) and whether the nucleic acid is single or double-stranded. Some viruses also acquire a capsule (envelope) made from virus-specific proteins and host membrane lipid and carbohydrate components.

Antiviral drugs are available in several classes. In immunocompetent individuals most viral infections can resolve using the host defences. Antiviral drugs are used to shorten the duration of the illness as well as the severity of symptoms. Such drugs are available to treat a limited number of viral infections such as hepatitis B and C, HIV, influenza and herpes viruses. Unlike antibiotics, antiviral drugs do not target the virus itself but target the steps involved in replication (Figure 23.6). This reduces the total number of viruses. Symptoms are reduced and pathogenicity is reduced and this allows the host defences to deal with the resulting viral infection.

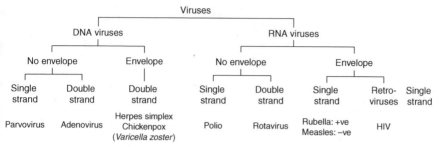

Figure 23.5 Simplified classification of viruses.

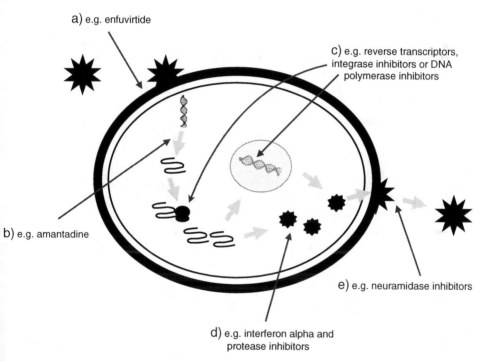

Figure 23.6 Summary of viral replication and points at which antiviral agents work; a) attachment and penetration, b) uncoating and release of nucleic acid, c) viral genome replication, d) protein synthesis and assembly of new virus, e) release of new virus from host cell.

Targets for Antiviral Drugs during the Replication Cycle

- Drugs affecting the attachment to and penetration of the host cell by the virus (e.g. enfuvirtide for HIV).
- Drugs that affect the uncoating of the viral nucleic acid and release into the host cell (e.g. amantadine).

- Drugs that affect the replication of the viral genome. This can be via reverse transcription (nucleoside and non-nucleoside reverse transcription inhibitors), DNA integration by integrase (integrase inhibitors) and nucleic acid inhibitors (DNA polymerase inhibitors).
- Drugs that interfere with protein synthesis and assembly of viral components. Protein synthesis by transcription and translation (interferon alpha) and protein processing by protease enzymes (protease inhibitors).
- Drugs affecting the release of new viruses from the host cell. This is known as viral budding and is reduced by neuraminidase inhibitors.

Aciclovir

Structure
Aciclovir is a nucleoside analogue.

Uses
Acyclovir is used to treat infection due to *Herpes simplex* (type I and II) and *Varicella zoster* as well as *Epstein-Barr Virus* (EBV). It does not eradicate the viruses.

Mechanism of Action
Acyclovir inhibits nucleic acid synthesis. Cells infected with *H. simplex* (HSV) or *V. zoster* contain a virally encoded thymidine kinase that converts aciclovir to aciclovir monophosphate. This is then converted to an active triphosphate that inhibits viral DNA polymerase and acts as a chain terminator. The thymidine kinase present in uninfected host cells has a low affinity for aciclovir meaning that the aciclovir only affects infected cells. Whilst useful against *H. simplex* and *V. zoster* it does not eradicate them and is only effective if given at the start of an infection. Thymidine kinase is not encoded by *Cytomegalovirus* (CMV) therefore aciclovir is ineffective in these situations. Mechanisms of resistance include reduced or absent thymidine kinase and reduced affinity for aciclovir.

Pharmacology
Aciclovir has a low oral bioavailability (15–30%) so the intravenous route is preferred in serious infections. It is eliminated unchanged in the urine via glomerular filtration and tubular secretion.

Special Points
Aciclovir is tolerated reasonably well by patients but acute renal failure and neurological toxicity have been reported, especially in those with dehydration or underlying renal dysfunction undergoing rapid injection. In suspected cases of viral encephalitis, the early use of high dose aciclovir (10 mg.kg^{-1}) may improve long-term neurological outcomes.

Related Drugs
Valaciclovir is a prodrug of aciclovir with improved oral bioavailability. Famciclovir is a prodrug of penciclovir, which has a profile similar to aciclovir.

Ganciclovir

Structure

Ganciclovir (and its ester valganciclovir) are nucleoside analogues.

Uses

Primarily used for cytomegalovirus (CMV) infections where acyclovir is ineffective, but it also has activity against herpes viruses.

Mechanism of Action

Ganciclovir and valganciclovir are converted intracellularly to an active monophosphate form. The viral kinase catalysing this reaction is produced in CMV-infected cells (in contrast to the thymidine kinase needed to convert aciclovir into the active form, which is not produced in CMV-infected cells). This makes ganciclovir and valganciclovir active against CMV-infected cells. Subsequently, cellular kinases catalyse the formation of ganciclovir diphosphate and ganciclovir triphosphate, which is present in 10-fold greater concentrations in CMV- or HSV-infected cells than uninfected cells.

Pharmacology

Ganciclovir is available orally and intravenously. It has a poor oral bioavailability which is significantly improved when administered as its prodrug valganciclovir. Ganciclovir is excreted unchanged in the urine and a dose adjustment is needed in renal failure. It is generally more toxic than aciclovir and has been associated with bone marrow suppression and renal toxicity.

Foscarnet Sodium

Foscarnet sodium is another antiviral drug used for CMV infections. It is a polymerase inhibitor and reverse transcriptase inhibitor that does not require activation by a viral kinase unlike aciclovir and ganciclovir. It has significant toxicity and can cause renal failure.

Neuraminidase Inhibitors

This class of drug consists of Zanamivir and Oseltamivir. Neuraminidase inhibitors reduce the release of new viral particles from infected cells (budding) and are used for influenza A and B to shorten duration of symptoms. Oseltamivir (oral) and zanamivir (inhaled) can be used for post exposure prophylaxis in influenza in high-risk individuals and is also used in a higher dose for the treatment of influenza in at-risk individuals if started within 48 hours of symptom onset. GI symptoms are common.

HIV Antiviral Treatment

The treatment of HIV infection involves the use of multiple antiviral drugs in combination. This is known as highly active antiretroviral therapy (HAART). Treatment usually involves two nucleoside reverse transcriptase inhibitors (NRTIs) and either a non-nucleoside reverse transcriptase inhibitor (NNRTI), or a protease inhibitor or an integrase inhibitor.

Nucleoside Reverse Transcriptase Inhibitors

Drugs in this class include zidovudine, lamivudine, emtricitabine, abacavir and stavudine. Zidovudine is converted by various kinase enzymes to zidovudine triphosphate, the active compound. This binds to HIV-reverse transcriptase and when it becomes incorporated into proviral DNA chain termination occurs. Its affinity for HIV-reverse transcriptase is 100 times greater than for host DNA polymerase.

Pharmacology

Zidovudine is given orally or intravenously and distributes widely. It is transported by the choroid plexus into the CSF where levels reach 50% of plasma levels. It is conjugated in the liver and up to 80% is excreted in the urine as the glucuronide. Accumulation occurs in renal failure and dose reduction is required. NRTIs require intracellular activation, and their efficacy is thus reliant on kinase availability and activity, which is variable.

Side Effects

- Haematological – anaemia and neutropenia.
- Gut – GI upset, anorexia, deranged liver function, steatorrhoea and lactic acidosis.
- Miscellaneous – headache, myalgia, paraesthesia and pigmentation of nail beds and oral mucosa. HIV-associated lipodystrophy – abnormal distribution of fat.

Non-Nucleoside Reverse Transcriptase Inhibitors

Drugs in this class include nevirapine and efavirenz. They act as non-competitive inhibitors of viral reverse transcriptase, not requiring intracellular activation. They are direct inhibitors.

Protease Inhibitors

Protease inhibitors include atazanavir, darunavir and ritonavir. They inhibit viral protease enzymes that ultimately result in the impairment of viral protein production by inhibiting protease-catalysed cleaving of viral polypeptides. The viral copies that are produced are immature and non-infectious. Protease inhibitors have been associated with the inhibition of insulin-dependent glucose transporters, impaired glucose tolerance and insulin resistance.

Integrase Inhibitors

These drugs inhibit viral integrase, an enzyme produced by HIV that incorporates the viral genome into the host cell DNA. Examples of these drugs include raltegravir and dolutegravir.

Fungi and Anti-Fungal Drugs

Structure and Function

Fungi are eukaryotic cells with cell walls. Fungal cell membranes have a unique sterol, ergosterol, which replaces cholesterol found in mammalian cell membranes. There are many classes of antifungal drugs, some of which are discussed below.

Polyenes

Structure

The polyenes possess a macrocyclic ring, one side of which has several conjugated double bonds and is highly lipophilic while the other side is hydrophilic with many hydroxyl groups. Amphotericin and nystatin are examples.

Use

Both drugs have a very low oral bioavailability. Amphoteracin is used for systemic fungal infections while nystatin is used for oral infections. It has a wide variety of activity.

Mechanism of Action

Polyenes specifically target fungal membranes (see Figure 23.7) and are ineffective against bacteria and viruses. They bind to ergosterol, which is the principal sterol in fungal membranes as opposed to cholesterol that is found in host membranes. This interference with membrane structure creates a transmembrane channel, and the resultant change in permeability allows leakage of intracellular components.

Amphotericin B

Amphotericin A and B were two anti-fungal agents isolated from soil samples in South America. Although very similar in chemical structure only amphotericin B has anti-fungal activity. It is a wide spectrum anti-fungal covering *Aspergillus*, *Candida* and *Cryptococcus*. It is often combined with flucytosine (see 'Flucytosine' below) for cryptococcosis and occasionally for systemic candidiasis. In common with most anti-fungal agents, resistance is seldom acquired during treatment.

Pharmacology

Amphotericin is only administered parenterally and is highly plasma protein-bound. Tissue penetration is poor and negligible levels are found in CSF or urine. It is metabolised by the

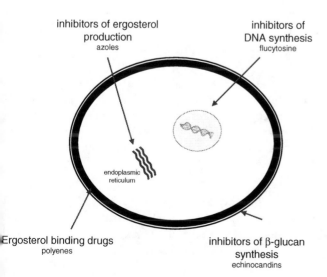

inhibitors of ergosterol production
azoles

inhibitors of DNA synthesis
flucytosine

endoplasmic reticulum

Ergosterol binding drugs
polyenes

inhibitors of β-glucan synthesis
echinocandins

Figure 23.7 Summary of mechanisms of some anti-fungal drugs.

liver and plasma levels do not rise in renal failure. However, due to its potential for nephrotoxicity, dose reduction is still considered in renal impairment. Liposomal preparations (e.g. AmBisome) are available that allow higher doses to be given with less renal toxicity.

Side Effects

It may provoke renal impairment which is only reversible if treatment is stopped early. Renal toxicity can be limited if the dose is gradually increased over the first 48 hours.

Azoles

Structure

This category can be further subdivided into triazoles (fluconazole and itraconazole) and imidazoles (ketoconazole and miconazole). They are active against a wide range of fungi and yeasts including species of *Candida*, *Coccidioides*, *Cryptococcus* and *Histoplasma*. Itraconazole and miconazole also cover *Aspergillus* infection. Resistance is rarely problematic, but isolates are known to demonstrate resistance to more than one agent.

Mechanism of Action

Azoles disrupt ergosterol production by interacting with 14-α demethylase, a cytochrome P450 enzyme necessary to convert lanosterol to ergosterol. As ergosterol is an essential component of the fungal cell membrane, inhibition of its synthesis results in increased cellular permeability causing leakage of cellular contents.

Pharmacology

These drugs are all absorbed well via the oral route with the exception of miconazole, which is available in a parenteral form. Fluconazole penetrates CSF well, is not metabolised and is excreted unchanged in the urine. Itraconazole, ketoconazole and miconazole are all highly protein-bound (99%) and do not penetrate CSF. Ketoconazole, itraconazole and miconazole are metabolised by the liver to inactive metabolites excreted in bile. Azole anti-fungals are very potent inhibitors of CYP450 enzymes in the liver and are involved in many important drug interactions including warfarin (raised PT) and cisapride (prolonged QT syndrome).

Echinocandins

Echinocandins interfere with the synthesis of the fungal cell wall by acting as a glucan synthase inhibitor that is important in the synthesis of β-glucan in fungal cell walls. The fungal cell wall is disrupted and results in cell death. Examples include anidulofungin, caspofungin and micafungin. They are active against *Aspergillus* and *Candida* being used to treat invasive disease with these species. They are not active against CNS infections.

Flucytosine

It is a pyrimidine antimetabolite that inhibits thymidylate synthase subsequently disrupting nucleic acid and protein synthesis and is only used in combination with other anti-fungals. It is synergistic with amphotericin. Often used in combination for systemic candidiasis and cryptococcal meningitis. Bone marrow suppression can limit its use.

Drugs Affecting Coagulation

Physiology

Haemostasis is complicated. Two models are currently used to explain what is thought to occur.

The Classical Model

This has three elements: platelets, the coagulation cascade and fibrinolysis. The first two are involved in preventing haemorrhage by thrombus formation, while fibrinolysis is an essential limiting mechanism.

Thrombus formation is initially dependent on platelet adhesion, which is triggered by exposure to subendothelial connective tissue. The von Willebrand factor, which is part of the main fraction of factor VIII, is essential in this process. Subsequent platelet aggregation and vasoconstriction is enhanced by the release of thromboxane A_2 (TXA_2) from platelets. Adjacent undamaged vascular endothelium produces prostacyclin (PGI_2), which inhibits aggregation and helps to localise the platelet plug to the damaged area. The localised primary platelet plug is then enmeshed by fibrin, converting it to a stable haemostatic plug.

The coagulation cascade is formed by an intrinsic and extrinsic pathway, which converge to activate factor X and the final common pathway (see Figure 24.1). The intrinsic pathway is triggered by the exposure of collagen, thereby activating factor XII, while the extrinsic pathway is triggered by leakage of tissue factors, activating factor VII.

Venous thrombus consists mainly of a fibrin web enmeshed with platelets and red cells. Arterial thrombus relies more on platelets and less on the fibrin mesh.

A crucial part of this process is its limitation to the initial site of injury. Circulating inhibitors, of which anti-thrombin III is the most potent, perform this function. In addition, a fibrinolytic system is activated by tissue damage, converting plasminogen to plasmin, which converts fibrin into soluble degradation products.

The Cell-Based Model

The cell-based model has been developed more recently in light of the perceived failings of the classical model, in particular its failure to explain haemostatic mechanisms in vivo.

For example, factor XII deficiency does not result in an increased bleeding tendency in vivo despite abnormal in vitro tests; the bleeding tendency surrounding factor XI deficiency is not closely related to in vitro tests.

The cell-based model places greater importance on the interaction between specific cell surfaces and clotting factors. Haemostasis is proposed to actually occur on the cell surface, the type of cell with its specific range of surface receptors allowing different cells to play specific roles in the process.

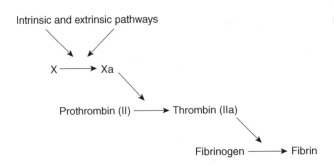

Intrinsic and extrinsic pathways

Figure 24.1 Final common pathway of the coagulation cascade.

The cell-based model proposes that coagulation is the sum of three processes each occurring on different cell surfaces rather than as a cascade. The three processes are **initiation, amplification** and **propagation**. Following vascular injury cells that bear tissue factor are exposed to the circulation and to circulating clotting factors thereby initiating the process. The limited amount of thrombin generated is crucial in amplifying the procoagulant signal and causes platelets to become covered in activated co-factors. The whole process is propagated by the activation of clotting factors on the surface of the tissue factor bearing cells and platelets. As a result, large amounts of thrombin are formed leading to the formation of fibrin from fibrinogen, which consolidates the platelet plug and forms a stable clot. It is this propagation phase that is so deficient in haemophilia despite relatively normal initiation and amplification phases because of insufficient platelet surface thrombin production.

Antiplatelet Drugs

Cyclo-Oxygenase I Inhibition
Aspirin

Uses
Aspirin reduces the risk of unstable angina progressing to acute myocardial infarction (MI) and reduces mortality following acute MI. The risk of stroke is also reduced for patients with transient ischaemic attacks.

Mechanism of Action
Aspirin acts by irreversible inhibition of cyclo-oxygenase (by acetylation) within the platelet, resulting in reduced production of TXA_2. This may be achieved with only 75 mg daily. Its effects and kinetics are discussed in Chapter 10.

Platelet Phosphodiesterase Inhibition
Dipyridamole

Uses
Dipyridamole has been used with limited success in conjunction with warfarin to prevent thrombus formation on prosthetic valves. There is some evidence that when combined with aspirin, dipyridamole may further reduce the risk of stroke, compared to aspirin alone.

Mechanism of Action

Dipyridamole inhibits platelet adhesion to damaged vessel walls (by inhibiting adenosine uptake), potentiates the effects of prostacyclin and at high doses inhibits platelet phosphodiesterase activity resulting in increased cAMP levels and lower intraplatelet calcium levels. Compared to aspirin it inhibits platelet adhesion to vessel walls more than platelet aggregation.

It is a potent coronary artery vasodilator and may be used in conjunction with thallium-201 during myocardial imaging.

Inhibition of ADP Binding
Clopidogrel

Clopidogrel is a prodrug, requiring hepatic CYP450 to convert it into its active form.

Uses

It is used to prevent atherothrombotic events in patients with peripheral vascular disease and when combined with aspirin it is also used to treat ST-elevation myocardial infarction (STEMI) and NSTEMI. It also forms a crucial part of post-coronary stent therapy with aspirin to prevent stent failure.

Mechanism of Action

Clopidogrel irreversibly binds to the $P2Y_{12}$ receptor (an ADP receptor) on platelets, which prevents the glycoprotein IIb/IIIa receptor from transforming into its active form and facilitating platelet activation and cross-linking.

Kinetics

An oral loading dose of 300 mg is followed by a maintenance dose of 75 mg. Antiplatelet effects are seen within 2 hours. Due to the irreversible binding to the $P2Y_{12}$ receptor its effects last for 7 days which is the recommended interval between the last dose and insertion of a neuraxial block. The majority of clopidogrel is hydrolysed by esterases to inactive derivatives, leaving only a small fraction to be oxidised by hepatic CYP450. This oxidation is a two-stage reaction, the final product being the active moiety that forms a disulfide bond with the $P2Y_{12}$ receptor. CYP3A4 and CYP3A5 are the primary isoenzymes but CYP2C19 is also involved. There are many genetic variants of CYP2C19 resulting in reduced or increased amounts of active drug and hence variable antiplatelet effect. In addition omeprazole, which is often prescribed alongside clopidogrel, has a CYP2C19 inhibitory effect and reduces the conversion of clopidogrel to its active form.

Prasugrel

Prasugrel, like clopidogrel, is also a prodrug. However, it is only licensed for percutaneous coronary intervention (PCI) in acute coronary syndrome and may be continued for 12 months with aspirin. It has a faster onset of action compared to clopidogrel and is more effective but also associated with more serious bleeding episodes. It appears to be less susceptible to the genetic polymorphism of the CYP450 system than clopidogrel, and is not affected by CYP450 inhibitors.

Ticagrelor

Ticagrelor is used in acute coronary syndrome in combination with aspirin. It has a bioavailability of 40%, is metabolised by CYP3A4 to active metabolites and excreted mainly in the bile. Other drugs that are metabolised by CYP3A4 or inhibit CYP3A4 may increase its plasma concentrations. It is an allosteric antagonist of ADP in that it antagonises ADP's binding to the $P2Y_{12}$ receptor by binding to a different site.

Glycoprotein IIb/IIIa-Receptor Antagonists

Abciximab is a monoclonal antibody with a high affinity for the platelet glycoprotein IIb/IIIa receptor. It has a plasma half-life of 20 minutes but remains bound in the circulation for up to 15 days with some residual activity.

Eptifibatide is a cyclic heptapeptide with a lower receptor affinity and a plasma half-life of 200 minutes. Fifty percent undergoes renal clearance.

Tirofiban has intermediate receptor affinity and undergoes renal (65%) and faecal (25%) clearance.

Uses

These drugs are used around the time of acute coronary events. They are used intravenously for a short duration during concurrent unfractionated heparin therapy with close control of the activated partial thromboplastin time (APTT) and/or the activated clotting time (ACT). They carry the rare but serious complication of thrombocytopenia.

Mechanism of Action

They act by inhibiting the platelet glycoprotein IIb/IIIa receptor and as such block the final common pathway of platelet aggregation. However, they do not block platelet adhesion, secretion of platelet products, inflammatory effects or thrombin activation.

Miscellaneous
Dextran 70

Dextran 70 is a polysaccharide that contains chains of glucose. It is produced by the fermentation of sucrose by the bacterium *Leuconostoc mesenteroides*.

Uses

It is used as prophylaxis against peri-operative venous thrombosis and as a plasma volume expander.

Mechanism of Action

The anticoagulant activity appears to depend on reducing platelet adhesiveness and a specific inhibitory effect on the von Willebrand factor. It also reduces red cell aggregation and provides a protective coat over vascular endothelium and erythrocytes. The dilution of clotting factors and volume expansion also improves micro-circulatory flow.

Other Effects

These include fluid overload, allergic reactions and anaphylaxis. Dextran 70 can impair cross-matching by rouleaux formation. Renal failure is a rare complication.

Epoprostenol (prostacyclin – PGI$_2$)

This is a naturally occurring prostaglandin.

Uses

Epoprostenol is used to facilitate haemofiltration by continuous infusion into the extra-corporeal circuit.

Mechanism of Action

Epoprostenol causes inhibition of platelet adhesion and aggregation by stimulating adenylate cyclase. The ensuing rise in cAMP reduces intracellular Ca^{2+}, effecting the change. It may also have a fibrinolytic effect. The recommended dose range is 2–12 ng. $kg^{-1}.min^{-1}$.

Side Effects

These relate to its vasodilator properties (hypotension, tachycardia, facial flushing and headache).

Heparins and Protamine

Unfractionated Heparin

Heparin is an anionic, mucopolysaccharide, organic acid containing many sulfate residues. It occurs naturally in the liver and mast cell granules and has a variable molecular weight (5000–25,000 Da).

Uses

Unfractionated heparin is used by continuous intravenous infusion to treat deep vein thrombosis (DVT), pulmonary embolus (PE), unstable angina and in critical peripheral arterial occlusion. Subcutaneous administration to prevent venous thrombosis peri-operatively and in the critically ill has largely been superseded by fractionated heparin, except in renal failure. It is also used in the priming of extracorporeal circuits. There has been limited use in disseminated intravascular coagulation (DIC).

Mechanism of Action

When anti-thrombin III combines with thrombin an inactive 'anti-thrombin–thrombin' complex is formed (see Figure 24.2). The rate of formation of this complex is increased thousand-fold by heparin. At low concentrations factor Xa is inhibited, while factors IXa, XIa and XIIa are progressively inhibited as heparin concentrations rise. Platelet aggregation becomes inhibited at high concentrations and plasma triglyceride levels are lowered due to the release of a lipoprotein lipase from tissues, which reduces plasma turbidity.

Side Effects

- *Haemorrhage* – this is the most common side effect and is due to a relative overdose.

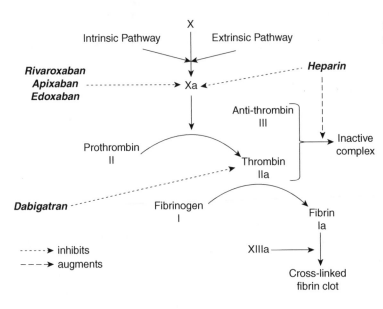

Figure 24.2 Actions of selected anticoagulants.

- *Thrombocytopenia* – a non-immune based thrombocytopenia (type I) occurs within 4 days of anticoagulant doses of heparin. This rarely has clinical significance and the platelet count recovers without stopping heparin.
- This contrasts with the more severe (type II) immune-mediated thrombocytopenia, which occurs within 4–14 days of starting intravenous or subcutaneous heparin (fractionated and unfractionated). Heparin complexes with platelet factor 4, which is bound by IgG causing platelet aggregation and thrombosis. Half of these patients develop serious thrombosis after the platelet count starts to fall and mortality is high, mainly from pulmonary embolus. In addition 20% get arterial thrombosis leading to stroke and limb ischaemia.
- *Cardiovascular* – hypotension may follow rapid intravenous administration of a large dose.
- *Miscellaneous* – osteoporosis, due to complexing of mineral substance from bone, and alopecia have been reported. Heparin (including low-molecular-weight heparins (LMWHs)) can cause hyperkalaemia, which may be due to inhibition of aldosterone secretion. Patients with diabetes mellitus and chronic renal failure are particularly susceptible and the risk increases with the duration of therapy.

Kinetics

As the potency of commercial preparations varies, unfractionated heparin is presented as units.ml^{-1} rather than mg.ml^{-1}. It is ineffective orally and may only be given subcutaneously or intravenously. It has a low lipid solubility and does not cross the blood–brain barrier or placenta. Owing to its negative charge it is highly bound in plasma to anti-thrombin III, albumin, proteases and fibrinogen. It is metabolised by hepatic heparinase and the products are excreted in the urine. During hypothermia (e.g. cardiopulmonary bypass) clearance is reduced. Its effects are reversed by protamine.

Low-Molecular-Weight Heparins
Enoxaparin, Dalteparin, Tinzaparin

These drugs are derived from the depolymerisation of heparin by either chemical or enzymatic degradation. Their molecular weights vary from 2000 to 8000 Da.

Uses

Low-molecular-weight heparins have proven benefit over unfractionated heparin in reducing the incidence of fatal PE after major orthopaedic surgery.

Advantages include:

- Single daily dose, due to a longer half-life
- Reduced affinity for von Willebrand factor
- Less effect on platelets
- Reduced risk of heparin-induced thrombocytopenia
- Reduced need for monitoring.

Mechanism of Action

Compared with unfractionated heparin, LMWHs are more effective at inhibiting factor Xa and less effective at promoting the formation of the inactive 'anti-thrombin–thrombin' complex.

Protamine is not fully effective in reversing the effects of LMWHs.

Monitoring Heparin Therapy

Unfractionated heparin is monitored by the activated partial thromboplastin time (APTT). It characterises coagulation affected by the intrinsic system factors (VIII, IX, XI and XII) in addition to the factors common to both systems. Phospholipid, a surface activator (e.g. kaolin) and Ca^{2+} are added to citrated blood. The clotting time varies between laboratories but is about 28–35 seconds.

Monitoring LMWH is difficult as its main effects are inhibiting factor Xa, so the APTT is not altered. Anti Xa activity can be measured in specialist laboratories.

Protamine

Protamine is a basic protein prepared from fish sperm. Its positive charge enables it to neutralise the anticoagulant effects of heparin by the formation of an inactive complex that is cleared by the reticulo-endothelial system. It is also used in the formulation of certain insulins.

It is given intravenously, 1 mg reversing 100 i.u. heparin.

Side Effects

- *Cardiovascular* – hypotension (due to histamine release), pulmonary hypertension (complement activation and thromboxane release), dyspnoea, bradycardia and flushing follow rapid intravenous administration.
- *Allergic reactions* – patients having previously received insulin containing protamine and those allergic to fish may be at increased risk of allergic reactions.
- *Anticoagulation* – when given in excess it has some anticoagulant effects.

Oral Anticoagulants

There has been a significant increase in the choice of oral anticoagulants in recent years. Their development has been driven largely by the potential to treat patients who are unable to tolerate warfarin and their predictable kinetics and therefore lack of monitoring.

Warfarin

Uses

Warfarin is a coumarin derivative and is used for the prophylaxis of systemic thromboembolism in patients with atrial fibrillation, rheumatic valve disease or prosthetic valves. It is also used in the prophylaxis and treatment of deep vein thrombosis (DVT) and pulmonary embolus (PE).

Mechanism of Action

Warfarin inhibits the synthesis of the vitamin-K-dependent clotting factors: II (prothrombin), VII, IX and X. The precursors of these clotting factors are produced in the liver and are activated by γ-carboxylation of their glutamic acid residues. This process is linked to the oxidation of reduced vitamin K. Warfarin acts by preventing the return of vitamin K to the reduced form (see Figure 24.3).

Circulating factors will not be affected by the actions of warfarin, which therefore takes up to 72 hours to exert its full effect.

Side Effects

- *Haemorrhage.*
- *Teratogenicity* – this is more common and serious in the first trimester. During the third trimester it crosses the placenta and may result in fetal haemorrhage.

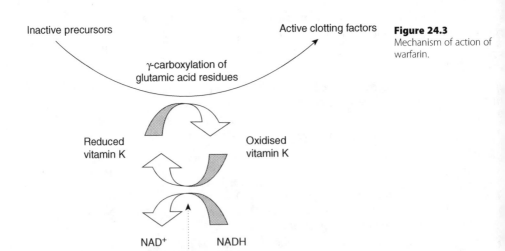

Figure 24.3
Mechanism of action of warfarin.

- *Drug interactions* – drugs that impair other aspects of coagulation (non-steroidal anti-inflammatory drugs (NSAIDs) and heparin) will potentiate the effects of warfarin. Competition for plasma binding sites (NSAIDs) and inhibition of metabolism (cimetidine, alcohol, allopurinol, erythromycin, ciprofloxacin, metronidazole and tricyclic antidepressants (TCAs)) lead to potentiation of warfarin's effects. Barbiturates, rifampicin and carbamazepine induce hepatic enzymes and antagonise the effects of warfarin. Cholestyramine interferes with the absorption of fat-soluble vitamins and thereby potentiates the action of warfarin. The effects of warfarin are rapidly reversed by fresh frozen plasma. Vitamin K (1 mg) will also reverse its effects but more slowly, while 10 mg vitamin K will prevent anticoagulation for a number of days. Spinal and epidural anaesthesia is contraindicated in patients anticoagulated with warfarin.

Kinetics

Warfarin is completely absorbed from the gut and highly protein-bound (> 95%). It undergoes complete hepatic metabolism by oxidation and reduction to products that are subsequently conjugated and excreted in the urine. Predictable genetic factors account for some of the variation in warfarin response, two genes, VKORC1 and CYP2C9, being particularly important. VKORC1 encodes the enzyme vitamin K epoxide reductase complex subunit 1, which is responsible for reducing vitamin K 2,3-epoxide to the active form. Less active mutations of VKORC1 leave patients more susceptible to bleeding. CYP2C9 is the main metabolic pathway for the more potent S-warfarin, so that reduced enzymatic activity can cause a significant increase in anticoagulant activity. Bleeding due to abnormal genetic polymorphisms is most significant at the start of therapy when a loading dose is used.

Monitoring Warfarin Therapy

Prothrombin time (PT) is a measure of the extrinsic system (VII) and factors common to both systems. Tissue thromboplastin (a brain extract) and Ca^{2+} are added to citrated plasma. Clotting normally takes place in 10–14 seconds. The international normalised ratio (INR) is a ratio of the sample PT to a control international standard PT. Warfarin treatment should aim to increase the PT so that the INR is raised to between 2.0 and 4.5 depending on the clinical situation.

Non-Vitamin K Oral Anticoagulants

Direct Thrombin Inhibitors

Dabigatran

Uses

Dabigatran was one of the first non-vitamin K oral anticoagulants (NOACs) to be licensed for venous thromboembolism (VTE) prophylaxis for arthroplasty at a dose of 220 mg od. Since then it has been licensed for atrial fibrillation (AF) using 150 mg bd.

Mechanism of Action

It is a competitive direct thrombin inhibitor. As it blocks a pivotal part of the final common pathway it is a very effective anticoagulant.

Kinetics

Dabigatran etexilate is a prodrug that is rapidly converted by plasma and liver esterases to the active dabigatran moiety. Less than 10% is metabolised in the liver by glucuronidation so that its elimination depends primarily on renal function. As a result the dose needs to be adjusted in the elderly and those with impaired renal function according to their eGFR which, if below 30 ml.min^{-1}.1.732 m^{-2}, contraindicates its use. It is advised that ketoconazole, rifampicin, phenytoin and carbamazepine are avoided and that the dose of amiodarone is reduced. Verapamil should be avoided for the 2 hours pre dabigatran. In addition proton pump inhibitors (PPIs) may reduce absorption by up to 25%. For these reasons and its efficacy profile it is not the most widely used of these new oral anticoagulants.

Side Effects

The predictable side effects include bleeding although this is less common compared to warfarin, especially for intracranial haemorrhage. The rather broad category of gastrointestinal (GI) upset may occur in up to 35% of recipients, which in the recovery phase of arthroplasty is tedious.

Direct Factor Xa Inhibitors

Rivaroxaban

Uses

Rivaroxaban is used for VTE prophylaxis (10 mg od) and treatment (15 mg bd for 21 days then 20 mg od) and in AF (20 mg od).

Mechanism of Action

Rivaroxaban is a direct Xa inhibitor, blocking the final common pathway of the clotting cascade.

Kinetics

With an oral bioavailability of 80–100% rivaroxaban has an onset of action similar to that of dabigatran of between 2–3 hours. As it undergoes 70% hepatic metabolism (CYP3A4 and CYP2J2) so renal function is less important compared to dabigatran, with no dose reduction required above an eGFR of 30 ml.min^{-1}/1.732 m^2. Like dabigatran, rivaroxaban has predictable kinetics that are not altered by age, weight or gender.

Drug Interactions

Rivaroxaban should be avoided with ketoconazole, used with caution with erythromycin and clarithromycin due to increased levels and with CYP3A4 inducers due to decreased levels, but unlike dabigatran there are fewer drug interactions to consider.

Side Effects

Haemorrhage, but favourable compared to warfarin. Like dabigatran, GI upset is common.

Apixaban

Uses

Apixaban is used for VTE prophylaxis (2.5 mg bd) and in AF (5 mg bd).

Mechanism of Action

It is a direct Xa inhibitor, blocking the final common pathway of the clotting cascade.

Kinetics

While apixaban's oral bioavailability is only 50%, in many other aspects its kinetics are similar to rivaroxaban with a predictable onset of action of a few hours, hepatic CYP3A4 metabolism and limited dependence on renal elimination (but a greater reliance on biliary elimination) requiring no dose adjustment above an eGFR of 30 ml.min^{-1}/1.732 m^2. Currently there is little data on drug interactions but CYP3A4 inducers may decrease levels.

Edoxaban

Uses

Edoxaban is a once daily alternative that displays no food–drug interactions. Unfortunately a number of relevant drug interactions may limit it's use. Ketoconazole, erythromycin, verapamil and cyclosporine inhibit the P-glycoprotein (P-gp) efflux transporter and concomitant use with edoxaban results in significant increases in plasma concentrations. Rifampin, a P-gp inducer, when administered along with edoxaban results in significantly lower concentrations.

Choosing between Dabigatran, Rivaroxaban and Apixaban

Compared to LMWH, there are differences in the efficacy of VTE prophylaxis and incidence of bleeding. While dabigatran is equivalent, rivaroxaban results in less VTE but more bleeding and apixaban results in less bleeding and equivalent VTE rates. Individual priorities will determine drug choice.

Monitoring and Overdose

While there are laboratory tests (chromogenic anti-factor Xa activity assays, diluted thrombin time and ecarin-based clotting tests) that can be used to measure the effects of these agents they are currently limited by the absence of validated therapeutic targets and a lack of standardisation. Where overdose is suspected, standard laboratory tests within the normal range can be used to exclude significant overdose, but when outside the normal range cannot be used to quantify the coagulopathy.

At the time of writing a number of agents have either become available or are being assessed, which are able to reverse NOACs.

Idarucizumab

Idarucizumab is a humanised monoclonal antibody fragment that binds irreversibly specifically to dabigatran and its metabolites. It works within 30 minutes and lasts for 24 hours in the majority of patients. It is used at a dose of 2.5 g intravenously which may be repeated once. Excretion is via the kidney so drug exposure is increased in the presence of renal impairment. However, as dabigatran is also eliminated primarily via the kidney its levels will also be raised. It is presented in a ready to use formulation but must be stored in a fridge and drug exposed to light used within 6 hours.

Andexanet Alpha

Andexanet alfa is a recombinant form of human factor Xa that has been modified to lack factor Xa enzymatic activity by substitution of the active serine site with alanine and removal of the gamma-carboxyglutamic acid domain. It binds and sequesters factor Xa inhibitors (rivaroxaban, apixaban and edoxaban) with a similar affinity compared with native factor Xa. In addition, it is also effective against indirect factor Xa inhibitors. It completely reverses fondaparinux which only acts on factor Xa, while it is partially effective against LMWH which also inhibits factor IIa. It is presented in 100 mg and 200 mg vials which need reconstituting prior to administration. It has a short half-life of 1 hour so it is used at a dose of 400 mg over 10 minutes followed by an infusion of 480 mg over 120 minutes. These doses may be doubled depending on the time and size of the last dose of factor Xa inhibitor. Serious prothrombotic effects have been observed in trials; DVT (6%), ischaemic stroke (5%), acute MI (3%) and pneumonia (5%), but not in healthy volunteers taking factor Xa inhibitors and andexanet alpha. It should be stored in a fridge.

Ciraparantag

Ciraparantag is a small, cationic, synthetic molecule which is being investigated as a potential 'universal antidote' to anticoagulants. It is currently in its trial phase of development but to date has been shown to bind unfractionated heparin, LMWH, direct thrombin inhibitors and direct factor Xa inhibitors. While its potential is obvious, much is still unknown about its kinetics, pharmacodynamics and ultimately its effectiveness in humans.

Neuraxial Anaesthesia and Oral Anticoagulants

As the number of oral anticoagulants increases so does the complexity of planning care when a neuraxial block is planned. The situation with warfarin is simple and an INR will confirm whether it is safe to proceed or not. However, the newer oral anticoagulants have no laboratory test that can be relied on and their half-lives (which are affected differently by renal impairment) are different. In addition, as the licensed indications have widened from the prophylaxis of VTE to include its treatment, and that of AF, the different doses need to be considered when deciding the duration to withhold drug. It is recommended that the most recent international guidelines are consulted.

Drugs Affecting the Fibrinolytic System

Fibrinolytics
Streptokinase

Streptokinase is an enzyme produced by group C β-haemolytic streptococci.

Uses

Streptokinase is used to dissolve clot in arterial (acute MI, occluded peripheral arteries and PE) and venous (DVT) vessels.

Mechanism of Action

Streptokinase activates the fibrinolytic system by forming a complex with plasminogen, which then facilitates the conversion of further plasminogen to active plasmin. The clot can then be lysed.

Side Effects

- *Haemorrhage* – streptokinase is contraindicated in patients for whom a risk of serious bleeding outweighs any potential benefit of therapy (i.e. active internal bleeding, recent stroke, severe hypertension).
- *Cardiovascular* – it may precipitate reperfusion arrhythmias and hypotension during treatment of acute MI.
- *Allergic reactions* may occur as it is very antigenic. Where high antibody titres are expected (5 days to 12 months from previous exposure to streptokinase), an alternative should be sought.

Kinetics

Streptokinase is administered intravenously as a loading dose followed by an infusion. The loading dose is sufficient to neutralise any antibodies that are often present from previous exposure to streptococcal infection. The streptokinase–antibody complex is cleared rapidly and the streptokinase–plasminogen complex is degraded to a number of smaller fragments during its action.

Alteplase (rt-PA, tissue-type plasminogen activator) is a glycoprotein that becomes activated only when bound to fibrin, inducing the conversion of plasminogen to plasmin. Because of its mode of activation, systemic fibrinolysis occurs to a lesser extent than with streptokinase.

Urokinase was originally extracted from human adult male urine but is now prepared from renal cell cultures. Recombinant DNA technology is currently used to produce pro-urokinase. It is not antigenic and is used in the lysis of clots in arteriovenous shunts and in hyphaema (anterior chamber haemorrhage with refractory thrombi).

Antifibrinolytics

Tranexamic Acid

Tranexamic acid (Figure 24.4) was first described in the 1960s and is a synthetic derivative of lysine It is available in tablet and intravenous formulations.

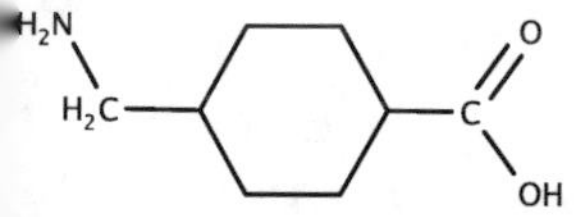

Figure 24.4 Structure of Tranexamic Acid

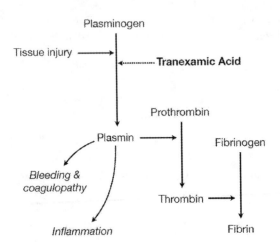

Mechanism of Action

Tranexamic acid competitively inhibits the activation of plasminogen to plasmin (Figure 24.5) by binding to the five lysine binding sites on plasminogen within its Kringle domain (so called after the Scandinavian pastry which it resembles; Kringle domains are autonomous protein regions that fold into large loops, are stabilised by three disulphide linkages, and are involved in the regulation of proteolytic activity). Tranexamic acid also displaces plasminogen from fibrin, and at high concentrations non-competitively blocks plasmin. Consequently, clot dissolution is inhibited. It is also thought to have a role in inflammation.

Uses

It is used in primary and secondary care to manage bleeding. Indications range from menorrhagia to major trauma and include elective arthroplasty, cardiac and obstetric surgery, although it should only be used in patients without risk factors for thrombosis.

Dose

In theatre it is given empirically as a slow intravenous bolus at 0.5–1 g, +/– a further 1 g over 8 hours.

Side Effects

Its prothrombotic potential has probably been overemphasised in those without significant risk factors. Seizures at high doses (> 10 mg.kg^{-1}) have been described following cardiac surgery, and suggested mechanisms have included inhibition at GABA receptors and cerebral vasoconstriction leading to ischaemia.

Aprotinin

Aprotinin is a naturally occurring proteolytic enzyme inhibitor acting on trypsin, plasmin and tissue kallikrein. It inhibits the fibrinolytic activity of the streptokinase–plasminogen complex. In addition it has been suggested that it preserves platelet function and decreases activation of the clotting cascade.

Concerns regarding increased morbidity and mortality lead to its worldwide withdrawal in 2007. However, in 2012 the European Medicines Agency (EMA) recommended its licence withdrawal should be lifted and that its use for patients undergoing coronary artery bypass grafting (CABG) at high risk of bleeding outweighed the risks.

Side Effects

- *Hypersensitivity* reactions including anaphylaxis.
- *Coagulation* – it prolongs the activated clotting time (ACT) of heparinised blood so that heparin/protamine protocols will need alteration during treatment with aprotinin.

Kinetics

Aprotinin is metabolised and eliminated by the kidney.

Chapter 25

Drugs Used in Diabetes Mellitus

Diabetes Mellitus Definition and Types

Diabetes mellitus is a group of metabolic disorders characterised by persistent hyperglycaemia. Diabetes mellitus is caused either by *deficient* endogenous insulin secretion or by *resistance* to the action of insulin. This leads to abnormalities of carbohydrate, fat and protein metabolism and subsequent damage to multiple body tissues and organ systems.

Type 1 diabetes mellitus and type 2 diabetes mellitus are the two most common classifications. In type 1 diabetes there is an *absolute* insulin deficiency caused by the destruction of β-cells in the pancreatic islets of Langerhans. Frequently caused by an autoimmune mechanism, the absolute deficiency in insulin production results in severe hyperglycaemia and dangerous disruption to many body systems. It appears frequently in children and early adulthood but can occur at any age. Type 2 diabetes mellitus is a chronic condition that is characterised by insulin *resistance*, as opposed to an absolute lack of insulin production. It typically develops later in life but can occur in children. Rarer types of diabetes include gestational diabetes that develops during pregnancy and resolves after delivery, and diabetes secondary to other conditions such as pancreatic destruction or damage, or use of certain endocrine, antiviral or antipsychotic drugs.

Insulin

Physiology

Human insulin is a polypeptide of 51 amino acids and is formed by the removal of a connecting or 'C' peptide (34 amino acids) from pro-insulin (see Figure 25.1). It has A and B chains, which are joined by two disulfide bridges. A third disulfide bridge connects two regions of the A chain.

Glucose forms the most potent stimulus for insulin release. It enters the β-cells of the islets of Langerhans in the pancreas, resulting in an increase in adenosine triphosphate (ATP), which closes K^+ channels. This causes depolarisation and Ca^{2+} influx through voltage-sensitive Ca^{2+} channels, which triggers insulin release. By way of negative feedback, the K^+ channels are re-opened.

In health there is a continuous basal insulin release, which is supplemented by bursts when plasma glucose levels rise. Following release, it is carried in the portal circulation to the liver (its main target organ) where about one-half is extracted and broken down, as glucose is converted to glycogen.

Insulin binds to the α subunit of the insulin receptor, which consists of two α and two β subunits that span the cell membrane. Once bound, the whole complex is internalised. The

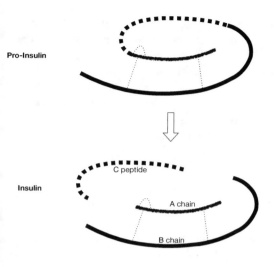

Figure 25.1 Conversion of pro-insulin to insulin and C peptide. (. . . . . = disulfide bridge).

mechanism by which this complex produces its effects is unclear but the tyrosine kinase activity of the β subunit appears important.

Insulin affects carbohydrate, fat and protein metabolism in an anabolic fashion. It promotes hepatic (and extrahepatic) uptake of glucose from the circulation and subsequently facilitates the actions of enzymes required to convert glucose into glycogen. Glycogenolysis is inhibited. The net result is that blood glucose levels fall. Fat deposition is also increased by the promotion of hepatic fatty acid synthesis and subsequent storage as triglycerides. Lipolysis is inhibited. The storage of amino acids as proteins is promoted and protein breakdown is inhibited. Insulin therapy in diabetes mellitus is given to reduce blood glucose levels to within the normal range thus preventing a wide variety of tissue damage throughout the body.

Preparations

Early insulins were extracted from porcine or beef pancreas, but modern preparations are almost entirely produced by recombinant DNA technology.

1. Human insulin
2. Insulin analogues
3. Animal insulin

Human insulins (also known as soluble insulins) are identical to endogenous human insulin, although produced by recombinant techniques. Human insulins may be modified to produce insulin analogues that have altered molecular structures resulting in different characteristics, such as onset of action and duration of effect. Animal insulins are no longer given to new patients but may still be in use by existing patients who are unable to make the change to a recombinant insulin.

Insulin cannot be administered by the gastrointestinal (GI) route because it is inactivated by gastric enzymes. It should be injected subcutaneously (or rarely intravenously) into an area with good subcutaneous fat stores. Absorption from subcutaneous injection can be highly variable based on blood flow, central or peripheral location of the injection site or any areas of lipodystrophy due to repeated use. If given intravenously, human soluble insulin has an almost immediate effect that lasts only for several minutes.

Insulin preparations can be categorised into groups based on their speed of onset and duration of effect profiles: short-acting insulins (including soluble insulins and rapid-acting insulin analogues), intermediate-acting insulins and long-acting insulins. There is considerable inter-individual variability in the above characteristics.

Short-Acting Insulins

These can be either human soluble insulin (e.g. Actrapid, Humulin S) or a rapid-acting insulin analogue (e.g. insulin aspart (Novorapid), insulin glulisine (Apidra) and insulin lispro (Humalog)).

Rapid-acting insulin analogues are injected subcutaneously and have an onset of action within 15 minutes and a duration of up to 5 hours. They are commonly used as part of a treatment regime involving pre-meal injections to replicate endogenous pancreatic insulin surges with meals and can be combined with a long-acting insulin to provide a background basal level of insulin ('basal bolus' regime). In addition to management of diabetes mellitus in the community, their rapid onset of action has led to them being recommended in the management of peri-operative hyperglycaemia.

Human insulins are used in a similar manner to insulin analogues. Despite the perhaps confusing trade name of one of this group (Actrapid) their onset after subcutaneous injection is slower (30 minutes) than rapid-acting insulin analogues. They are most commonly used as part of variable rate *intravenous* insulin infusions (VRIII) where they have a rapid onset (minutes) and much shorter duration of action compared to administration via the subcutaneous route.

Intermediate-Acting Insulins

These are designed to mimic the effect of endogenous basal insulin. Onset when given subcutaneously is 1–2 hours, peaking at 3–12 hours with a duration of 11–24 hours. A number of different preparations exist. They are manufactured with the addition of substances such as zinc or protamine which reduce solubility and prolong the absorption. In addition, they can be combined with rapid acting insulins and taken immediately before meals.

Long-Acting Insulins

These are manufactured in a similar way and last up to 36 hours. Onset is slow requiring several days use to achieve constant insulin levels (aiming to mimic the basal insulin production by the pancreas). At steady state there are minimal, if any, peaks or troughs in insulin levels. Often combined in a basal bolus regime where the patient takes a long-acting insulin once or twice per day to cover basal requirements, and then administers a rapid-acting insulin analogue immediately prior to meals.

Safe Use of Insulin

Insulin is a lifesaving medication, but it also has the potential to be extremely dangerous. Insulin errors are a frequent cause of harm and death. The standard insulin concentration in the UK is 100 units per ml. When drawing up insulin it is vital that a dedicated insulin syringe is used, and one that is calibrated to 100 units per ml. Using the scale on the correct syringe, the correct number of units can be administered. Some patients with type 2 diabetes mellitus are extremely resistant to exogenous insulin and can be taking several hundred units per day. To facilitate this, manufacturers produce highly concentrated insulins of 200 or 300 units per ml and the potential for error here is obvious.

Care must be taken when prescribing to write the number followed by the word 'units'. Abbreviations such as 'U' or 'IU' have led to serious administration errors.

The following recommendations have been used to promote the safe use of insulin.

- Prescribe using the brand name written out in full
- Avoid abbreviations
- Where insulin is prescribed the treatment of hypoglycaemia must also be prescribed
- The use of protocols and guidelines is recommended
- When prescribed and used intravenously, a supply of substrate must be continuously and simultaneously infused to prevent hypoglycaemia (as in a variable rate intravenous insulin infusion).

Side Effects

When calorie or substrate intake is insufficient hypoglycaemia will ensue. If untreated this will lead to coma and death. All insulins are immunogenic but, despite this, immunological resistance is rare. Beef insulin has three different amino acids compared to human insulin while pork insulin has only one; the latter is therefore less immunogenic.

Non-Insulin Glucose-Lowering Drugs

The number of drugs in this group, used to treat mainly type 2 diabetes mellitus, has expanded dramatically over the last few years to include eight different classes.

- Alpha glucosidase inhibitors
- Biguanides
- Dipeptidyl peptidase-4 inhibitors (gliptins)
- Glucagon-like peptide-1 receptor agonists (GLP-1)
- Meglitinides
- Sodium glucose co-transporter 2 inhibitors (SGLT-2)
- Sulfonylureas
- Thiazolidinediones (TZDs).

Alpha Glucosidase Inhibitors

Acarbose is a competitive inhibitor of intestinal α-glucosidase with a specific action on sucrase. Polysaccharides are therefore not metabolised into their absorbable monosaccharide form. This delay in intestinal glucose absorption reduces the post-prandial hyperglycaemia seen commonly in diabetics. Acarbose is not absorbed significantly and has few other systemic effects. Owing to an increased carbohydrate load reaching the bacterial flora in the large bowel, patients may experience borborygmi, flatulence and diarrhoea. Hepatic transaminases may be transiently raised. It may enhance the hypoglycaemic effects of insulin and other drugs. Oral glucose, but not polysaccharides, can be used to treat hypoglycaemia in these patients.

Biguanides

Metformin is the only currently available biguanide in the UK.

Mechanism of Action

There are several mechanisms including delayed uptake of glucose from the gut, increased peripheral insulin sensitivity (increasing peripheral glucose utilisation) and inhibition of hepatic and renal gluconeogenesis. It requires the presence of endogenous insulin to increase the peripheral utilisation of glucose and therefore is only effective in patients with some functioning islets of Langerhans.

Other Effects

Gastrointestinal disturbances including diarrhoea sometimes occur but are generally mild. More significant is its ability to precipitate severe lactic acidosis (metformin associated lactic acidosis). The mechanism of this phenomenon is understood if one considers the physiology of lactate production.

Metformin-Associated Lactic Acidosis

In health, the body produces pyruvate by glycolysis. Pyruvate from glycolysis enters the Krebs cycle (after conversion to Acetyl Co-A catalysed by the pyruvate dehydrogenase enzyme) resulting in ATP production. Pyruvate is in equilibrium with lactate, catalysed by the enzyme lactate dehydrogenase. Traditionally, the conversion of pyruvate to lactate only occurs under anaerobic conditions however, it has been demonstrated that lactate is produced in health, at a ratio of 10:1 lactate to pyruvate. In normal conditions, 20 mmol. $kg.day^{-1}$ of lactate is produced and subsequently metabolised. Lactate is a vital metabolic fuel, especially in times of metabolic stress, where it is metabolised in a variety of locations (brain, kidney, liver etc.) at very high rates by a variety of pathways, including gluconeogenesis.

In states of metabolic stress, the amount of glucose entering glycolysis increases (due to sympathetic activation) and hence the amount of pyruvate (and lactate) increases. The Krebs cycle has limited capacity to incorporate the increased pyruvate and a significant amount is converted to lactate. Lactate can therefore accumulate unless its metabolism increases in other ways.

The capacity of the Krebs cycle to accommodate the increased pyruvate can be further reduced in thiamine deficiency (an essential co-factor for pyruvate dehydrogenase), resulting in even more lactate build-up. In a patient taking metformin, the following factors contribute to an elevation in plasma lactate levels:

- Increased supply of glucose for glycolysis due to increased cellular glucose uptake – resulting in an increase in pyruvate and lactate production.
- Reduction in lactate metabolism/clearance due to inhibition of gluconeogenesis.

Risk factors for metformin-associated lactic acidosis reflect conditions whereby there is an imbalance between production and clearance of lactate:

- Poor renal function (reduced metformin clearance) – particularly related to hypovolaemia.
- Impaired hepatic and renal metabolism of lactate (reduced lactate clearance) caused by a variety of disease states.
- Increased production from sepsis, hypoperfusion, sympathetic activation and metabolic stress states (glycolysis overactivity).
- Reduced capacity to channel pyruvate into the Krebs cycle (thiamine deficiency – malnourished or alcohol users).

Kinetics

Metformin is slowly absorbed from the gut with a bioavailability of 60%. It is not bound by plasma proteins and is excreted unchanged in the urine. Renal impairment significantly prolongs its actions.

Dipeptidyl peptidase-4 Inhibitors (Gliptins) and Glucagon-Like Peptide-1 Receptor Agonists

These drugs work by modulating the actions of the incretin hormone system within the gut. In health, the presence of glucose in the gut lumen results in the release of several hormones, including glucagon-like peptide-1 (GLP-1) from L cells in the gastric mucosa. GLP-1 has several effects:

- Increase in insulin secretion from the β-cells in the pancreas
- Reduction in glucagon secretion from the alpha cells in the pancreas
- Delayed gastric emptying and subsequent slower delivery of glucose to the gut from the stomach
- Reduced appetite and increased satiety (reducing overall glucose intake).

GLP-1 is quickly inactivated by the dipeptidylpeptidase-4 (DPP-4) enzyme. In patients with type 2 diabetes mellitus the incretin system is impaired with marked reductions in GLP-1 levels. GLP-1 receptor agonists and DPP-4 inhibitors are therefore helpful in the management of individuals with type 2 diabetes and have been associated with improvements in glycaemic control, weight loss and improved cardiovascular profiles.

Glucagon-Like Peptide-1 Agonists

Currently available GLP-1 agonists include dulaglutide, exenatide, liraglutide, and lixisenatide. Endogenous GLP-1 is rapidly degraded within the gut so the GLP-1 agonists must be administered via the subcutaneous route where they have a much longer duration of action. Some preparations are administered weekly and their effect can persist a considerable length of time after discontinuation. They are frequently used in combination with other non-insulin glucose-lowering drugs and may provoke hypoglycaemia. Nausea is a common side effect and they have been associated with pancreatitis. All are contraindicated in moderately impaired renal function.

Dipeptidyl Peptidase 4 Inhibitors (Gliptins)

Currently available dipeptidyl peptidase 4 (DPP-4) inhibitors include sitagliptin, linagliptin and alogliptin. When given orally they increase the duration of action of endogenous GLP-1, thus increasing the effect of endogenous insulin. They can be administered as monotherapy or in combination with other non-insulin glucose-lowering drugs. Generally, dose modification is needed in renal dysfunction (except linagliptin) and they have been associated with pancreatitis.

Meglitinides
Repaglinide and Nateglinide

Meglitinides are oral antidiabetic agents that may be of most use in treating patients with erratic eating habits as they are relatively short acting. They are taken just before meals.

Mechanism of Action

Meglitinides block the potassium channels in pancreatic β-cells, closing the ATP-dependent potassium channels and opening the cells' calcium channels. The resulting calcium influx causes the cells to secrete insulin.

Kinetics

Repaglinide has an oral bioavailability of 50%, is 98% plasma protein-bound and is metabolised in the liver by CYP3A4 and therefore is potentially susceptible to drug interactions. Its elimination half-life is 1 hour.

Sodium Glucose Co-Transporter 2 Inhibitors

Glucose freely passes into the ultrafiltrate in the kidneys and in health virtually all is reabsorbed in the proximal convoluted tubule via the sodium glucose linked transporter 2 mechanism (SGLT-2). Consequently, inhibitors of the SGLT-2 mechanism reduce this reabsorption and therefore blood glucose. The side effects are the expected polyuria, polydipsia and dehydration.

There have been reports of serious, sometimes life-threatening cases of diabetic ketoacidosis in patients on SGLT-2 inhibitor treatment for type 1 and type 2 diabetes. The presentation is often atypical and has been described as a euglycaemic ketoacidosis due to the absence of markedly raised plasma glucose levels (potentially causing diagnostic confusion).

Patients on SGLT-2 inhibitors should be tested for ketones when they present with symptoms of acidosis in order to prevent delayed diagnosis.

Sulfonylureas

Two generations of sulfonylureas exist and have slightly different characteristics:

- First generation – tolbutamide
- Second generation – glibenclamide, gliclazide, glipizide.

Mechanism of Action

In general, these drugs work at the pancreas by displacing insulin from β-cells in the islets of Langerhans. For this reason, they are ineffective in insulin-dependent diabetics who have no functioning β-cells. They may also induce β-cell hyperplasia, while reducing both glucagon secretion and hepatic insulinase activity. During long-term administration they also reduce peripheral resistance to insulin.

Kinetics

Sulfonylureas are all well absorbed from the gut and have oral bioavailabilities greater than 80%. Albumin binds these drugs extensively in the plasma. A significant fraction is excreted unchanged in the urine and in the presence of renal failure its half-life is prolonged. The other drugs in this class are extensively metabolised in the liver to inactive metabolites (with the exception of glibenclamide whose active metabolites are probably of little clinical significance), which are subsequently excreted in the urine. Cimetidine inhibits their metabolism and, therefore, potentiates their actions. Drugs that tend to increase blood sugar (thiazides, corticosteroids, phenothiazines) antagonise the effects of the sulfonylureas and make diabetic control harder.

The second-generation sulfonylureas bind to albumin by non-ionic forces in contrast with tolbutamide that binds by ionic forces. Thus, anionic drugs such as phenylbutazone, warfarin and salicylate do not displace second-generation drugs to such an extent and may be safer during concurrent drug therapy.

Other Effects

Tolbutamide has been associated with cholestatic jaundice, deranged liver function and blood dyscrasias.

Thiazolidinediones
Pioglitazone

Pioglitazone is the only remaining thiazolidinedione available in the UK. It is an oral antidiabetic agent with a high oral bioavailability. The effects may take weeks to be fully established due to their mechanism of action. Other drugs in the class (including rosiglitazone) were withdrawn in the UK after an association with heart attacks and strokes. Pioglitazone is associated with an increased risk of heart failure when combined with insulin, especially in patients with predisposing factors. Patients who take pioglitazone should be closely monitored for signs of heart failure and those with the condition should not receive the drug.

Mechanism of Action

Pioglitazone activates peroxisome proliferator-activated receptor γ (PPARγ, situated within the cell nucleus) and thereby regulates several genes involved in glucose and lipid metabolism. As a result, it acts to improve insulin sensitivity.

Kinetics

It is extensively metabolised by hepatic cytochrome P450. Some of the pioglitazone metabolites are active and are excreted in faeces and urine.

Peri-Operative Care of the Diabetic Patient

Comprehensive guidelines have been published on this topic and a full discussion here is beyond the space available. However, a few points are worth highlighting:

- Insulin infusions should be referred to as variable rate intravenous insulin infusions (VRIII), rather than 'sliding scales'.

- Management of diabetic medications should follow established guidelines and protocols.
- Management depends on the number of missed meals and current diabetic control.
- If there is only one missed meal (a short starvation period) a VRIII is often not required.
  - Long-acting insulins can be taken at a reduced dose (20% reduction) the day before.
  - Intermediate- and short-acting insulins need no dose adjustment the day before.
  - On the day of surgery, the time of the operation affects the modification of insulin doses.

- If the starvation period is longer (more than one missed meal) most patients will need a VRIII.
  - If a VRIII is indicated and the patient usually takes a long-acting insulin, this should be continued alongside the VRIII to reduce rebound hyperglycaemia when the VRIII ends (20% dose reduction).

- Regarding the non-insulin glucose lowering drugs:
  - All can be taken normally the day prior to surgery.
  - On the day of surgery, GLP-1 agonists, DPP-4 inhibitors, and pioglitazone can be taken as normal if only one missed meal. All others are suspended.
  - Metformin is controversial, it may be continued for day surgery patients with good renal function and not receiving intravenous contrast, albeit at a reduced dose. Many hospitals recommend it is suspended regardless for all surgery.
  - If a VRIII is being used all drugs are suspended except GLP-1 agonists.

Chapter 26

Corticosteroids and Other Hormone Preparations

Glucocorticoids

The adrenal cortex releases two classes of steroidal hormones into the circulation:

- Glucocorticoids (from the zona fasciculata and zona reticularis)
- Mineralocorticoids (from the zona glomerulosa).

The main endogenous glucocorticoid in humans is hydrocortisone. Synthetic glucocorticoids include prednisolone, methylprednisolone, betamethasone, dexamethasone and triamcinolone. They have **metabolic, anti-inflammatory** (see Table 26.1) and **immunosuppressive** effects.

Metabolic Effects

Glucocorticoids facilitate gluconeogenesis (i.e. synthesis of glucose from a non-carbohydrate source, e.g. protein). Glycogen deposition and glucose release from the liver are stimulated but the peripheral uptake of glucose is inhibited. Protein catabolism is stimulated and synthesis inhibited.

When exogenous glucocorticoid is given in high doses or for prolonged periods, the altered metabolism causes unwanted effects. Increased protein catabolism leads to muscle weakness and wasting. The skin becomes thin leading to striae, and gastric mucosa becomes susceptible to ulceration. Dietary protein will not reverse these changes. Altered carbohydrate metabolism leads to hyperglycaemia and glycosuria. Diabetes may be provoked. Fat is redistributed from the extremities to the trunk, neck and face. Bone catabolism leads to osteoporosis.

Anti-Inflammatory Effects

Glucocorticoids reduce the production of tissue transudate and cell oedema in acute inflammation. Circulating polymorphs and macrophages are prevented from reaching inflamed tissue. The production of inflammatory mediators (prostaglandins, leukotrienes and platelet-activating factor) is suppressed by the stimulation of lipocortin, which inhibits phospholipase A_2. Normally phospholipase A_2 would facilitate the breakdown of membrane phospholipids to arachidonic acid, the precursor of inflammatory mediators, in particular prostaglandins.

These effects may reduce the patient's resistance to infection (latent tuberculosis may become reactivated), and the normal clinical features usually present may be absent until the infection is advanced.

Table 26.1 Anti-inflammatory potential of various steroids

Drug	Relative anti-inflammatory potency	Equivalent anti-inflammatory dose (mg)
Hydrocortisone	1	100
Prednisolone	4	25
Methylprednisolone	5	20
Triamcinolone	5	20
Dexamethasone	25	4

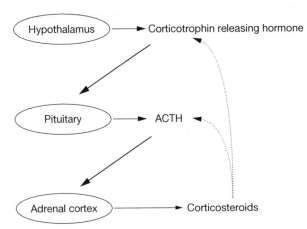

Figure 26.1 Feedback loops affecting corticosteroid production. ──►, Stimulates; ┈┈►, inhibits.

Immunosuppressive Effects

Glucocorticoids depress macrophage function and reduce the number of circulating T-lymphocytes. The transport of lymphocytes and their production of antibodies are also reduced. Interleukin 1 and 2 production is inhibited, which reduces lymphocyte proliferation.

Other Effects

- *Adrenal suppression* – during long-term steroid therapy there is adrenal suppression due to negative feedback on corticotrophin-releasing hormone and adrenocorticotrophic hormone (ACTH) (see Figure 26.1). The adrenal gland becomes atrophic and remains so for many months after treatment has stopped. As a result the adrenal cortex cannot produce sufficient glucocorticoid when exogenous glucocorticoid is withdrawn abruptly or during periods of stress, that is, infection or surgery. If supplementary hydrocortisone is not administered in such patients peri-operatively, they are at risk of hypotension and possibly cardiovascular collapse (see 'Peri-Operative Steroid Supplementation' below).
- *Fluid retention* – glucocorticoids have only weak mineralocorticoid activity. However, some do act on the distal renal tubule, leading to Na^+ retention and K^+ excretion. In very large doses, water retention may cause oedema, hypertension and cardiac failure.
  Mineralocorticoid (sodium retaining) activity is greatest with hydrocortisone and cortisone, lesser with prednisolone and least with methylprednisolone and dexamethasone.

- *Vascular reactivity* – glucocorticoids have a 'permissive action' on vascular smooth muscle, allowing them to respond efficiently to circulating catecholamines. Therefore, glucocorticoid deficiency leads to an ineffective response by vascular smooth muscle to circulating catecholamines. In sepsis there may be an inappropriately reduced production of cortisol so that higher levels of inotropic support are required. This may be improved by the administration of intravenous hydrocortisone.

Other 'permissive actions' of glucocorticoids include the calorigenic effects of glucagon and catecholamines, and the lipolytic and bronchodilator effects of catecholamines.

Peri-Operative Steroid Supplementation

Patients with adrenal insufficiency (AI) require peri-operative steroid supplementation. AI may be Primary (adrenal gland disease / failure), Secondary (deficient ACTH or CRH production) or most commonly Tertiary (the result of glucocorticoid therapy, sometimes classified within Secondary). Peri-operative steroid supplementation is in addition to the patient's usual steroid medication. Recent guidelines highlight that doses as low as 5 mg prednisolone and standard doses of inhaled glucocorticoids taken for more than 1 month can cause an inadequate response to the short synacthen test. As the side effects of peri-operative steroid supplementation are minimal compared to an inadequate glucocorticoid stress response it is recommended that this group of patients has peri-operative steroid supplementation. Tables 26.2 & 26.3 summarise the recommendations.

Table 26.2 Steroid cover for Primary and Secondary Adrenal Insufficiency

	Intra-operative	Postoperative
Surgery (under regional or general anaesthesia)	Hydrocortisone: 100 mg iv at induction, followed immediately by an infusion of 200 mg over 24 hrs	Hydrocortisone 200 mg iv over 24 hrs for patients with PONV or NBM (alternatively, hydrocortisone im 50 mg qds)
		On resumption of oral route – double hydrocortisone doses for 24-48 hrs or for up to a week following major surgery
Bowel procedures requiring laxatives / enemas	Bowel prep under clinical supervision. Consider iv fluids & iv/im glucocorticoid, especially for fludrocortisone or vasopressin-dependent patients Hydrocortisone 100 mg iv/im at start of procedure	Post procedure, double hydrocortisone dose for 24 hrs
Labour & vaginal delivery	Hydrocortisone: 100 mg iv at onset of labour, followed by 200 mg iv over 24 hrs Alternatively, Hydrocortisone: 100 mg im followed by 50 mg im qds	Post delivery on resumption of oral route, double hydrocortisone doses for 48 hrs

Table 26.3 Steroid cover for Tertiary Adrenal Insufficiency (those on ≥ 5 mg prednisolone or equivalent)

	Intra-operative	Postoperative
Major surgery (including Caesarian Section)	Hydrocortisone: 100 mg iv at induction, followed immediately by an infusion of 200 mg over 24 hrs	Hydrocortisone 100 mg iv over 24 hrs for patients with PONV or NBM (alternatively, hydrocortisone im 50 mg qds)
	Alternatively, dexamethasone 6-8 mg iv will suffice for 24 hrs	On resumption of oral route – return to normal pre-operative dose or double if recovery is complicated for up to a week
Body surface and Intermediate surgery	Hydrocortisone: 100 mg iv at induction, followed immediately by an infusion of 200 mg over 24 hrs	On resumption of oral route – double normal pre-operative dose for 48 hrs then return to normal dose if recovery is uncomplicated
	Alternatively, dexamethasone 6-8 mg iv will suffice for 24 hrs	
Bowel procedures requiring laxatives / enemas	Continue normal glucocorticoid dose, but use iv route if needed. Consider treating as per Primary AI if clinically indicated	
Labour & vaginal delivery	Hydrocortisone: 100 mg iv at onset of labour, followed by 200 mg iv over 24 hrs	
	Alternatively, Hydrocortisone: 100 mg im followed by 50 mg im qds	

It should be noted that dexamethasone is not recommended in Primary AI due to its lack of mineralocorticoid effect.

Drugs Used in Thyroid Disease

Thyroid Replacement

Thyroxine (T_4)

The thyroid gland synthesises triiodothyronine (T_3) and thyroxine (T_4) by combining iodine with tyrosine residues present in thyroglobulin. The release of T_3 and T_4 is controlled by the hypothalamic thyrotropin-releasing hormone (TRH) and thyrotropin (TSH), which are inhibited in the presence of T_3 and T_4 (see Figure 26.2).

Uses

Replacement hormone is required to treat hypothyroidism, which may be due to thyroid, hypothalamic or pituitary disease. Synthetic T_4 (Levothyroxine) is the mainstay of oral replacement therapy but L-triiodothyronine (T_3) may be given intravenously (5–50 μg according to response) in hypothyroid coma as it has a faster onset. T_3 may also be given orally.

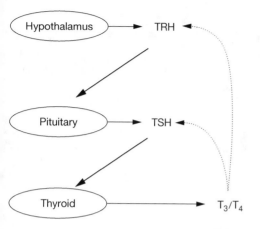

Figure 26.2 Feedback loops affecting thyroid hormone production. ———▶, Stimulates; ·········▶, inhibits.

Mechanism of Action

Free T_4 enters the cell via a carrier mechanism where most is converted to the more active T_3. Their main intracellular targets are receptors on the mitochondria and cell nucleus to which they bind inducing a conformational change.

Effects

- *Cardiovascular* – thyroid hormones exhibit positive inotropy and chronotropy. The cardiac output increases, while a reduced peripheral vascular resistance often leaves the mean arterial blood pressure unchanged. The increased myocardial oxygen demand may cause ischaemia in those with ischaemic heart disease.
- *Respiratory* – owing to an increased metabolic rate the minute volume increases.
- *Central nervous system* – they act as central stimulants and may evoke tremor. They also act to inhibit thyroid-stimulating hormone (TSH) and thyrotropin-releasing hormone (TRH) by negative feedback.
- *Metabolic* – T_3 affects growth, development, lipid metabolism, intestinal carbohydrate absorption and increases the dissociation of oxygen from haemoglobin by increasing red blood cell 2,3-diphosphoglycerol (2,3-DPG).

Kinetics

When administered enterally both T_3 and T_4 are well absorbed from the gut. Once in the plasma they are more than 99% bound to albumin and thyroxine-binding globulin. Some T_4 is converted within the liver and kidneys to T_3 or to the inactive reverse T_3. Metabolism occurs in the liver and the conjugated products are excreted in bile. Up to 40% may be excreted unchanged in the urine.

Drugs Used in the Treatment of Hyperthyroidism

Carbimazole

Carbimazole is a prodrug, being rapidly converted to methimazole in vivo.

Mechanism of Action

Carbimazole prevents the synthesis of new T_3 and T_4 by inhibiting the oxidation of iodide to iodine and by inhibiting thyroid peroxidase, which is responsible for iodotryrosine synthesis and the coupling of iodotyrosines. Stored T_3 and T_4 is unaffected and so treatment with carbimazole requires weeks before the patient becomes euthyroid.

Side Effects

These include rashes, arthralgia and pruritus. Agranulocytosis occurs rarely and may be heralded by a sore throat. It crosses the placenta and may cause fetal hypothyroidism; however, it is not contraindicated during breastfeeding as only tiny amounts enter the breast milk.

Kinetics

Carbimazole is well absorbed from the gut and completely converted to methimazole during its passage through the liver. It increases the vascularity of and is metabolised within the thyroid gland. It is minimally plasma protein-bound.

Propylthiouracil

This oral preparation blocks the iodination of tyrosine and partially blocks the peripheral conversion of T_4 to T_3. There is no parenteral formulation and it is reserved for those patients intolerant of carbimazole. It has a slightly higher incidence of agranulocytosis.

Propranolol

Propranolol is a β-blocker with negative inotropic and chronotropic activity. It will help control the sympathetic effects of a thyrotoxic crisis. However, it also blocks the peripheral conversion of T_4 to T_3 and blocks hypersensitivity to the actions of catecholamines. It is relatively contraindicated for patients with heart failure or reversible airflow limitation.

Iodides

Iodide has been given as potassium iodide orally, sodium iodide intravenously and iodide containing radiographic contrast dyes. It is concentrated in the follicular cells where peroxidases oxidise it to iodine, which is then combined with tyrosine residues.

Iodide is required for normal thyroid function and, when levels are too low or too high, thyroid function becomes abnormal. Large doses cause inhibition of iodide binding and hence reduced hormone production. This effect is greatest when iodide transport is increased, that is, in thyrotoxicosis. Iodide also reduces the effect of TSH on the thyroid gland and inhibits proteolysis of thyroglobulin. Thyroid vascularity is decreased, which is useful pre-operatively, but iodide is not used for prolonged periods as its actions tend to diminish with time.

Lithium may be considered in those with iodide sensitivity.

Oral Contraceptives

The oral contraceptive pill (OCP) takes two forms: a combined oestrogen/progesterone preparation and a progesterone-only preparation. The former is taken for 21 consecutive days followed by a 7-day break, while the latter is taken continuously.

Mechanism of Action

The combined preparation inhibits ovulation by suppressing gonadotrophin-releasing hormone and inhibiting gonadotrophin secretion. The progesterone-only pill prevents ovulation in only 25% of women and appears to work by producing an unfavourable endometrium for implantation.

Side Effects

- *Major* – these include cholestatic jaundice and an increased incidence of thromboembolic disease. The following are considered a contraindication for the combined OCP: a history of thromboembolism, obesity, smoking, hypertension or diabetes mellitus.
- *Minor* – these include breakthrough bleeding, weight gain, breast tenderness, headache and nausea. Hirsutism and depression may occur following the combined OCP. Side effects are lower in the progesterone-only pill.

Hormone Replacement Therapy

Hormone replacement therapy (HRT; oestrogen or oestrogen/progesterone combinations) is used to relieve menopausal symptoms, reduce osteoporosis and reduce the risk of cardiovascular disease.

Side Effects

- *Endometrial cancer* – oestrogen therapy alone increases the risk of endometrial cancer and is therefore reserved for those who have had a hysterectomy. Women with a uterus require combined oestrogen/progesterone therapy.
- *Breast cancer* – concerns have been raised regarding HRT and breast cancer and there may be a slightly higher risk of breast cancer with combined oestrogen/progesterone therapy compared to oestrogen alone.
- *Deep vein thrombosis* – HRT may increase the risk of deep vein thrombosis although the absolute risk is low. The mechanism is unclear, but HRT may provoke changes in relation to the haemostatic system, increasing age of patients and unmasking of thrombotic traits.

Peri-Operative Hormone Replacement Therapy

There is no evidence to support stopping HRT in the peri-operative period provided the usual thromboprophylaxis protocols are followed.

Oxytocic Drugs

Oxytocin

The posterior pituitary gland secretes two peptides each of nine amino acids (seven similar, two different): oxytocin and vasopressin. Oxytocin has central and peripheral actions. The peripheral actions are well understood and are critical to breastfeeding (via the letdown reflex) and uterine contraction.

Presentation

Oxytocin is presented as a clear liquid in 1 ml vials containing 5 or 10 mg and in combination with ergometrine as syntometrine.

Uses

It is used to induce or augment labour and to increase uterine tone following delivery to facilitate delivery of the placenta. Controlled intravenous infusions are used due to its short plasma half-life (3–5 minutes).

Mechanism of Action

Oxytocin binds to oxytocin G-coupled receptors in the uterus and promotes calcium release thereby activating uterine contraction. Due to its similarity to vasopressin it has weak anti-diuretic-like effects which are only significant during prolonged infusions.

Side Effects

Tachycardia may follow bolus doses and headache is also common.

Carbetocin

Carbetocin is a synthetic oxytocin analogue, used to control bleeding by stimulating contraction of the uterus. Due to its long shelf life of 3 years (at <30°C), it may be preferred where cold storage of oxytocin is not possible.

It acts by stimulating oxytocin receptors in the uterus and due to its long duration of action only a single dose of 100 μg is required.

It has a high incidence of nausea and vomiting, and is contraindicated during labour and in those with high blood pressure and cardiovascular disease.

Ergometrine

Ergometrine is an ergot alkaloid with a chemical structure similar to that of LSD. It is used to facilitate delivery of the placenta and to prevent postpartum bleeding. The mechanism by which it stimulates strong uterine contractions is unknown.

It may cause headache, nausea and hypertension. As a result it is contraindicated in pre-eclampsia.

Uterine contraction is seen a few minutes after intramuscular injection and lasts for up to 6 hours. It is metabolised by the liver and excreted in the bile.

Carboprost

Carboprost is a synthetic prostaglandin analogue of $PGF_{2\alpha}$. It is used to treat postpartum haemorrhage resistant to treatment with oxytocin and ergometrine. An initial intramuscular dose of 250 μg may need to be followed by further doses at 90-minute intervals up to a maximum of 2 mg.

It is contraindicated in pregnancy, cardiorespiratory disease and pelvic inflammatory disease.

Side effects include nausea and vomiting, flushing and bronchospasm. Cardiovascular collapse has been reported.

Index

Printed in the United States
by Baker & Taylor Publisher Services